Door-to-Door Collectibles
Salves, Lotions, Pills & Potions from W.T. Rawleigh

C.L. Miller

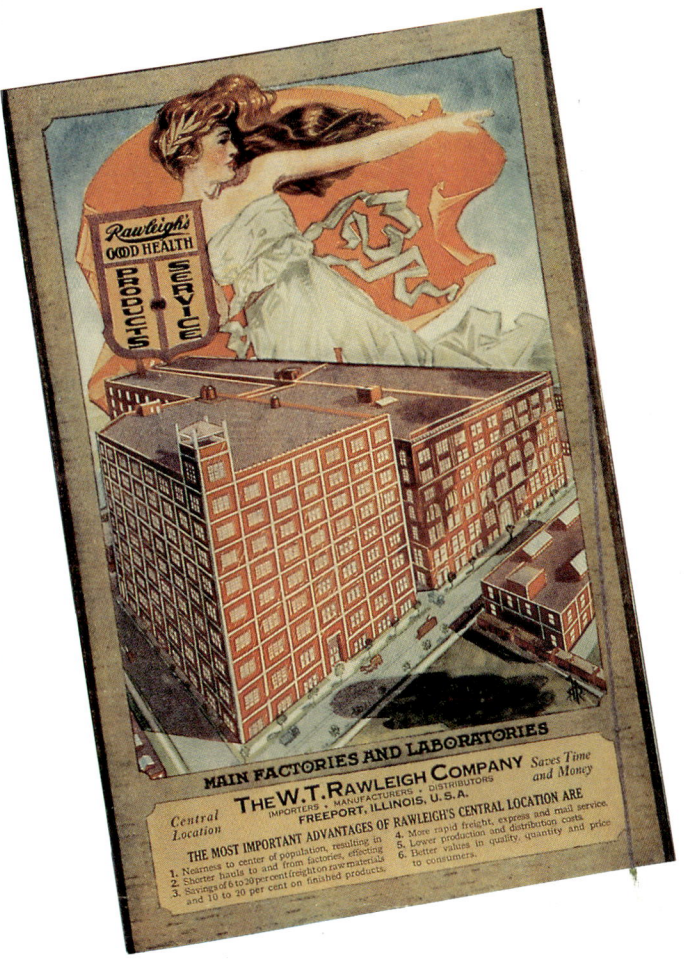

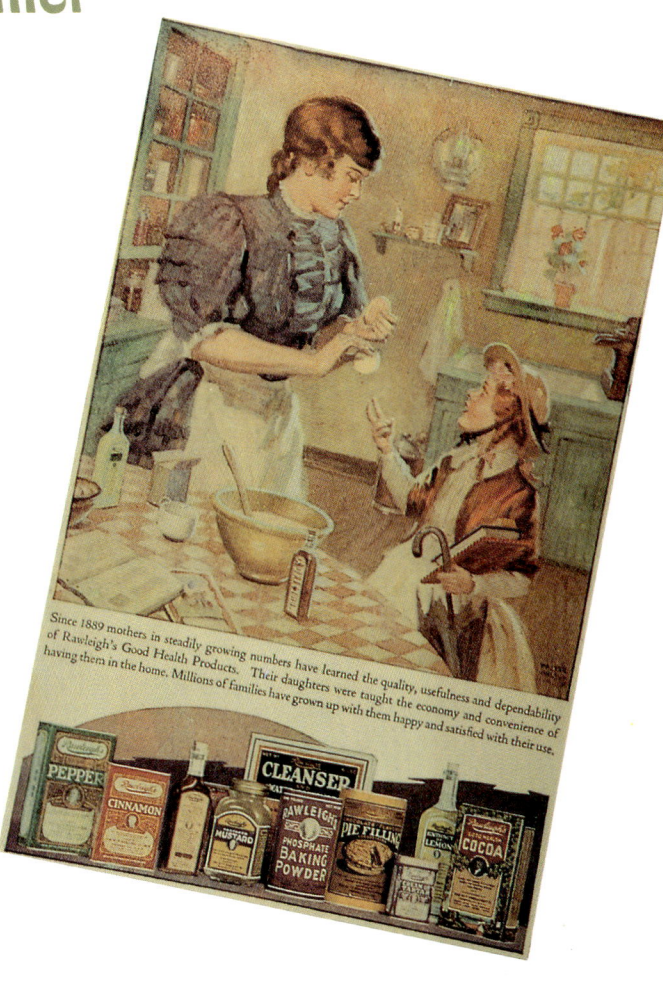

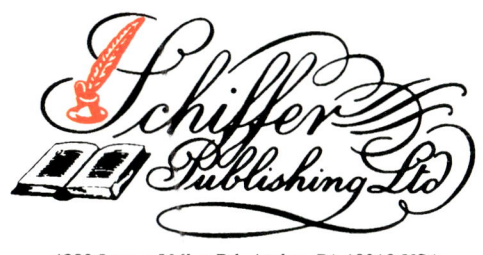

4880 Lower Valley Rd. Atglen, PA 19310 USA

Library of Congress Cataloging-in-Publication Data

Miller, C.L. (Charles L.), 1941-
  Door-to-door collectibles : salves, lotions, pills & potions from W.T. Rawleigh / C.L. Miller.
      p. cm.
  Includes bibliographical references and index.
  ISBN 0-7643-0331-7
  1. Household supplies--Collectors and collecting--Catalogs. 2. Cosmetics--Collectors and collecting--Catalogs. 3. Toilet preparations--Collectors and collecting--Catalogs. 4. Patent medicines--Collectors and collecting--Catalogs. 5. Farm supplies--Collectors and collecting--Catalogs. 6. W.T. Raweigh Compay--Catalogs. I. Title
TX303.M55   1998
640'.75--dc21   97-31799
                                                             CIP

Copyright © 1998 by C.L. Miller

All rights reserved. No part of this work may be reproduced or used in any form or by any means—graphic, electronic, or mechanical, including photocopying or information storage and retrieval systems—without written permission from the copyright holder.

Designed by Bonnie M. Hensley

ISBN: 0-7643-0331-7
Printed in China
1 2 3 4

Published by Schiffer Publishing Ltd.
4880 Lower Valley Road
Atglen, PA 19310
Phone: (610) 593-1777; Fax: (610) 593-2002
E-mail: Schifferbk@aol.com
Please write for a free catalog.
This book may be purchased from the publisher.
Please include $3.95 for shipping.

Please try your bookstore first.
We are interested in hearing from authors
with book ideas on related subjects.

Dedication

To Lon and Lynda Lemons, for their confidence, encouragement, past patronage and their cherished friendship during this and my future endeavors. My **Love** to you both.

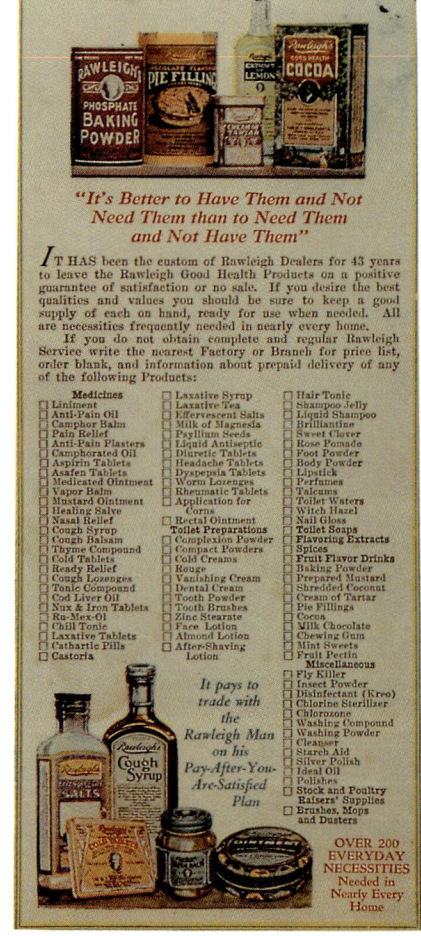

"It's Better to Have Them and Not Need Them Than to Need Them and Not Have Them. Over 200 Everyday Necessities Needed in Nearly Every Home." *Rawleigh 1932.*

Contents

Acknowledgements --------- 4
Foreword --------- 4
Introduction --------- 5
Chapter 1. History --------- 9
   Founder W.T. Rawleigh --------- 9
   Quality the First Consideration --------- 11
   An Institution of Unusual Utility --------- 12
   The Rawleigh-Schryer Company --------- 12
   Big Commodity --------- 13
   The Rawleigh Organization --------- 14
   Policies and Business Practices --------- 15
   New Branch's --------- 15
   The Minneapolis Branch --------- 17
   The Richmond, Virginia, Branch --------- 17
   Inside Rawleigh's Factories --------- 18
   Rawleigh Retailer --------- 21
   Your Recruiting Opportunity --------- 25
   The Rawleigh Foundation --------- 26
   Golden Pride International™ --------- 26
Chapter 2. Rawleigh Methods and Health Products --------- 28
   How Rawleigh Used Them --------- 28
   Why Rawleigh Retailers Served You Best --------- 28
   Why Rawleigh Made Their Own Tablets --------- 30
   Road to Health the Rawleigh Way --------- 30
   Packing Half a Million Tablets Daily --------- 32
   Why Mothers Prefer Rawleigh Products --------- 32
   Rawleigh Health Products --------- 32
Chapter 3. Rawleigh's Paper Memorabilia --------- 51
   Paper Care --------- 51
   Rawleigh's Printing Department --------- 51
   Good Health Guide and Almanac --------- 52
   Cookbooks --------- 74
   Calendars --------- 75
Chapter 4. Trading in Foreign Countries --------- 84
   Tropics to Table --------- 87
Chapter 5. Collecting Rawleigh Products --------- 88
   Food Products --------- 88
   Spices and Extracts --------- 89
   Miscellaneous --------- 111
   Care of Your Products --------- 117
Chapter 6. Cosmetics, Toiletries and Work Savers --------- 118
Chapter 7. Rawleigh Brushes, Mops, Dusters, and Toothbrushes --------- 154
Chapter 8. Rawleigh's Experimental Farm --------- 157
   Originators of the All-Medicine Mixtures --------- 160
   Livestock and Poultry Losses --------- 161
   Care of Livestock the Rawleigh Way --------- 161
   Farm and Gardening Products --------- 163
Bibliography --------- 174
Index --------- 175

Acknowledgements

My appreciation to Betsy Stockdill, Executive Vice President of GOLDEN PRIDE INTERNATIONAL™ for permitting me to develop this Rawleigh publication and for the support and contributions of collectors and interested individuals. If I have overlooked anyone, I apologize at this time. I wish to extend my thanks to Dan W. Andrews, Mark A. Baker, Murray C. Barron, Dan and Debbie Breeding, Ronald A. Breeding, Taylor Gregory Breeding, Phil and Maureen Bond, Kevin and Lynn Burkett, Garry F. and Betty J. Bushue (Independent Distributors), Neal and Patti Byerly, Ronald and Norma Chappell, Russ and Donna Colwell, Evelyn L. Miller Cox, Ann C. Davis, Douglas B. Dupler, Earl F. and Mary Edler, Patty Elwood, Freeport Journal Standard, Diane Foster, Carolyn Haas, Heritage on High Antique Mall, David H. Jentgen (Captured Images Studio), Russell Keith, Kurt Koester Studio, Phillip L. Krumholz, Casey and Chris McGowan, Jack and Sarah Miller, Ralph and Linda Miller, Tommie Miller, Carl and Bonnie Riddlebarger, Mike and Cindy Schneider, Joseph H. and Mary Ann D. Shepard, Linda Simonton, Norm Storkel, N.L. Truessel, Randy and Marsha Vogel, and to my family and friends.

To Freeport residents, Ronald and Joan Pasch, I appreciate their phone calls, letters, friendship, and support in locating many of the various products that appear throughout this publication.

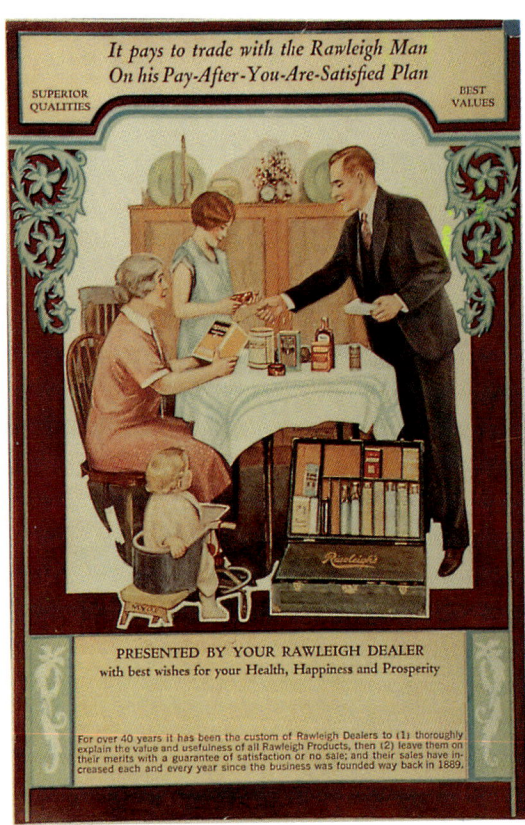

The advertisement, "It pays to trade with the Rawleigh Man On his Pay-After-You-Are Satisfied Plan", appeared in a 1931 Rawleigh publication.

Foreword

The Rawleigh Organization

Entering its nineteenth year in business in 1914, The W.T. Rawleigh Medical Company of Freeport, Illinois, was recognized as one of the greatest manufacturers and distributors of over one hundred farm and household products. Their line included medicines, ointments (for both man and beast), extracts, spices, cosmetics, sewing machine oil, stock medicines, stock feed, and stock disinfectants.

The W.T. Rawleigh Medical Company, which changed its name to The W.T. Rawleigh Company in approximately 1916, began work by gathering its raw materials from remote parts of the world and ended its service with the delivery of pure and fresh products to the customer's door. Each year the company continued to grow larger and to extended its business across the nation.

From the best markets of the world, the company brought hundreds of carloads of raw materials and manufactured a line of goods extensive enough to compete with any single manufacturer in the United States. A mammoth organization was built, delivering finished products directly to millions of doors. Facets of the company included domestic and foreign buying connections, factories, branch houses and warehouses, and a selling organization extending from the Hudson Bay to the Gulf of Mexico, and from the Atlantic to the Pacific.

Rawleigh was the largest buyer in the world of thousands of raw materials necessary in the manufacturing of the largest line of products sold from roughly two thousand salesmens' horse-drawn wagons. To buy them at the lowest cash prices, Rawleigh sought the best markets in the world. From these, samples were gathered by expert buyers and tests were made by the Rawleigh Analytical Department for purity and strength. This was followed by placing large carloads of orders, often by cable, with those who supplied Rawleigh from the greatest foreign and domestic markets.

In 1914, Rawleigh owned and operated three factories. The company had about three hundred and fifty factory and warehouse employees whose wages and salaries amounted to around $150,000 a year. This was approximately $430.00 per year per employee. Approximately one to two thousand additional workers were given indirect employment producing Rawleigh bottles, medicine wagons, tins cans, paper boxes, shipping cases, engravings, and other supplies.

From 1913 to 1914, half a million dollars had been expended for facility improvements which included several large, fire proof factory buildings, and a variety of new modern machinery and equipment. Rawleigh management was confident that no other organization had any advantage over their organization in buying, selling, or manufacturing. Their claim was based on their capital and resources of over two million dollars in property, the company's centrally located modern factories, plus a rapidly growing sales organization of over two thousand salesmen traveling by horse and wagons in nearly every state and throughout Canada. Rawleigh management boasted that with their experience, they were able to serve their customers as well as — or better than — anyone else in the WORLD.

Introduction

"With Rawleigh, service came first, profits were only secondary. 'He profits most who serves best.'"
—Rawleigh's 1928

Of all the home delivery companies' names in our country's history, The W.T. Rawleigh Medical Co., of Freeport, Illinois (a.k.a. The W.T. Rawleigh Company) is perhaps the most well known and recognized. For collectors who specialize in advertising and promotional items, Rawleigh has rapidly become one the most collected memorabilia in the secondary market. These items of pure nostalgia are available from most flea-markets, antique shows, shops, and yard sales. Only recently has this company's simple household and farm products — carrying the famous founder's signature (and often his photograph) — escalated in price and demand.

Collectible Rawleigh products are known for their consistency. Seldom did Rawleigh's packaging change in design or style. The contents and/or ingredients always remained the same. Many of the vintage advertising items have become so rare and expensive that the novice must forgo the purchase of such items.

William Thomas Rawleigh in 1889 began selling a small line of Good Health Products as a "one-man" concern. He left his products with prospective customers on approval with his guarantee of satisfaction or no sale. His dependable service, honest methods, and free trials soon gained the confidence, good will, and the patronage of thousands of families who became both his steady customers and his friends.

Within just a few years, Rawleigh's became one of the largest retail businesses of its kind in the country and was incorporated on January 11, 1895. The most substantial evidence of the superiority of its products that the W.T. Rawleigh organization could point to was in the enduring quality of those products and in the services rendered.

Before long, over one hundred of Rawleigh's steady customers became dealers in Illinois, Wisconsin, Iowa, and throughout the Mississippi Valley states. The growth of this small factory to home service - from producers to consumers - was unparalleled — sales rapidly increased as the business was extended from Freeport, Illinois, into all the Eastern, Southern, and later the Pacific Coast States.

At the time of his death in 1951, William T. Rawleigh's credentials were impressive and his small line of Good Health Products sold regionally had increased to an extensive line sold worldwide.

To meet the increasing demand for Rawleigh Products, large factories were built at Memphis to supply the Southern States. Then the business was extended into Canada, with state-of-the-art factories constructed at Montreal and Winnipeg.

As the Company grew into an international organization, management sent their buyers to the most remote corners of the world, importing vast quantities of raw materials and converting them into useful products in one of those three immense factories in Freeport, Memphis, and Winnipeg. The company's ability to procure massive loads of raw materials from around the globe allowed it to produce uniform and reliable products in vast quantities and at low costs.

This international business expanded to a world-wide organization. Rawleigh had a tremendous sales increase when the company began manufacturing in Australia and New Zealand as well. There the business was the oldest and the largest of its kind in the Far East.

In 1889, great-grandparents were learning the usefulness and quality of "Rawleigh's Good Health Products." They were discovering the practical service of having those products left at their homes on a trial basis with the retailer's guarantee of satisfaction.

Seventy-five years ago grandmothers showed good judgment in keeping stocks of these necessities ready to use when needed. In millions of homes their daughters considered their usefulness in their daily lives. They said they couldn't keep house without them, liked the easy way of buying at home and the completeness of the service given them by "The House of Rawleigh" and their business methods. They welcomed the arrival of the Rawleigh retailer, talked over their needs and had him leave stocks of everything they may have needed.

Then the children of those generations began learning that health, enjoyment and satisfaction go with Rawleigh's Good Health Products and Service.

Today collectors seek these products that were once acquired by all those mothers, grandmothers, and great-grandparents. As their progenitor had discovered "Tis Better To Have Them and Not Need Them Than To Need Them And Not Have Them." The continued use of Rawleigh products by the descendants of those first families proved that they were reliable and adequate. In the United States alone it is estimated that over 800,000 collectors maintain collections and/or deal in vintage advertising tins and historical products. Approximately 150 - 800 advertising products are in an average collection and this number is rapidly increasing.

Throughout this publication various Rawleigh products, historical photographs, and original advertisements appear. However, many dates are not certain, as my collection and other sources of Rawleigh publications are limited. If I have misled anyone or have made mistakes, I apologize at this time. If you should have historical information or products in your collection that are not shown in this publication, I would appreciate hearing from you. Direct all correspondence to Schiffer Publishing Ltd. Their address appears in the front of this publication.

Included in this book are many original Rawleigh advertisements that I have rescued from deteriorating publications. The oldest original print material presented here, RAWLEIGH'S ALMANAC, COOKBOOK and MEDICAL GUIDE, is dated ©1906. These publications provided an abundance of historical documentation. Presently, the Rawleigh Almanac, Cookbook and Medical Guide and/or paper documents of all sorts are moderately priced and readily available to any collector.

Central Location

Near the center of the population in the United States — Freeport, Stephenson County, Illinois — W.T. Rawleigh built his empire. With that central location in Freeport, the company had the following advantages: 1) lower freight rates in and out; 2) a shorter haul; 3) quicker service; and 4) lower production and distribution costs.

Over 30,000 tons or more than two thousand carloads of freight were handled in and out annually at the W.T. Rawleigh Company. Freight charges were in excess of $275,000. This covered raw materials shipped into the plant and finished products shipped from factories and branches. Rawleigh bought more raw materials and shipped more medicines, household products, and veterinary preparations than any other industry in the world.

The majority of merchandise received in Freeport came from the eastern and southern regions. Many thousands of dollars and much time were saved when shorter hauls — giving quicker freight, express, and mail service — were provided. Shorter hauls saved days on all outgoing shipments from Freeport to points

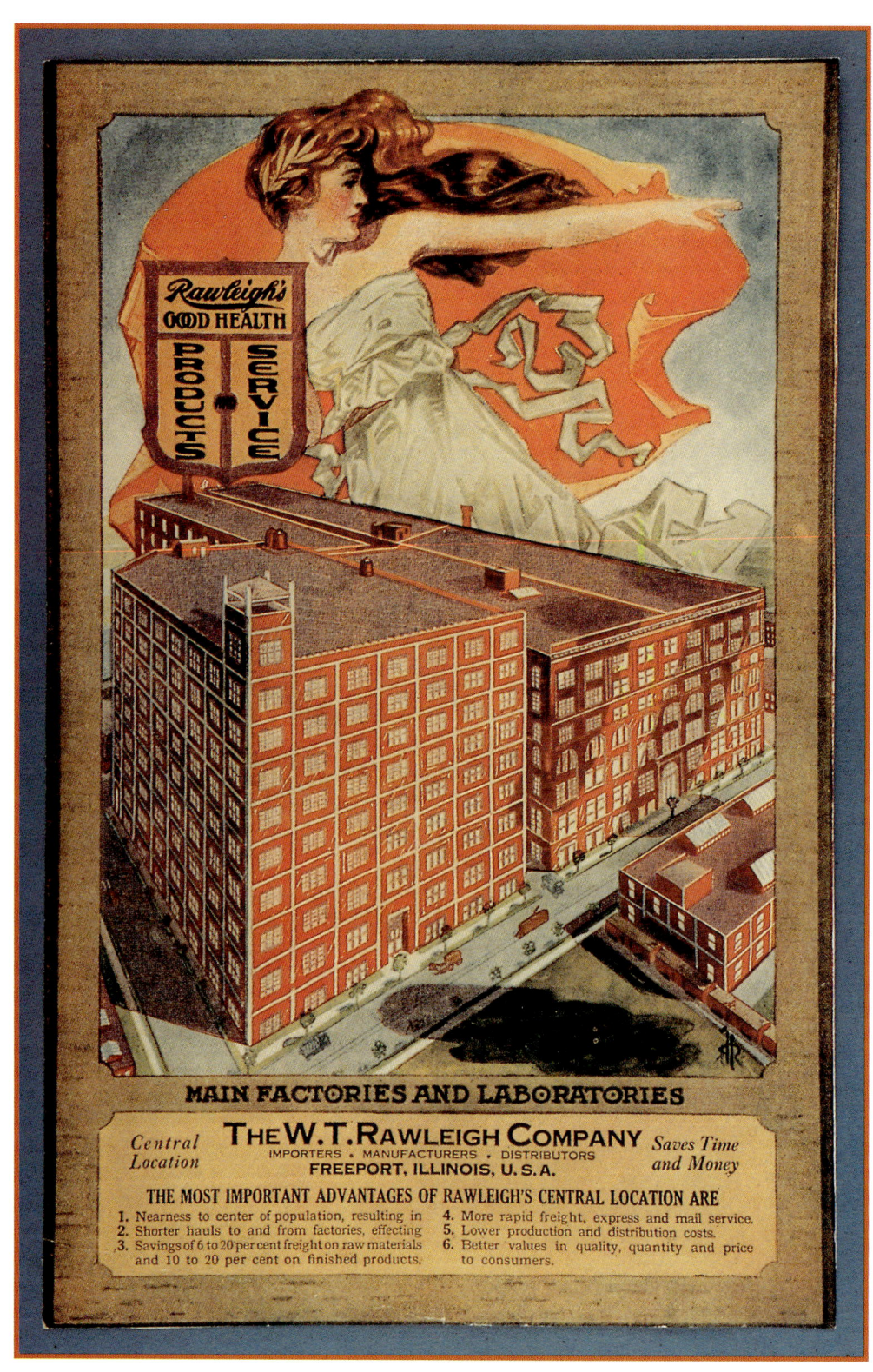

Shown above an original 1920s publication "The Most Important Advantages of Rawleigh's Central Location are." "Saves Time and Money."

west and southwest. For Illinois, Indiana, Kentucky, Ohio, and Michigan, the service was quick with shorter hauls. The Illinois Central, St. Paul, Northwestern, and Great Western railroads dispersed in nine different directions from Freeport, Illinois.

Close proximity to the Chicago outer belt line was a great advantage for the freight-car system in the United States, as well as Chicago being the greatest railroad center in the world.

The W.T. Rawleigh Company manufactured their own products. While materials and supplies were received from all over the world, most were from the eastern and southern regions.

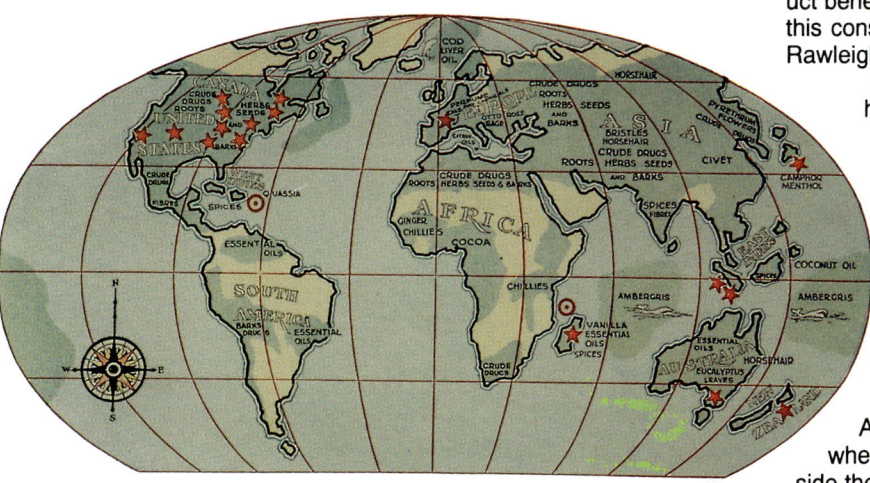

All the different countries where raw materials were secured by the Rawleigh industries are shown in the green portions on the map. The buff coloring indicates the parts of the world where no materials were secured by the industry. Red stars indicate Rawleigh factories and branches in the United States, Australia, Canada, Dutch East Indies, France, Japan, Madagascar, and New Zealand. Rawleigh plantations indicated by the red circles were in the West Indies and on the Grand Comore Island. Rawleigh industries obtained only the best qualities and values at the lowest costs in all the world's markets.

In 1924, Rawleigh's had the largest, most complete and best equipped factories with the largest number of products in this type of business. Rawleigh's made all their products complete with the exception of a few items like toothbrushes, bottles, and cans. They were fully equipped to make many things that other companies could not make at all. Later they would manufacture their own line of toothbrushes and construct a facility for the production of bottles.

In 1932, over a million bottles of Rawleigh's Liniment were sold. This was the oldest Rawleigh home remedy and was first named "Rawleigh's Mountain Herb Liniment." Second in sales and serviceability was Rawleigh's Anti-Pain Oil introduced into the product line in 1896. If you should have "Rawleigh's Mountain Herb Liniment" in your collection, I would appreciate hearing from you.

W.T. Rawleigh started his company in the family home with little capital. He made **SERVICE** the fundamental principle in his business structure and strove to provide his customers with the largest and best line of "Good Health Products" obtainable any-

where. A devotion to this ideal, correct and current business methods of the day, superior laboratories, the most modern manufacturing facilities, factory location, large resources and conservative management made The W.T. Rawleigh Company one of the foremost of its kind.

To the consumer, Rawleigh not only supplied reliable medicines, food flavors, spices, extracts, soaps, toilet accessories, washing compounds, cleaners, polishes, insecticides, veterinary remedies, and stock and poultry preparations, but also dispensed information on healthful living and disease prevention. The company claimed that those who used a Rawleigh laboratory product benefited in the greatest degree from such service, and that this consumer benefit was the dominant aim of "The House of Rawleigh."

Throughout the text, only a small portion of Rawleigh history, policy, and business practice is covered. Among the materials presented is an ad a would-be Rawleigh retailer might have answered in February 1934:

"WANTED: Man with car. Hustler can start earning $35 weekly and increase rapidly. Nothing new. Now over 8,200 Rawleigh Routes. Many doing $5,000 - $12,000 annual business in necessities for home - farm. All backed by $17,000,000 worldwide industry. Stocks, equipment, supplied on credit. Write for information how to start in business on our capital. **W.T. RAWLEIGH CO., Dept. B-43-FAF, Freeport, Ill.**

An illustration of this original advertisement appears elsewhere in this publication, as Rawleigh also advertised outside the company for dealers.

It is impossible to list or photograph every Rawleigh product or document that was available to the consumer. Many were lost to time. I have provided those made available to me through other sources and those in my private collection.

Welcome "To The House of Service," where "The Rawleigh Man Sells the Greatest Number and Largest Variety on Rawleigh's Pay-After-You-Are-Satisfied Plan." Explore Rawleigh's Printing Department, examine Rawleigh Paper Memorabilia, and discover facts about Preserving Documents. Discover "Why Rawleigh Retailers Served You Best," "Why Mothers' Preferred Rawleigh Products," and "Collecting Rawleigh Products." Discovered Rawleigh service of today through the Golden Pride International.™ Examine Rawleigh's Experimental Farms and inspect Rawleigh Farm Products. It's all part of Rawleigh's history and well worth preserving.

As with any collection, old paper items, historical documents, and photographs are highly sought by collectors. When purchasing Rawleigh items, it is wise to study each product carefully before you purchase. The "Condition Factor" is very important.

Here is a clue as to the date of Rawleigh collectibles. A five digit zip code number was put into use by the United States Post Office in 1959. Zip codes appearing on any product indicate a date after 1959.

Author's Note: The fate of the Freeport, Illinois vacant Rawleigh factory is unknown as of this writing. In June 1996, to reduce overcrowding in the Stephenson County jail, modular jail cells may have been placed within the vacant factory.

Any collector interested in starting a national Rawleigh collectors' organization may write to my attention. As previously stated, please direct your correspondence to Schiffer Publishing Ltd.

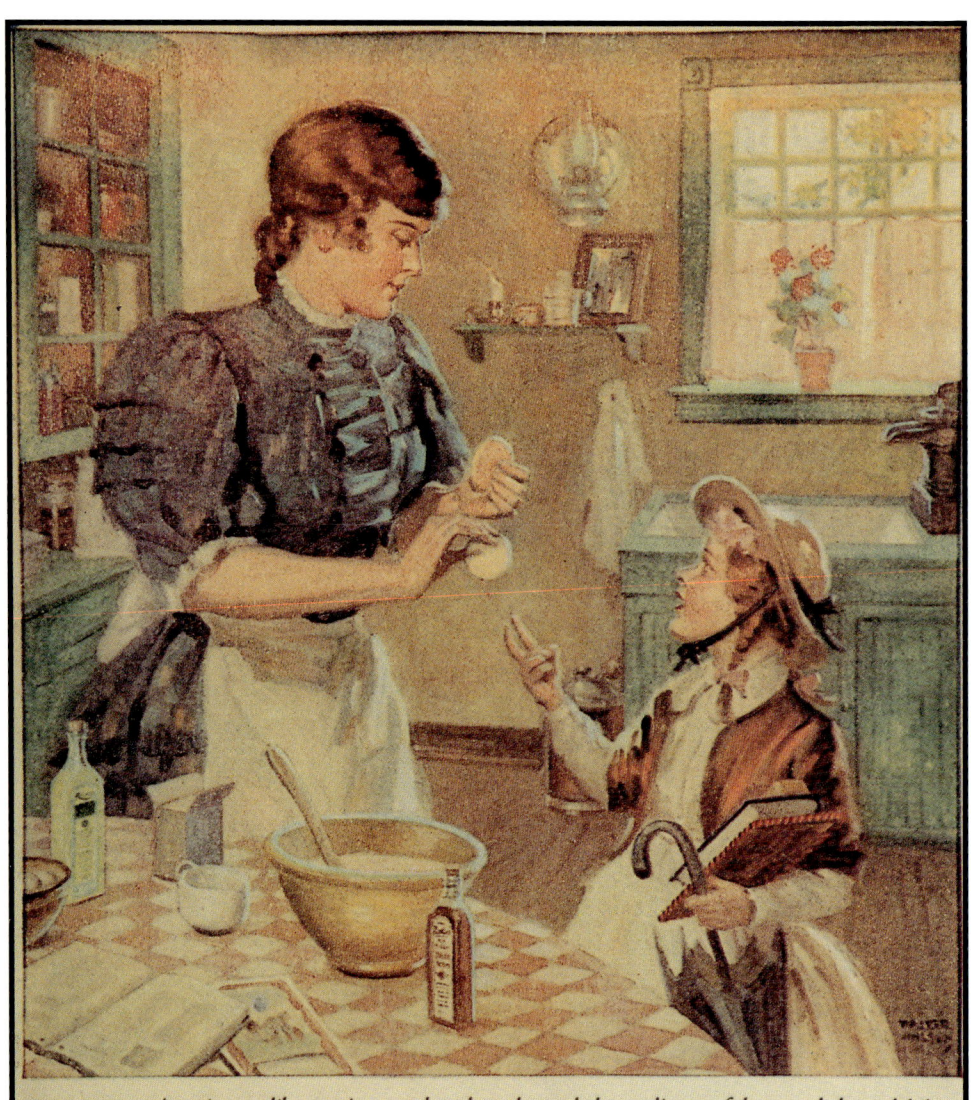

Since 1889 mothers in steadily growing numbers have learned the quality, usefulness and dependability of Rawleigh's Good Health Products. Their daughters were taught the economy and convenience of having them in the home. Millions of families have grown up with them happy and satisfied with their use.

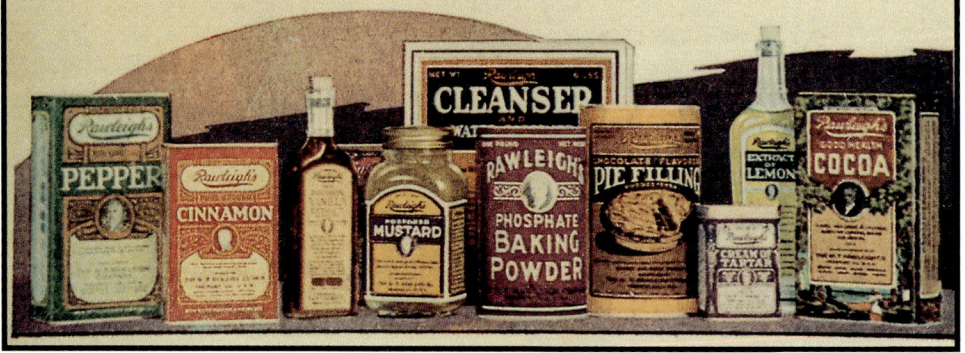

Daughters were taught the economy and convenience of having Rawleigh products in their home. *Rawleigh's 40th Anniversary 1929.*

Chapter 1. History

A FRIEND OF THE FAMILY®
Founder W.T. Rawleigh

William Thomas Rawleigh was not even eighteen years old when he tied his horse and mortgaged buggy to a post near the residence and — taking his sample case containing four different kinds of medicines, a few brands of extracts, and essences — walked up to the front door of his first customer. Little did this young lad know that his ability as a salesman would attract attention and that his name "W.T. Rawleigh" would become recognized around the world.

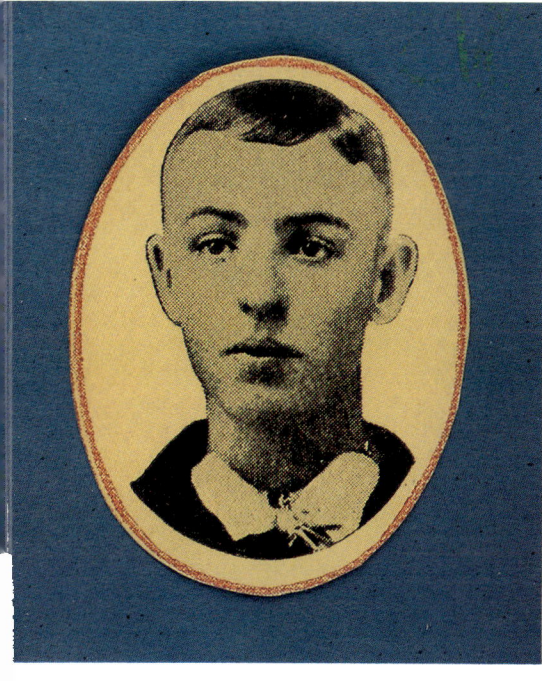

The young William T. Rawleigh (born December 3, 1870 - died January 23, 1951).

It was April 6, 1889, when W.T. Rawleigh drove his buggy into Stephenson County, Illinois, from his parents farm near Mineral Point, Wisconsin. At this Illinois farm house he made his first sale of liniment and salve.

W.T. Rawleigh began with little capital; his only business experiences were in selling the book "Deeds of Daring by Blue and Gray" — short stories of the Civil War, and in making ink (at the age of 15 which he sold to school mates and country stores) and his own medicines which he sold to neighbors and friends.

He was born December 3, 1870 to Charles and Sarah (Babcock) Rawleigh and was the eldest of eight children. Raised on the farm, he helped with chores during the summers months and attended school in the winter.

At the age of 17, he talked his father, Charles Rawleigh, into helping him launch the business venture which would be built into a successful private company of which he and his family were the sole owners.

W.T. Rawleigh was an acquaintance of J.R. Watkins, founder of The J.R. Watkins Medical Company of Winona, Minnesota. For a brief period of time, Rawleigh traveled as a salesman for Mr. Watkins in 1889, just prior to selling his own "Good Health Products" line. It is understood that Rawleigh discussed his plans for starting his own medical company with Watkins.

In 1890, twenty-year-old William T. Rawleigh married Minnie B. Trevillian. They had three children: Anna May, Wilbur Thomas Rawleigh who died during World War I, and Lucille. W.T. Rawleigh later married Marguerite Schneider. Both wives preceded him in death.

Records indicate that William Thomas and Minnie B. Rawleigh turned their kitchen into a part-time factory where they produced liniment until W.T. could get enough money together to rent a small building on East Exchange Street. In 1891, Rawleigh began manufacturing poultry powder, and later other medicines, some of which were made, bottled, and labeled in his own home. These items were sold at wholesale and retail with a positive guarantee of satisfaction or no sale.

In 1895, W.T. Rawleigh founded the Dr. Blair Medical Company, later to become known as The W.T. Rawleigh Medical Company. Rawleigh soon hired additional salesmen to sell his products using the "direct-to-customers method" which Rawleigh had first used himself. Within three years, his sales technique was leading the way throughout the country.

W.T. Rawleigh recognized that correct, economic business principles were absolutely essential for his success, so that year he went **straight** to the farmer. Rawleigh passed by the jobber and the dealer, taking the shortest route to the greatest market. Rawleigh was among the first pioneer manufacturers to offer a free trial and guarantee absolute satisfaction or no sale.

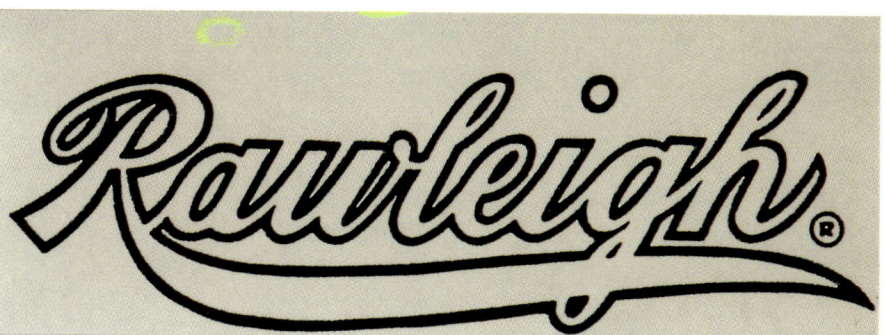

The name "Rawleigh" became a symbol and a guarantee of the highest merit and integrity, value, good faith, and of genuine service.

The "Rawleigh" symbol became synonymous with service directly to the home and farm. Over the years Rawleigh would meet the continuing need of products of practical usefulness. The two-fold purpose of the firm, and Rawleigh's personal determination, was to make the best products and to deliver them to consumers in the most direct, economical, and convenient way while at the lowest possible price and on terms that guaranteed full satisfaction and protected against disappointment and loss of time or money.

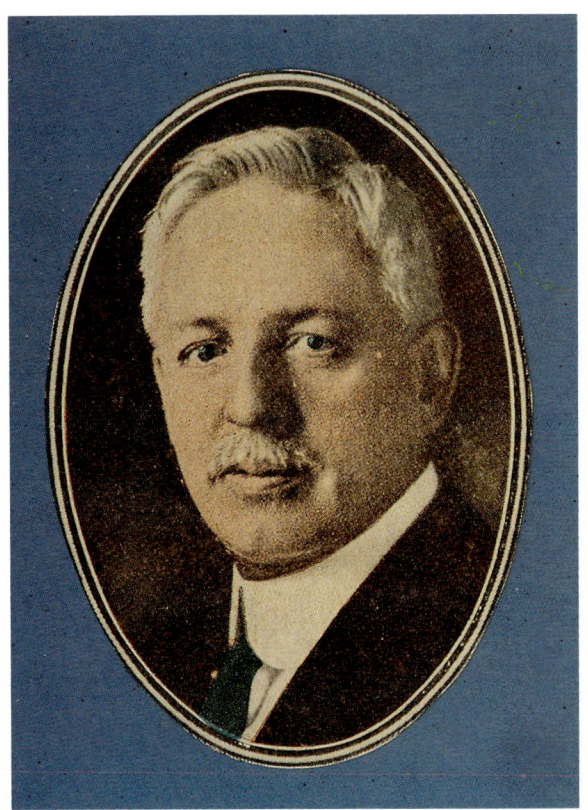

W.T. Rawleigh in a later photograph, that appears on many Rawleigh products and in numerous publications. Very seldom did Rawleigh products change in packaging.

Incorporated January 11, 1895, manufacturing began on a larger scale. The process was slow at first, but with each year a larger number of reliable workers, including W.T. Rawleigh, went in person to farmers and explained the uses of the Rawleigh line. Each salesman provided a free trial offer on the company's "Pay-After-You-Are-Satisfied" plan.

In 1898, on the corner of Douglas Avenue and Powell Street, the first brick factory was built, but soon found inadequate. In 1901 a larger addition was built providing fourteen times as much floor space as was required at the time the company was organized six year before.

From 1902 to approximately 1916, the company's name was changed to "The W.T. Rawleigh Medical Company." Packaging marked "The W.T. Rawleigh Medical Co." can be dated to this period.

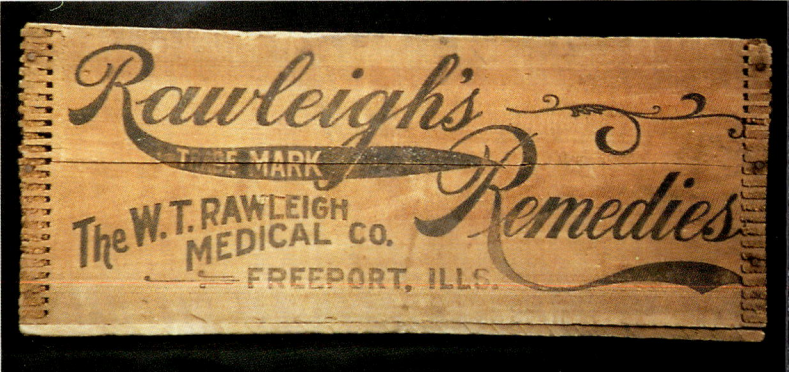

The wooden crate is marked "Rawleigh's Remedies. TRADEMARK THE W.T. RAWLEIGH MEDICAL CO. FREEPORT, ILLS." The side panel indicated "GLASS BE VERY CAREFUL" and Shannon, Ill. *See additional wooden crates in this publication.* $75-$100.

Between the years 1908 and 1911, W.T. Rawleigh served as President of the Citizens' Commercial Association, Mayor of Freeport, Member of the Legislature, Bank Director, Owner and Editor of a daily newspaper, and as President of the Rawleigh-Schryer Company.

On the morning of January 23, 1951, William Thomas Rawleigh, at age 80, died at the local hospital following an extended illness. He was buried in Freeport's Oakland Cemetery.

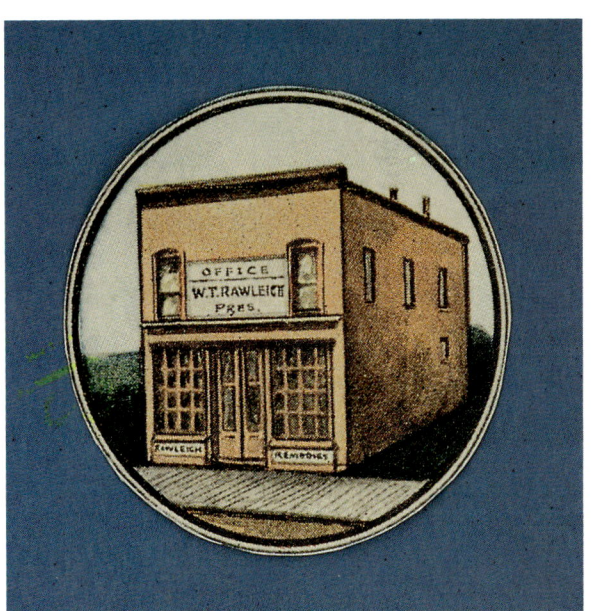

The first Rawleigh factory in 1895, started with three employees in a rented building. One employee was believed to have been Rawleigh's brother-in-law, James R. Jackson. By 1896, thirty men were selling products within the Freeport area and factory space was doubled.

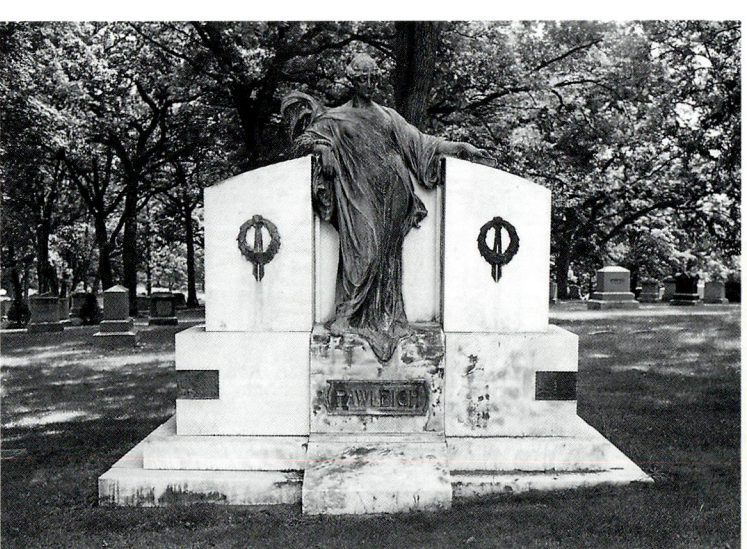

The massive monument in Oakland Cemetery chiseled with the prestigious name "RAWLEIGH."

Quality the First Consideration

During his early selling experience, Rawleigh observed that, while a good salesman could sell most anything ONCE, that to satisfy customers and hold their patronage year after year every product must be scientifically made, reliable, and of an unusually high degree of quality. To improve Rawleigh products to meet the highest degree of efficiency and to guarantee uniform quality, the company's first Analytical Laboratory was installed in 1898. This laboratory was enlarged numerous times and in 1915 it was valued at thousands of dollars and produced the results required by W.T. Rawleigh. It was recognized for its standard of excellence by many millions of customers.

The first of many large buildings was constructed in 1904, filled with modern equipment in all departments. Many Rawleigh customers never realized the enormous magnitude of the Rawleigh business, either in size, in the completeness of its three factories, or in the number and extent of its branches and warehouses.

Rawleigh's growth was rapid, and real estate was constantly being purchased. Buildings once considered too large were found to be inadequate in less than two years.

Within ten years the high quality of Rawleigh Preparations, the honesty of their plan of selling, and the unquestioned character of the management, brought Rawleigh's up to the forefront of medical manufacturers. Rawleigh's capitalization was one million dollars ($1,000,000.00) in 1906. Their floor space was measured by acres; their work force was nearly a thousand strong.

Around 1905, W.T. Rawleigh purchased the "Freeport Standard" newspaper, and continued to publish it until his responsibilities in other connections made the publication of the "Standard" difficult. It was then acquired by Dwight B. Breed and James R. Cowley who were former newspaper men.

In 1906 Rawleigh's was in every state and territory in the country, satisfying hundreds of thousands of homes where they carried - "HEALTH, HAPPINESS AND PROSPERITY." By 1908, sixty-six times more floor space was occupied than in the original factory of nine years prior. In 1909, it was necessary to add extra space onto the building in Freeport and purchase more real estate for storage purposes to provide for the growth of the business. During this period, the company originated its pure, all-medicine mixtures which gradually took the place of weaker and inferior animal stock foods offered by other manufacturers.

W.T. Rawleigh also served as mayor of Freeport, Illinois, from 1909 to 1911. Rawleigh began his administration with an empty treasury and by 1911 a balance of $22,029 was shown.

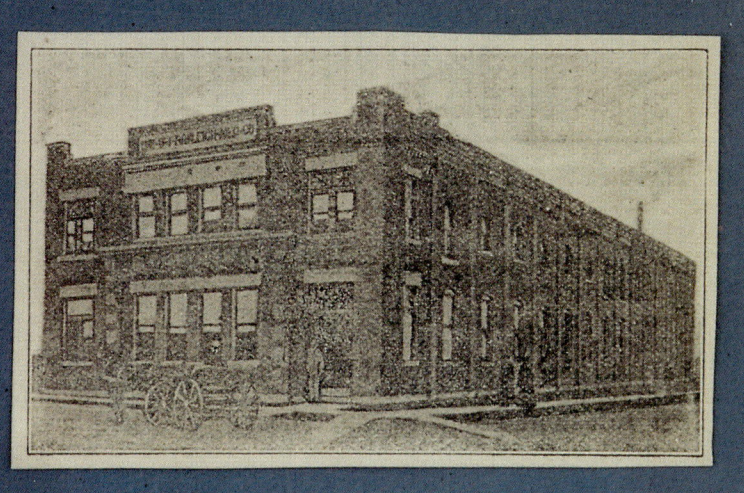

The Powell Street factory, 1898 - 1901.

Shown above a section of the 1911 enlargement to the Rawleigh factory.

The Chester, Pennsylvania Branch House built in 1911.

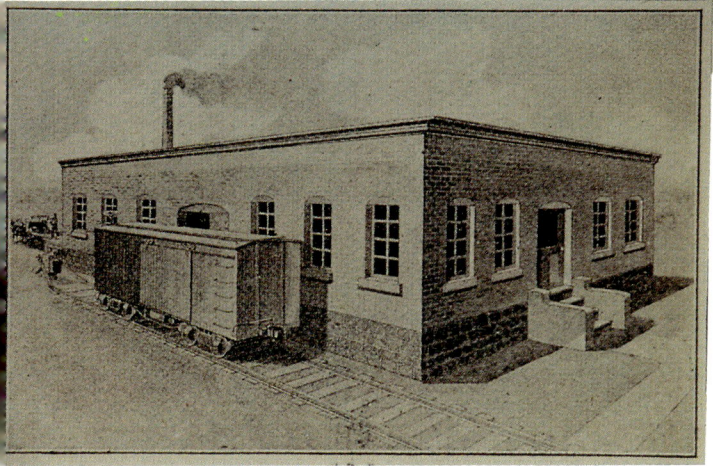

PART RAWLEIGH'S ENLARGED FACTORIES IN 1911

In 1911, Rawleigh management confirmed to W.T. Rawleigh that the four and six-story buildings they had erected between 1904 to 1909 was insufficient due to the demand for Rawleigh products throughout the Central States. W.T. Rawleigh and management found it necessary to construct another new six-story building and to add two more stories to the main building, completing an immense structure 120 ft. wide by 252 ft. long, 6 stories high with a full basement. The main power house was also rebuilt to accommodate larger engines and additional boilers were installed because of the growth of the business.

On March 13, 1919, the Rawleigh Band was organized and financial support was given by W.T. Rawleigh. The band conductor was Willard Rubendall and had eighteen fully uniformed musicians.

An Institution of Unusual Utility

By 1924, the company was referred to as "An Institution of Unusual Utility," built on a sound foundation. Following correct but progressive policies, the W.T. Rawleigh Company became the fastest-growing industry of its kind. The company was also the most recognized leader among direct-selling organizations; it was considered to be the largest, most substantially complete, experienced, best equipped, and the most productive.

All along, Rawleigh had designed his products to fill some universal need. He firmly believed "The power to satisfy human wants is utility." According to Rawleigh literature, his company came to be seen as an institution of great and unusual utility that held an enviable record, worthy of their confidence, deserving of their patronage, and capable of giving the most complete service and satisfaction. It became known as "The House of Service," conscious of the responsibilities of leadership and prepared for a future whose limits were only time and a faithful devotion in service. The trademark became a symbol of that guaranty and of a genuine service.

W.T. Rawleigh established a 240 acre experimental stock farm west of Freeport during the early 1920s, known as "Ideal Farms." (*See* Chapter 8, "Rawleigh's Experimental Farms," for additional information.) Later he would have his estate, which he called "Countryside," built across from Ideal Farms. This estate was "a site of many well-landscaped acres" that would remain his residence until the last years of W.T. Rawleigh's life.

With 12 million dollars in assets in 1925, Rawleigh paid cash for everything. With no debt to hamper the growth or cost increase and expenses of doing business, Rawleigh's was financially the strongest organization of its kind, free from bonded indebtedness.

The Rawleigh-Schryer Company

Incorporated in 1909, and with a capital and resources of approximately $200,000, was "The Rawleigh-Schryer Company" of Freeport, Illinois — manufacturers of modern high grade gasoline and kerosene engines adapted for general farm use. That year, W.T. Rawleigh, an acquaintance of Schyer's, became president of the corporation, providing his experience in manufacturing, selling, counseling, and financial assistance in the development of "The Rawleigh-Schryer Company."

The large and modern buildings that composed "The Rawleigh-Schryer Company" were located on a six acre tract of land in the manufacturing and shipping district of Freeport. Constructed of fireproof concrete, the machine shop was 80 ft. wide by 180 ft. long and $30,000 was invested in its modern machinery. This did not included over $10,000 worth of wood and metal patterns and tools which enabled the company to produce engines.

All of the castings were made in their own foundry, which they also operated. The company grouped their warehouses and storerooms, which were large and close together, making it the most modern and complete plant of its kind.

The Rawleigh-Schryer engines were noted for their simplicity, reliability, surplus power, balance, and fuel economy. They were sold by dealers throughout the United States and in the Eastern and Western Provinces of Canada.

The Rawleigh-Schryer Company offered a 32 page, copyrighted, fully illustrated booklet entitled "How To Choose A Gas Engine." In 1915, a two-cent postage stamp brought it free to all Rawleigh customers. (*Also see* Chapter 8. Rawleigh's Experimental Farm.)

Paul F. Schryer, who became General Manager of the business, was a pioneer builder, designer, and the originator of many improvements in gasoline engines. He built his first engine of his own design in 1897.

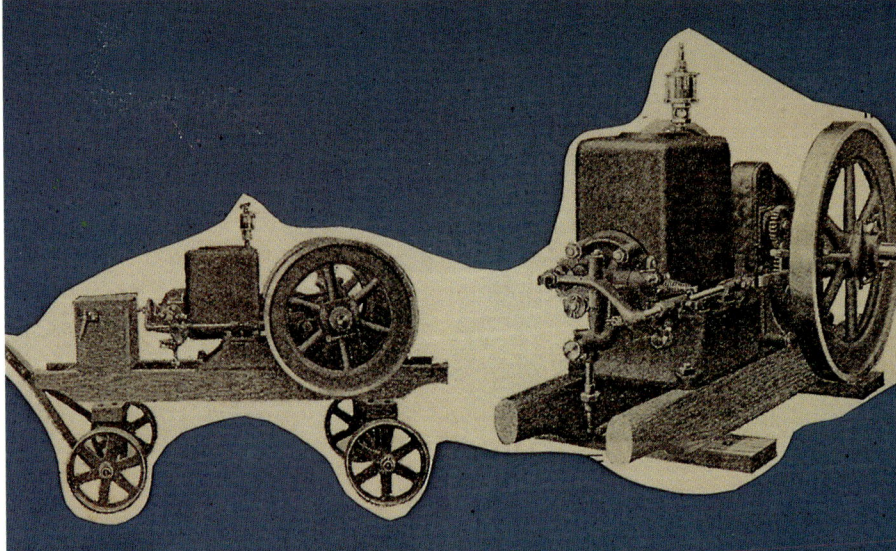
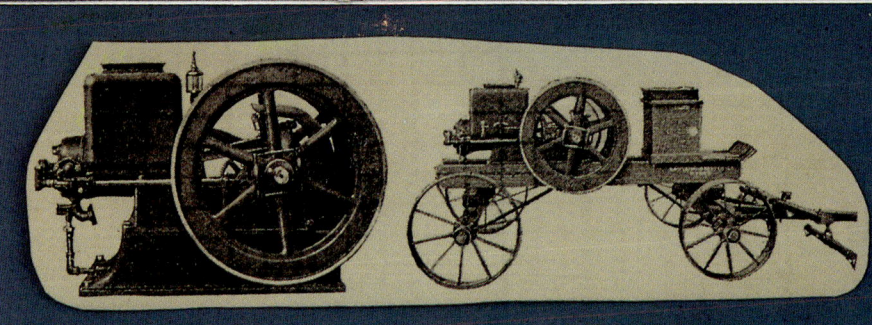

The Rawleigh-Schryer Company engines.

Big Commodity

Service was the big commodity in which Rawleigh greatly excelled. He believed that "Leadership" came to those who excelled (which Rawleigh did) and that as they became better qualified, they were ready to grasp any opportunities. When Rawleigh had seen a need, he was ready to fill it and was not afraid of responsibility, never turning away from work or duty. "Leadership" came through the service and in the end it was proven that his management team could lead.

As Rawleigh's growth continued, the company held onto its "Leadership" position by serving customers and consumers better than any other similar industry. With its continuing success, in 1926, the W.T. Rawleigh Company built a factory in Freeport to produce glass containers for their products.

At the turn of a switch — power, lights, steam, heat, water, ventilation, and automatic machinery began to produce newly made bottles twenty-four hours a day. Presses printed 125 carloads of paper. The company facilities were equipped with machine, wood, electrical, and steam fitting shops, laundry, and a first aid department. The W.T. Rawleigh Company also had laboratories, a veterinarian, a dietitian, and the farms. These were just the highlights in a complete industry.

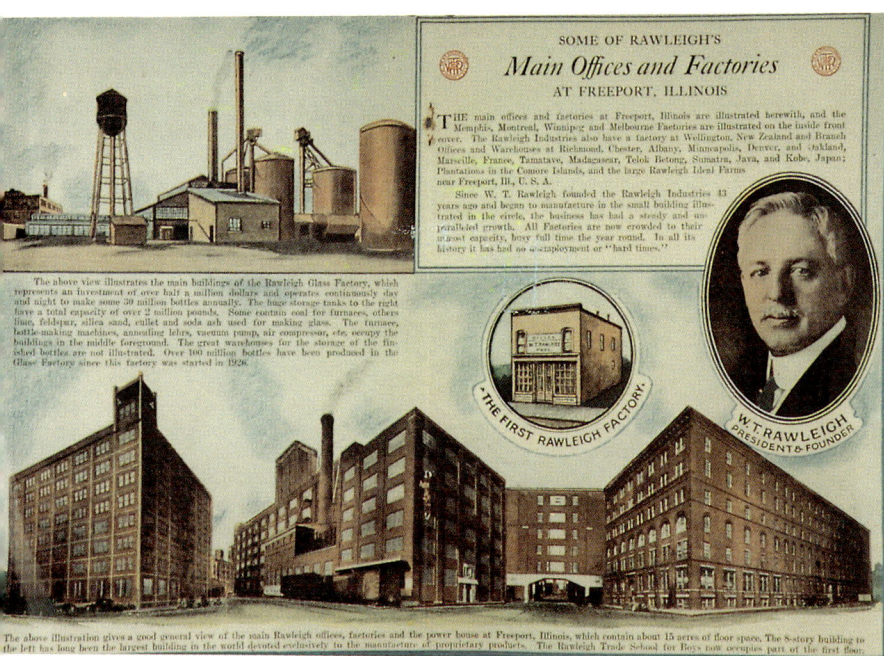

In the left corner are the main buildings of the Rawleigh Glass Factory, circa 1932. This factory represented an investment of over half a million dollars and operated continuously day and night, making over 30 million bottles annually. On the right, storage tanks had a total capacity of over two million pounds, containing coal for furnaces, along with lime, feldspar, silica sand, cullet, and soda ash used in the production of glass. The buildings in the foreground housed the furnace, bottle-making machines, annealing lehrs, vacuum pump, and air compressor. The warehouses for the storage of the finished bottles are not illustrated. From 1926 to 1932, over 100 million bottles had been produced in this factory. Also shown are the first Rawleigh factory, W.T. Rawleigh (president and founder), and a general view of the main Rawleigh facilities. In 1932, the Rawleigh Trade School for Boys occupied part of the first floor.

A present day view of the former 223 East Main Street Rawleigh factories and office in downtown Freeport, Illinois. The building to the left was the largest of its kind devoted to the manufacture of proprietary products. In 1989, Harry W. Hersey purchased the W.T. Rawleigh Company. The buildings were not purchased by Hersey in the acquisition. *Kurt Koester Photograph*

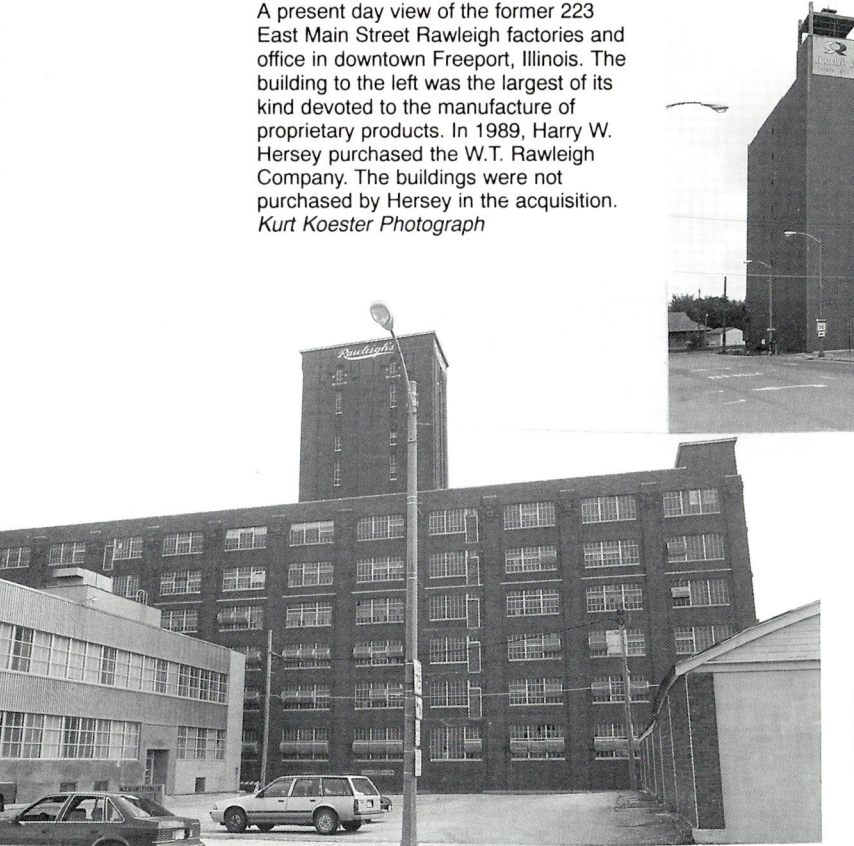

A view of the former print shop at the Rawleigh factories and office building complex in Freeport. *Kurt Koester Photograph*

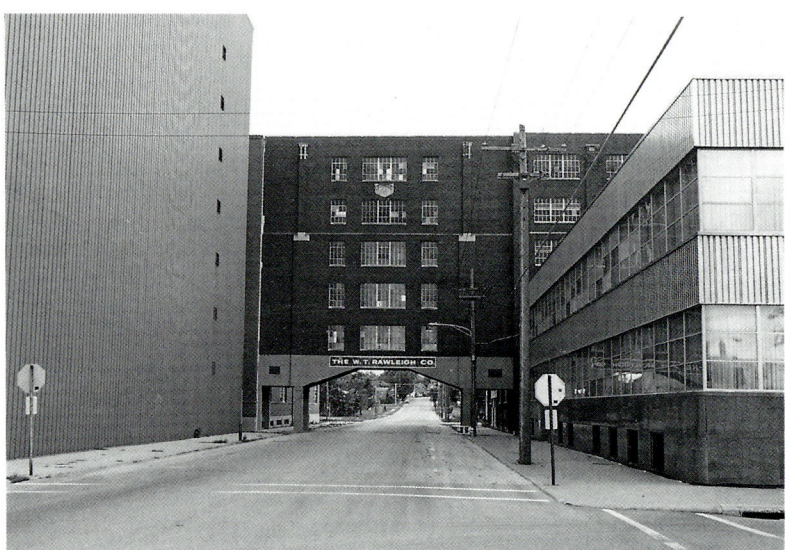

The W.T. Rawleigh Co. facilities in Freeport, Illinois. *Kurt Koester Photograph*

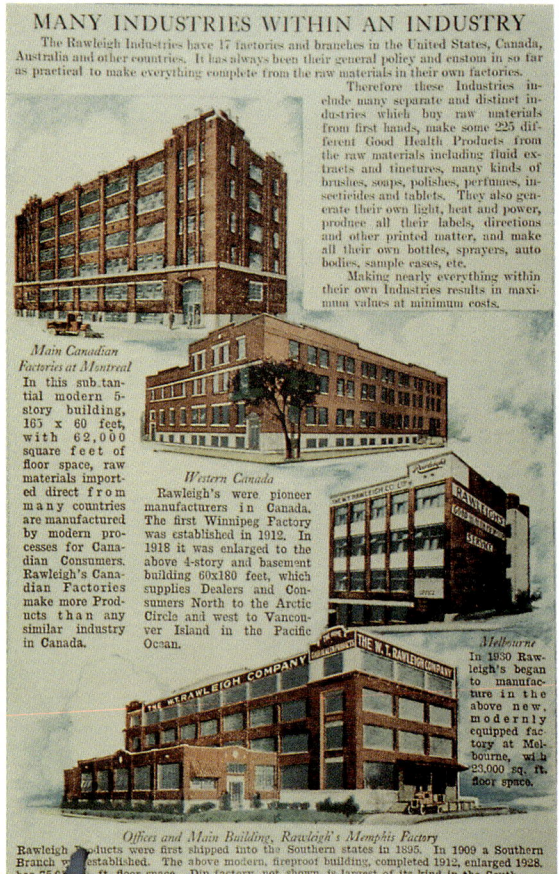

The original promotion "Many Industries Within An Industry" from a 1932 Rawleigh publication.

Within their 40 years of business prior to 1929, the construction of new factories and branches had reached across North American and as far away as Australia. Over 1,000 employees and 7,000 Rawleigh retailers made and delivered 35,000,000 products a year.

Rawleigh buyers bought raw materials from foreign branches of the company and at tropical plantations that grew vanilla. Over 2,000 tons of raw materials valued at $2,000,000 were imported in a year and hundreds of producers supplied 1,200 different materials fillings 1,834 carloads a year.

Rawleigh firmly believed in the continued study, experience, methods, ideals, devotion, and obligation to doing things better in providing better quantity. The firm provided value and satisfaction from within "The House of Service."

The Rawleigh Organization

A photograph taken at the main offices and factories in Freeport, Illinois. This group of employees represents some of the officers, managers, superintendents, engineers, chemists, correspondents, and executives that were located in Freeport.

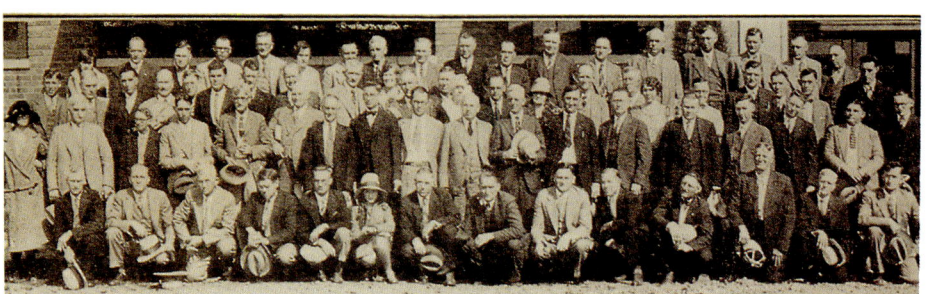

W.T. Rawleigh had taught the organization that service was the function of business and basis of progress and that QUALITY goes with service and progress. Proper materials, methods, facilities, production, and fulfillment of needs were all necessary to meet the Rawleigh's excellence requirements.

The Freeport, Illinois, organization was made up of experienced, dependable and highly trained employees. Many had been with the company from five to twenty years and longer. The majority of these employees were experts with years of experience, and specialists in their trade.

Any new employee not familiar with the operation of the organization was trained to be thorough, careful, and painstaking in everything they were to do. Careful employee training made the Rawleigh organization most reliable.

Among the company's highly skilled occupations and professions during the early 1920s were: accountants, advertising men, artists, bacteriologists, bill clerks, bindery men, bookkeepers, branch managers, cabinet makers, carpenters, cashiers, chemists, city sales managers, compositors, cost accountants, designers, dietitian, Dictaphone operators, draftsmen, electricians, engineers, executives, factory managers, filing clerks, firemen, foreign buyers, foremen, freight handlers, industrial engineers, layout men, librarians, linotype operators, machinists, mailing clerks, managers, mechanics, multigraph operators, night watchmen, officer managers, painters, plumbers, press feeders, pressmen, printers, purchasing agents, receiving clerks, recruiting managers, sales director, sales managers, secretaries, shipping clerks, steam fitters, stenographers, stock clerks, tablet makers, telephone operators, traffic managers, and typists. With the help of these employees, the W.T. Rawleigh Company bought all the raw materials used in the manufacturing of Rawleigh's Products and distributed the finished goods from seven factories and branches throughout the United States and Canada.

In 1931, Harland H. Hoppock was brought into the W.T. Rawleigh Company in Freeport, Illinois. Harland was a buyer of raw materials such as spices in Europe, Africa and the Far East. His wife, Yvonne, was a native of Marseilles, France.

Mr. Hoppock was responsible for gathering many of the Rawleigh Museum's valuable artifacts during his travels abroad. Other Rawleigh buyers also purchased artifacts wherever they went.

W.T. Rawleigh traveled extensively in various European countries, studying business, political, and economic conditions. Throughout his travels he acquired a vast collection of paintings, rugs, and statuary that was returned to his "Countryside" estate and to the city of Freeport.

I understand many of these pieces are now displayed in the Freeport public library and art museums while others remain in private collections.

Policies and Business Practices

As a privately owned corporation, the W.T. Rawleigh Company was independent and kept free from entangling alliances, price fixing, and other trade agreements. They were against unlawful profiteering schemes which often destroyed essential independence and freedom in the conduct of business. They opposed all local, state, and national combinations, monopolies, trusts, and other illegal practices that increased the cost of living and caused burdens upon consumers.

Rawleigh believed in the intelligent cooperation between producer and consumer, eliminating all unnecessary middlemen, and in encouraging free, open markets and exchange of trade between individuals and nations. They believed strongly that no restrictions should be put upon the rights of anyone and were against adding unnecessary expenses to the cost of producing or selling any necessity of life.

After World War I, Rawleigh Retailers were able to undersell their competitors because they sold hundreds of thousands of dollars worth of their old stock on hand, bought at low prices before the war, without raising their wholesale prices. The benefit of these stocks were given to the retailers and consumers.

When Rawleigh was faced with the increased cost of nearly all materials, supplies, labor, and other expenses, they found it necessary to increase their wholesale and retail prices on all of their products. This took place during the early 1920s.

The Company would continue its independent and competitive policies, do its best to obtain raw materials at the lowest costs, and try to keep manufacturing and selling expenses down. They would continue to improve their quality, sell at the lowest wholesale prices, and provided the best values in everything at the lowest prices.

In 1922, 648 carloads, (approximately 10,000 tons) of products were shipped from Rawleigh factories to branch houses at the lowest rates and sold in wholesale quantities to retailers, who sold them direct to the consumer.

New Branches

In 1895, Mississippi received its first Rawleigh's shipment. By 1897, salesmen started to deliver in Arkansas, Texas, Alabama, Georgia, and Tennessee. It was not until 1909 that the southern trade had grown to such large proportions that W.T. Rawleigh felt it necessary to provide other buildings. Real estate was acquired and a 26 foot wide by 140 foot long warehouse was constructed, opening the company's first branch in Memphis, Tennessee.

By April 1, 1911, the staff of 66 salesmen had increased to about 300 and the Memphis headquarters was too small. That fall construction began on the large Memphis factory which was completed in 1912. It was the most artistic factory in Memphis, sitting back from the street and surrounded by shrubbery. This factory doubled the number of people employed in all similar Memphis factories combined.

In 1912, the Rawleigh's building was the largest of its kind in Memphis, a fireproof structure 63 ft. wide by 183 ft. long and five stories high. It was constructed of solid steel and concrete and trimmed with substantial face brick and stone.

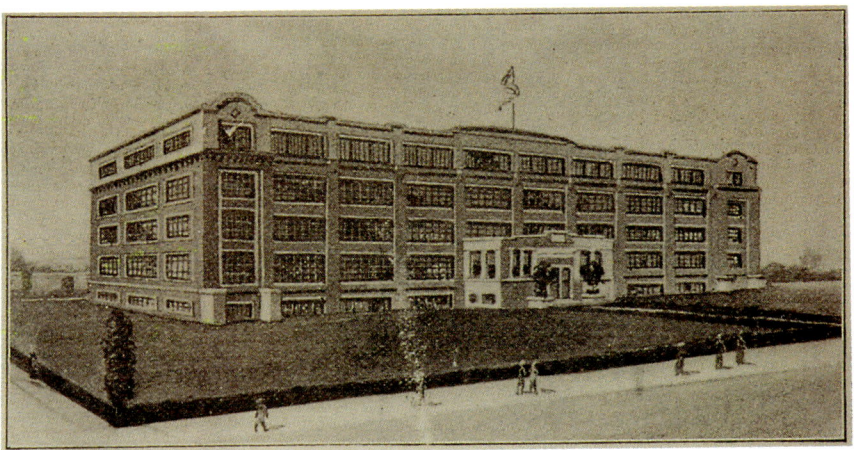

Rawleigh's Memphis factory was completed in 1912.

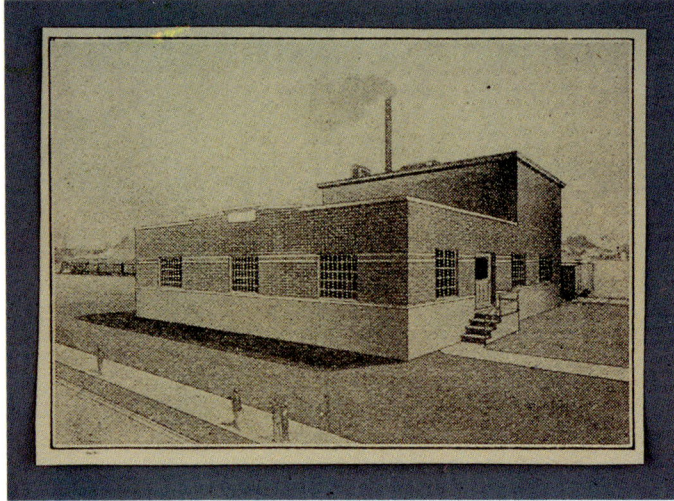

In 1913, Rawleigh's Memphis Stock Dip Factory was constructed.

In 1896 Rawleigh's Products went westward, first into Iowa and Nebraska. The first small shipment was made into California the year before, in 1895; however, it would not be until 1898 that Rawleigh's products reached Utah and Idaho. In 1897, shipments were first made into Kansas, Arkansas and Missouri.

In 1898, the first shipments of Rawleigh's Products were made into Pennsylvania, Massachusetts, New York, Vermont, New Hampshire, Maine, the Virginias, the Carolinas, and other Atlantic coast states.

On September 1, 1912, the first factory of its kind in the Dominion was built in Winnipeg. This was the third factory established by Rawleigh and it was stocked with raw materials and equipped with enough machinery to make every Rawleigh's Product sold in Canada at a total outlay of over $100,000.

Thousand of dollars were spent for raw materials and new machinery and equipment before the manufacturing began. The Canadian factory grew so fast that another building was constructed in 1914, providing an additional 46 by 70 feet of space.

On April 1, 1914, the Toronto Branch opened and supplied products to Ontario, Quebec, Nova Scotia, New Brunswick, and Prince Edward Island; within two years Rawleigh's Products were available in every Province. All products were manufactured in the Winnipeg Branch.

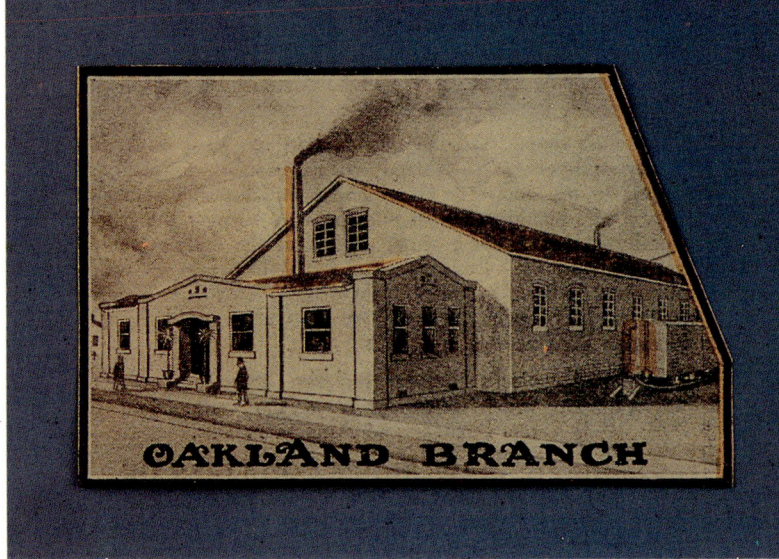

The Oakland, California branch — in 1922 the company shipped everything in carload lots from the main factories to the Oakland branch. From there, products were distributed to customers by rail, ocean freight, and river freight.

An original 1920 promotion for "Six Other Factories and Branches."

In 1900, the business spread from California into Oregon and Washington. Because of high freight rates and the slow service, Rawleigh made no effort to increase the Pacific coast trade; however, the increased volume of business became so fast that the Oakland, California Branch was established on June 1, 1914. This completed a branch house system of distribution, beginning with three factories located at the central points, and extending from the Atlantic to the Pacific and from the Hudson Bay on the north to the Gulf of Mexico on the south.

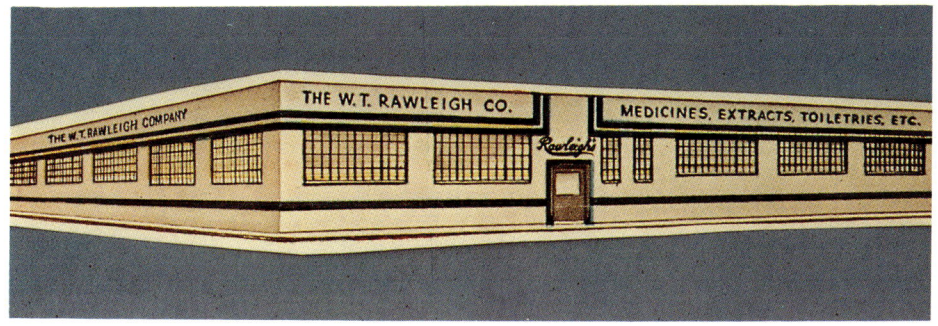

In 1949 Rawleigh announced their new Los Angeles branch, shown above. The vast movement of people into this area and the rapidly expanding business of Rawleigh dealers in Southern California and Arizona prompted Rawleigh to erect a new branch office and warehouse in order to improve their service.

The Minneapolis Branch

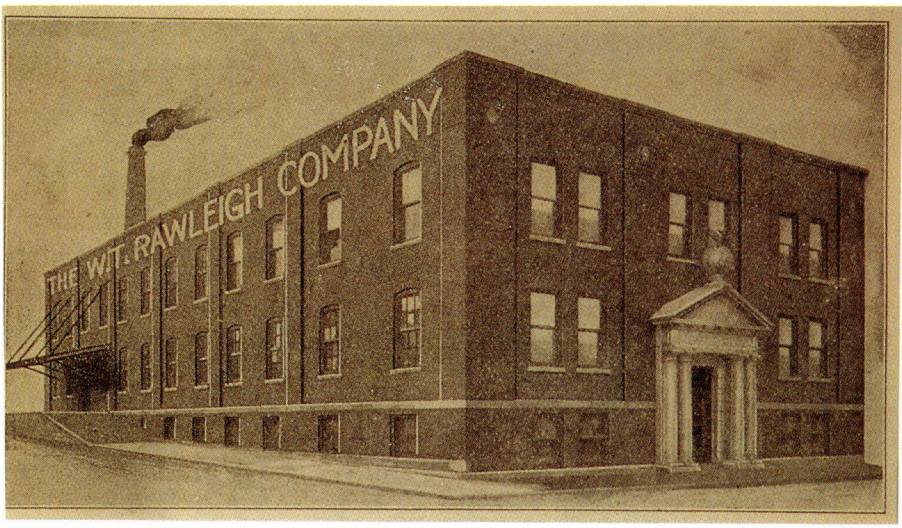

The new Minneapolis branch was opened in January 1916, providing retailers (who sold in Northern Wisconsin, Minnesota, the Dakotas, and Montana) lower freight rates, along with quicker and better service.

Constructed at the corner of 701 Third Street North and Tenth Avenue, the new fire-proof building was centrally located near the working districts and the principal freight depots in Minneapolis. The two story construction with basement was 152 feet long by 60 feet wide and had 27,600 square feet of floor space. It was designed to withstand a load of 300 pounds per square foot and constructed so that additional stories could be added when needed. Rawleigh owned additional land surrounding the building.

The main walls were made with hard pressed vitrified brick and Bedford stone trimmings. Fenestra steel window sashes provided the offices with adequate light and ventilation.

A 5000-pound modern power elevator and scales provided quick freight handling. Private sidings accommodated carloads of shipments from the main factories. On a 10 x 40 foot platform, incoming and outgoing freight of less than a carload lot was handled.

The advantages of the Minneapolis branch to the Northwest Rawleigh retailers and consumers were seen in cheaper, quicker, and better freight handling through express and parcel post service.

The Company maintained a complete selling organization at this executive branch which provided additional valuable service.

The Richmond, Virginia, Branch

The Richmond, Virginia, branch was completed and opened in 1924. The building was 80 x 165 feet in size and the two floors offered 26,400 square feet. Two freight cars could be unload at a private siding that was also equipped with a freight elevator. Located at the rear of the main building was a 30 x 30 foot fire-proof garage used for trucks and autos.

In order to open this branch, it took 14 carloads of Rawleigh's Products valued at $110,000 as the initial stock. This location provided the advantage of giving quicker, cheaper and better shipping service than could be obtained anywhere else in its district. Rawleigh's was constantly bringing production closer to consumers and making improvements and additions in their interests.

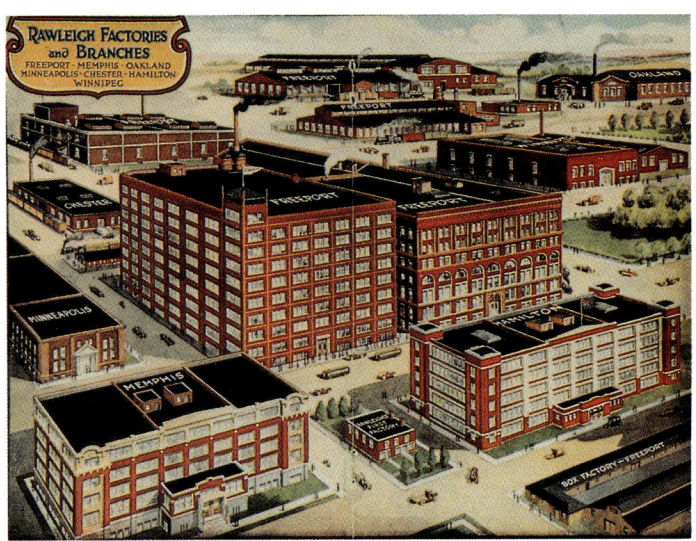

Rawleigh advocated their factories and branches located in Freeport, Memphis, Oakland, Minneapolis, Chester, Hamilton and Winnipeg in the original advertisement.

Inside Rawleigh's Factories

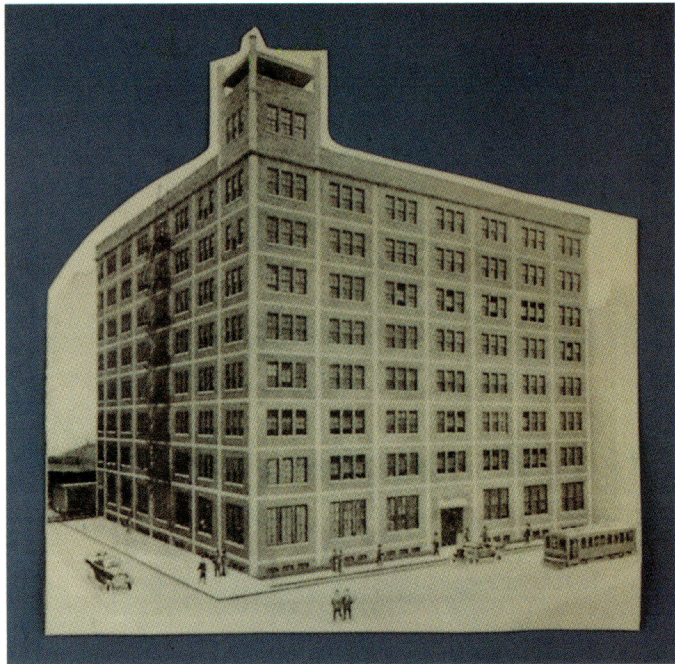

The largest building in the world devoted exclusively to making proprietary products. The 1914 addition to the Rawleigh Freeport factories included over 300 tons of steel, approximately 15,000 barrels of Portland cement, 800 carloads of sand and gravel, one-half million bricks, and about 50 carloads of other essential materials and supplies. The building is 120 ft. wide by 146 ft. long, eight stories high, with a basement underneath, and a tower above. The total floor area was 157,000 square feet.

The W.T. Rawleigh Company of Freeport, Illinois, often welcomed thousands of visitors from across the United States. Visiting Rawleigh's factories was interesting because of the great variety and enormous quantities of supplies they had gathered from far and near. Also of interest to the visitor was the variety of sizes and shapes of packaging that had arrived from domestic and European markets. It took the average visitor two hours to see all the features of the factories. The largest freight elevators ascended to the eighth floor, then visitors climbed two additional flights of stairs into the tower to see the view of Freeport from the town's highest point. One would take in the view of the railroads radiating in all directions and the large size of the plant.

From the tower view, visitors could see The Rawleigh-Schryer factories which also provided tours. Rawleigh guides accompanied all tourist throughout the factories. Leaving the tower, the tour visited the enormous steam jacketed heaters, conveyers, and special equipment where 33,500 cans of Rawleigh's Antiseptic Healing Salve, Medicated Ointment, and Pomade were manufactured and made ready for shipment.

In 1981, the Rawleigh tradition was emphasized by the reintroduction of authentic containers originally created eighty years ago for Rawleigh's Medicated Ointment and Antiseptic Salve. These two products were big sellers for almost the entire history of the Rawleigh Company, made with natural ingredients from an early American formula. (These products are also shown elsewhere in this text.)

On the sixth floor, visitors could see the immense storage barrels, boxes, and cans containing large quantities of drugs, oil, roots, barks, and seeds in their original packages just as they were gathered by the growers. In an adjoining room, visitors could see the large equipment and copper vacuum stills used in extracting the active medicinal elements of the Rawleigh drugs. This was where chemists tested and standardized everything before anything was used. This room was considered an interesting and rare sight. Rawleigh was the only manufacturer at that time that made the fluid extracts they used.

The guide pointed out the thirty-three glass-lined, steel tanks ranging in size from 1,000 to 4,000 gallons capacity used for the aging and storing of only eight of the manufactured articles. Thirteen vats of 650 to 4,000 gallons each were kept in constant use for compounding Rawleigh's Liniment — one of the oldest, reliable, general-purpose remedies. This liniment had such a large sale that over 20,000 gallons of the finished product were kept in stock.

Next on the tour was the great store-room. On 1,464 shelves, 2,400,000 bottles and packages of Rawleigh Products awaited shipment.

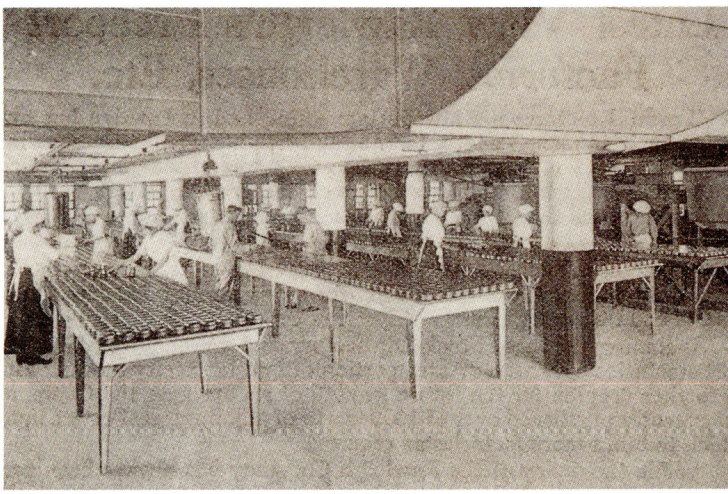

In one day 33,500 cans of salve, ointment and pomade were manufactured.

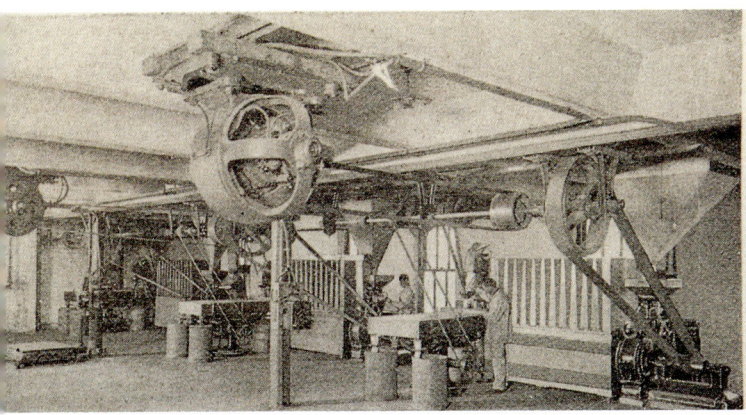

The room where Rawleigh's spices were ground and granulated.

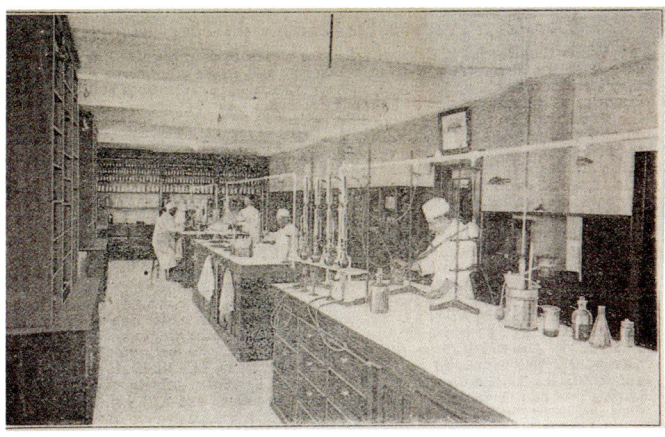

Rawleigh's Analytical Laboratories, Freeport, Illinois. This photograph appeared in a 1917 Rawleigh's Good Health Guide.

In the large spice storage room, visitors saw where one million pounds of whole spices gathered from Africa, India, China, The Dutch East Indies, and other countries were kept in stock. Visitors saw the twelve mills with a daily capacity of 20,000 pounds and three machines that were capable of breaking coarse spices and drugs equal to one railcar. There were numerous smaller machines also used for manufacturing spices and drugs.

On the third floor of the largest building was located the Bottling Room where liquid preparations were bottled. Here visitors observed three 13-tube machines filling bottles at the rate of 45,000 to 85,000 bottles per nine hour day. On large storage tables 25,000 to 50,000 bottles of medicines and extracts were ready to be labeled and packaged. Approximately 43 carloads of manufactured extracts and flavors were kept regularly in stock.

All of two floors of the Freeport buildings were used in the making of Rawleigh's Stock Tonic, Poultry, and All-Medicine Mixtures. Annual sales were 200 carloads.

All of the grinding, mixing, and packaging was done by machinery. Two large rooms were used for the storage of 30,000 pails of these preparations, packed and ready for shipment. This did not include branch house stocks and thousands of pounds packed in drums ready to ship.

A year's supply of raw materials used by the Rawleigh Company required 25 train loads of 30 cars each, not including the thousands of articles received in smaller quantities which amounted to many millions of pounds.

Visitors were often detained because of the immense volume of traffic moving in and out of the factories daily; many areas were also off-limit to visitors. In 1915, Rawleigh records showed that over 1,700 full carloads of freight were handled annually.

In 1915, combined real estate, factories, and warehouses at Freeport, Memphis, Chester, and Winnipeg, equipment, stocks of merchandise, supplies, and other handling's, gave The W.T. Rawleigh Medical Company over three million dollars worth of tangible property, making it one of the strongest institutions of its kind in the world. The company had no bonded indebtedness or preferred stock obligations. They paid cash for everything they bought, and owed no one.

The W.T. Rawleigh Company carried no Fire or Accident Liability Insurance but did create Insurance Reserve Funds for its own protection against such losses. For all of its 20 years as a company in 1915, Rawleigh's management had been conservative, progressive, absolutely independent, and competitive. Its great resources, factories and branches, enormous volume, and the wide extent of its business were all indisputable evidence of substantial continued growth.

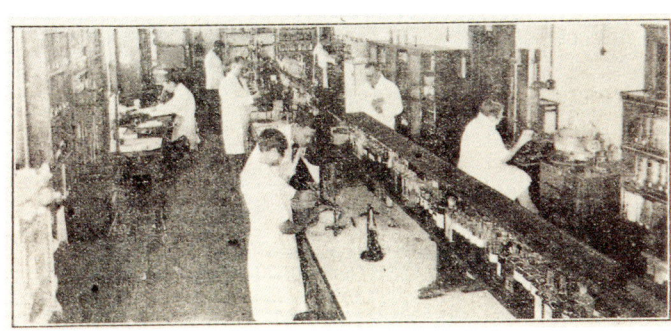

The Rawleigh laboratories, where chemists, pharmacists, and biologists tested both raw materials and finished products. The extensive scientific equipment was used to improve qualities and values.

Superior quality products could not be made from inferior raw materials. Therefore, the Rawleigh Industries had a large staff of chemists and pharmacists working in modern and scientifically equipped laboratories used for testing raw materials, controlling material quality, and for conducting the most extensive research.

Another fundamental policy was that no Rawleigh product was officially recommended on the labels and directions for any other purpose than the particular use for which they were scientifically compounded by experienced chemists and pharmacists who were in charge of manufacture at all Rawleigh's factories. The consumer depended on Rawleigh Quality Products being scientifically made and reliable. Customers expected these products to be useful for everything for which they were officially recommended because all such products were manufactured, packaged and distributed strictly in harmony with local, state, federal, and provincial laws, rules and regulations.

Rawleigh Industries positively guaranteed their products to be of the highest quality of their respective kinds; scientifically made from carefully selected drugs, roots, herbs, essential oils, chemicals, and other raw materials by the most modern methods. Products were shipped fresh and pure, in full weight and measure. They contained no narcotics or habit-forming drugs, and when used as directed were absolutely safe for children and adults.

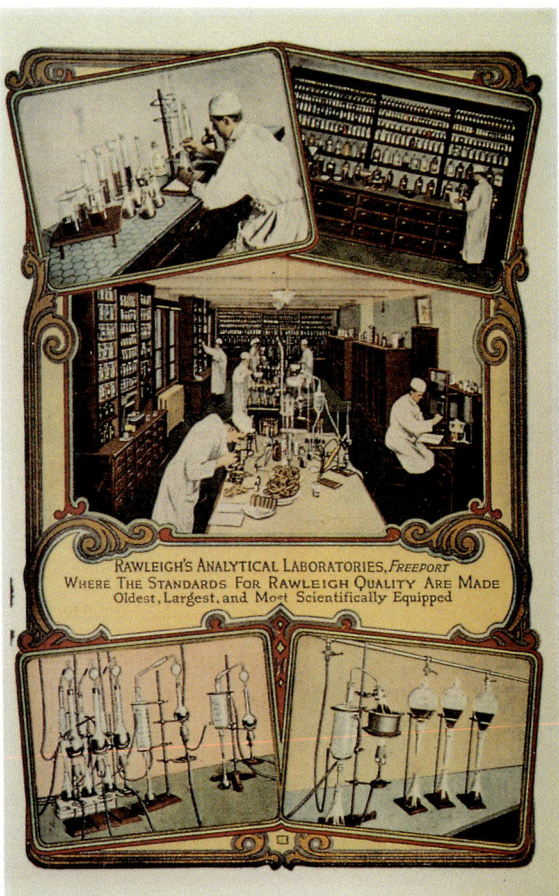

Rawleigh provided customers nine **GOOD HEALTH RULES** to avoid sickness and doctor's bills:
1. **Eight hours' sleep** with lots of fresh air.
2. **A daily cold shower,** in the morning if possible.
3. **At least 2 warm cleansing baths** weekly.
4. **A good substantial breakfast.**
5. **Regular meals.**
6. **At least a pint of milk a day,** but preferably a quart.
7. **Plenty of fresh fruit and vegetables** but a moderate amount of meat.
8. **All the exercise possible.**
9. **Clean warm clothing** but not too much.

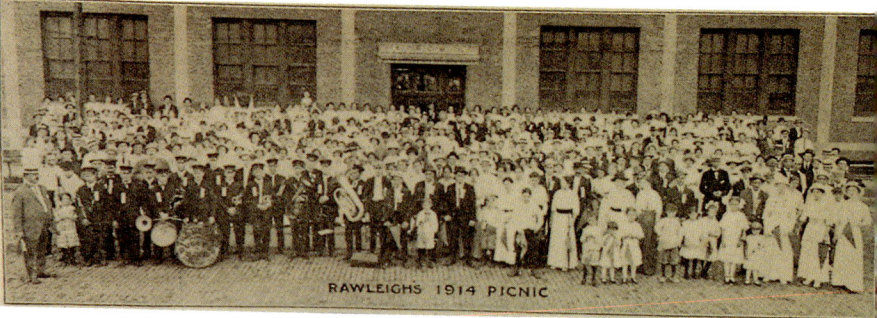

In 1914, over 300 people employed by The W.T. Rawleigh Medical Company at its factories and branches were photographed before boarding cars for their 1914 picnic. They arrived in Freeport in eight special rail cars over the Rockford and Interurban line.

A staff of Rawleigh scientists — experienced in the science of pharmacy, chemistry, bacteriology, and dietetics — were employed in the Rawleigh Laboratories in 1931 to examine, test and analyze botanical drugs, roots, herbs, seeds, spices, chemicals, citrus oils, natural and synthetic perfumes, and other raw materials.

Finished products were tested to make sure that they met the "Rawleigh Standard of Quality." The most delicate and complicated testing apparatus included: microscopes to identify bacteria, the polariscope, refractometer, specific gravity balances for testing essential oils, electric ovens, furnaces, and refrigerators to ascertain the moisture, age, and other physical contents of botanical drugs. This equipment registered temperatures from 23 degree Celsius up to 200 degree Fahrenheit while supersensitive analytical balances weighed with precision up to 1/200,000 part of an ounce.

The Rawleigh experimental diet kitchen in the Freeport factories, where scientific studies and experiments were made to improve the value and usefulness of "Rawleigh's Good Health Products." In this 1931 kitchen, selected recipes were tested and approved for publication in Rawleigh handbooks. Rawleigh's kitchen personnel is presently unknown.

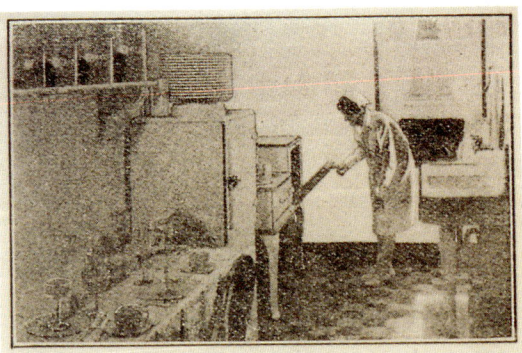

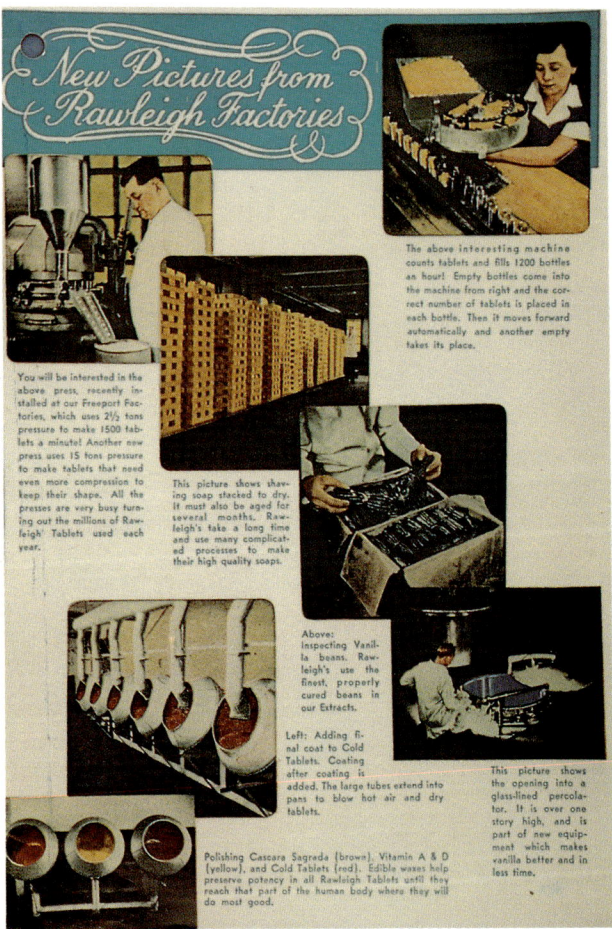

An original page entitled "New Pictures from Rawleigh Factories" from *Rawleigh's 61st Year Good Health Guide Almanac Cook Book 1950.*

Rawleigh Retailer

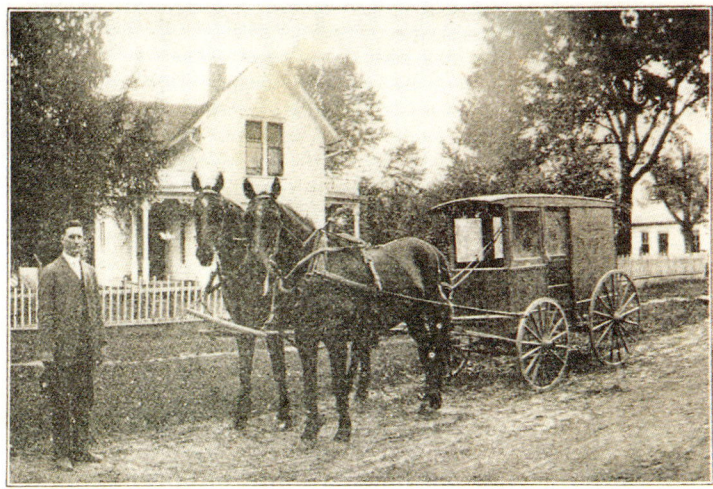

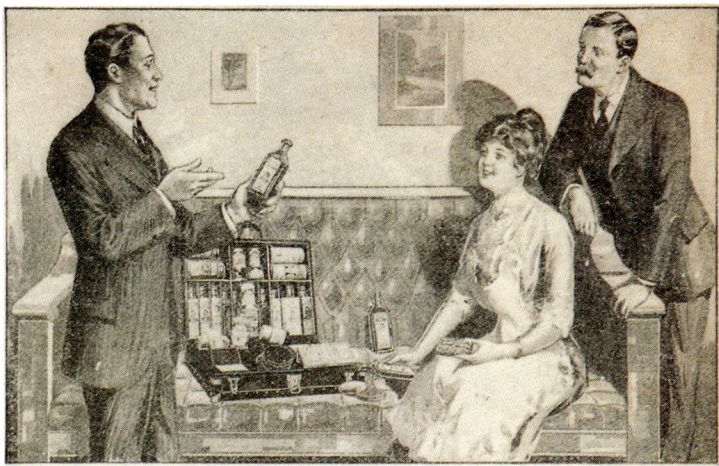

"Buying In Your Own Home!" In 1915, the Rawleigh Retailer was the only man between the customer and the Rawleigh Company. He was the connecting link between Rawleigh's factories, the farm, and your home.

It was the custom of Rawleigh Industries to be very careful in choosing only "reliable and worthy personnel of steady habits" for Rawleigh Dealers. Interested persons were required to give business men as references. All applicants were carefully investigated before they were accepted by Rawleigh Industries.

Most Dealers lived within the localities and districts where they worked, provided their own outfits, carried a good stocks of products, and many owned their own homes and paid taxes like other citizens.

Dealers were the sole owners and managers of their business. All furnished contracts or letters of credit signed by a responsible relative or friend as sureties that enabled them to buy products on time at low wholesale prices, carry all the items they required in stock, and to sell their products to their customers on time and trial, and wait for their pay until after the products had been used and found satisfactory.

Dealers understood that they were expected to call on every family within their respective localities and districts. These dealers were expected to make frequent, regular, and dependable service calls necessary to secure each customer's respect, good will, and repeated patronage.

Rawleigh Dealers offered many other important advantages to their customers, including the lowest independent and competitive prices, free trials of any medicines or other products that a customer had not used before with a guarantee of satisfaction or no sale, ample time to test their value and usefulness, and payment only after one was satisfied that each and every product was the best and most reliable obtainable.

The Rawleigh Company explained that, "The Rawleigh Dealer **SHOULD** always be welcomed when he called, and he was required to explain the usefulness of his products, of keeping the customers well supplied with all necessities which were frequently needed and used in every home."

As the Rawleigh Industries were building new factories and branches and constantly extending their business into more rural localities, cities, and towns every year, the dealer's business was pleasant, dignified, and profitable. The company assured prospective dealers that only a small capital was required for outfitting and starting expenses.

Anyone interested in becoming a Rawleigh Dealer and thought they qualified could write directly to the company or request that *their* Rawleigh Dealer provide full details and then decide for themselves. Rawleigh always had openings for persons of good character and habits who could qualify and be depended upon to give their business the much needed time and attention it required.

This 3-1/2" x 6" "List of TERRITORY VACANT AND TAKEN" was issued August 10, 1907. The object of this 36 page booklet was to serve those seeking positions as Rawleigh salesmen. They were to use it as a guide in the selection of their territory. States and territories were arranged in alphabetical order; under each state an alphabetical list of counties, population, and square miles was given. Counties marked with a (*) were taken, those marked with a dagger indicated that a county was only partly taken or that the entire county was likely to fall vacant. This booklet was issued monthly by THE RECRUITING DEPARTMENT. THE W.T. RAWLEIGH MEDICAL COMPANY FREEPORT, ILLINOIS. U.S.A. $50-$60.

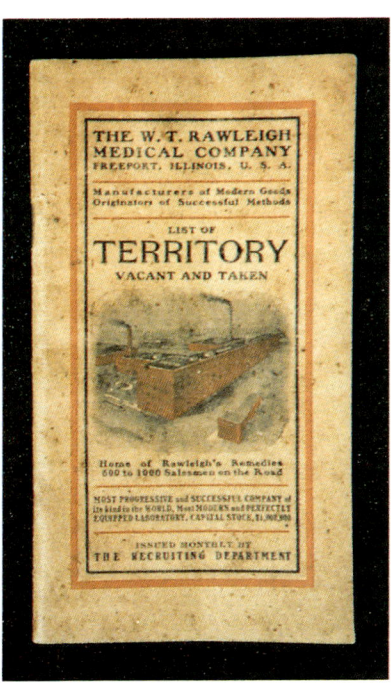

Rawleigh Industries advertised for dealers nationwide and through their own publications and other sources.

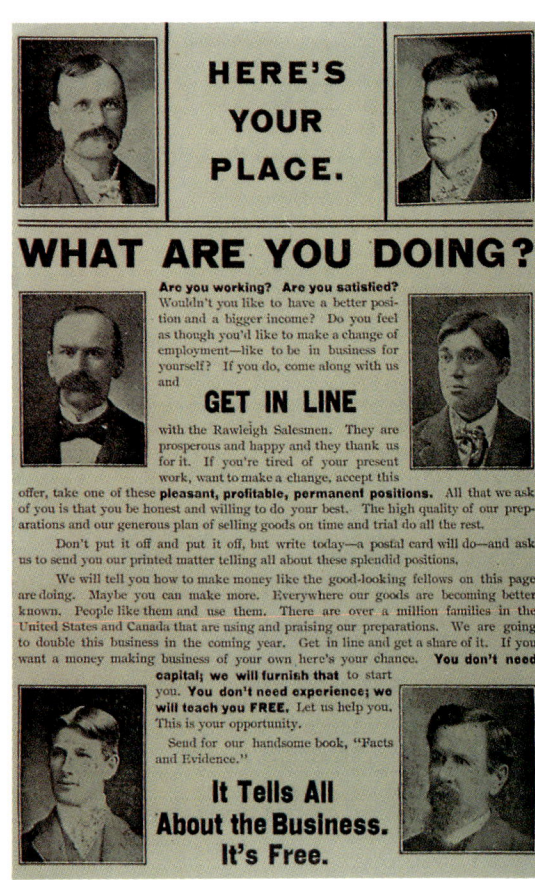

This original "WHAT ARE YOU DOING?" advertisement appeared in *Rawleigh's Almanac Cook Book & Medical Guide*, Compiled and Published by THE W.T. RAWLEIGH MEDICAL CO., FREEPORT, ILL., U.S.A. COPYRIGHT BY THE W.T. RAWLEIGH MEDICAL CO., 1905.

The Rawleigh man who delivered the products of the Rawleigh's Factories to the home was not an agent, peddler, or hired man. Every Rawleigh Retailer was the manager of his own business, purchasing his stocks at wholesale and retailing it to his own customers. He knew that to gain and *retain* his customers confidence and patronage, his business conduct and habits must be above reproach. In order for him to be successful, he must be honest, industrious, and attentive to his business. He called upon his customers several times each year — frequent dependable service was expected of all successful Rawleigh men. In order to support himself and his family, he depended upon the business patronage he secured from his customers.

He was required to cover the territory he served, to be courteous in conduct, honest in all his dealings, correct in his habits, and to give careful attention to all the details of his business. Customers were to report any discourtesy, dishonesty, or business neglect upon the part of any Rawleigh Retailer. All Rawleigh Retailers realized that their success depended upon their industry and regular, frequent, dependable service to every home.

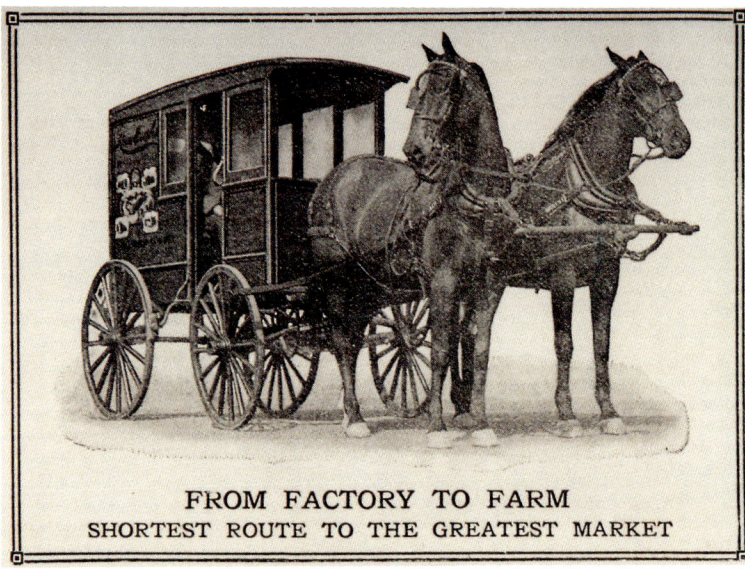

"FROM FACTORY TO FARM SHORTEST ROUTE TO THE GREATEST MARKET" appeared in a 1916 Rawleigh's Almanac. $1-$2.

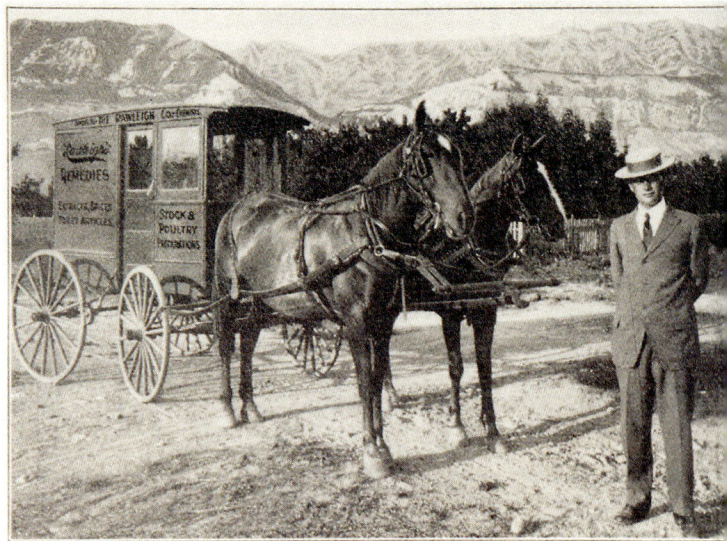

A typical Rawleigh wagon is captured in this photograph taken in Utah in approximately 1916. Route No. 326 was a regular traveling store, carrying 107 different products from the factory to the farm.

The Rawleigh Retailers offered free trials on any medicines which their customers had not used before and, as always, positively guaranteed everything or there was no sale. Each Retailer had hundreds of customers. He knew the average needs of a family and was expected to provide the right advice. He often left copies of "Good Health Guides and Bulletins" when scientific information was needed in regaining health if he heard of ailing family members or friends.

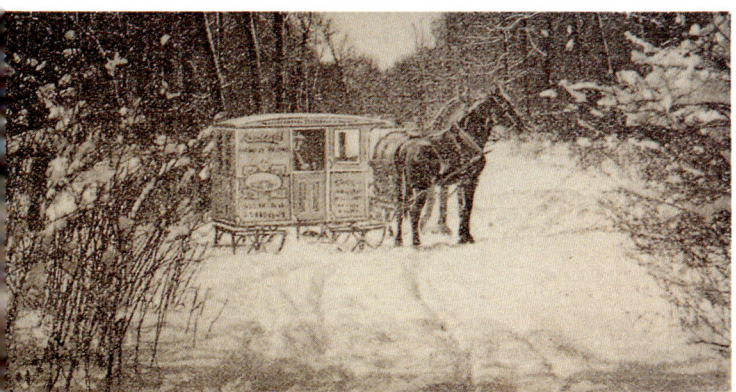

Winter weather obstructs the movement of the Rawleigh sleigh in this 1916 illustration.

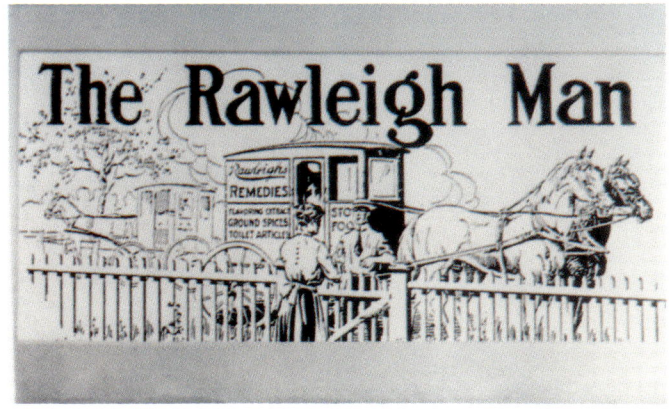

"The Rawleigh Man" illustration was presented to Walter Keith, a former Arkansas Rawleigh dealer. Until the early 1920s, Mr. Keith sold and delivered Rawleigh products out of a wagon pulled by a team of horses. He retired to his country farm in the 1940s. *Courtesy Russell Keith.*

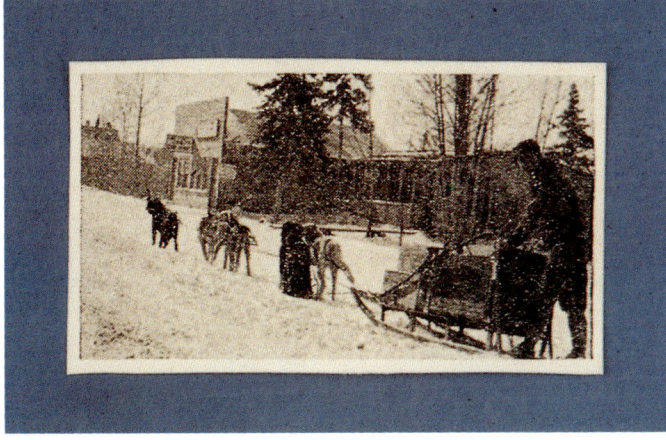

A Rawleigh dealer in the far northern region of Canada providing service via dog sled during the winter.

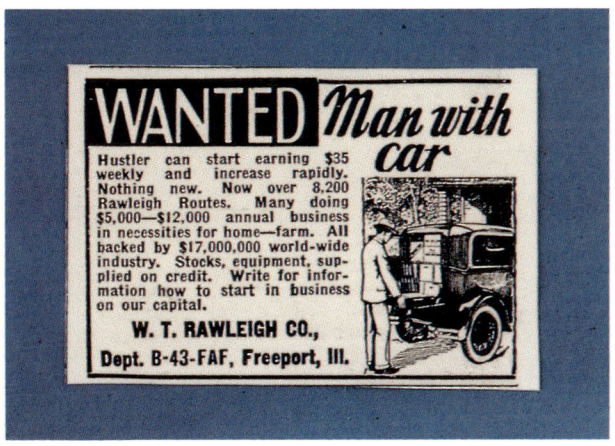

An original Rawleigh advertisement that appeared in a February 1934 issue of "THE Country Home," a magazine for farm, garden, and home. *Dupler Collection.* $1-$2.

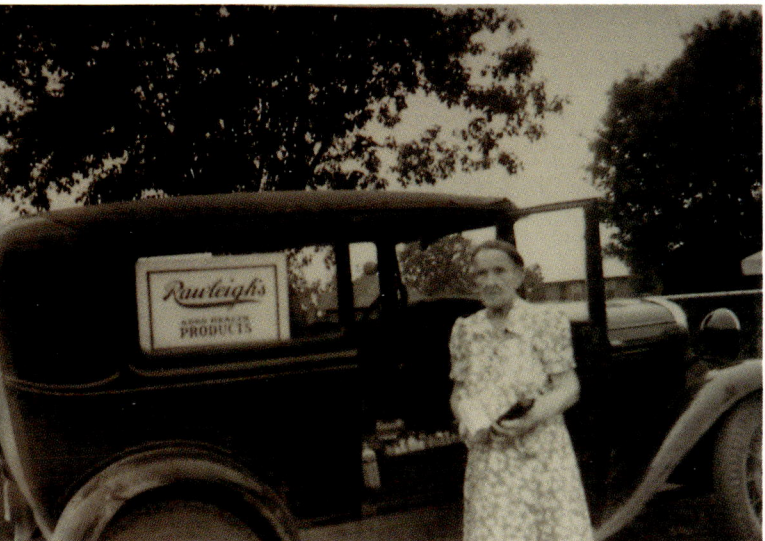

Mrs. Alexander, a Rawleigh customer of Murray C. Barron of Pefferlaw, Ontario, Canada. Murray has served as a Rawleigh dealer for fifty years. Born September 30, 1911 to Charlie and Delilah Barron, Murray began his career with the Rawleigh company on April 12, 1944. Mr. Barron continues to sell Golden Pride International™ products as of this writing; he doesn't have time to retire or even to think about it. *Barron Collection.*

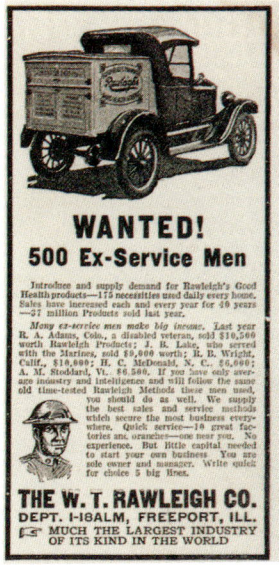

"WANTED! 500 Ex-Service Men." An original advertisement appearing in "The American Legion Monthly" magazine, circa 1927. This ad used the same illustration of the Rawleigh truck that appeared in the 1927 "Rawleigh's Good Health Guide." $1-$2.

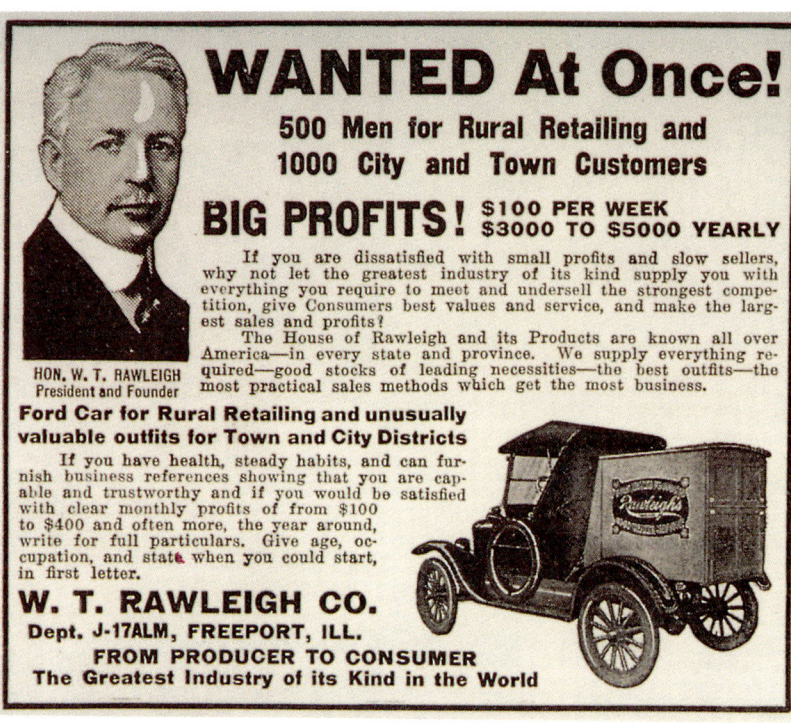

"WANTED At Once!" original advertisement appeared in an unknown magazine, circa 1927. $1-$2.

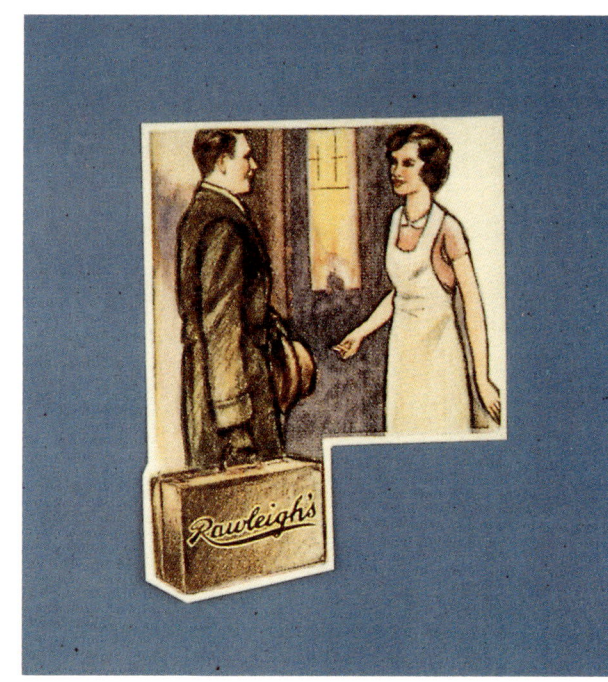

A section from Rawleigh's 1939 GOOD HEALTH GUIDE, COOK BOOK & ALMANAC. The dealer brought his products direct to the home, showing them, and as he demonstrated tehm he explained their sericeability an left them on their merits.

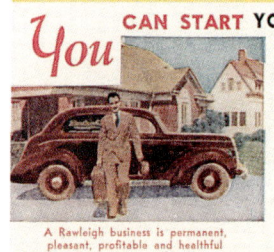 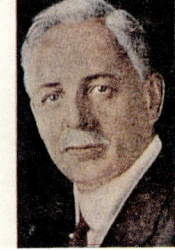

"You Can Start Your Own Business on Credit." Circa 1950.

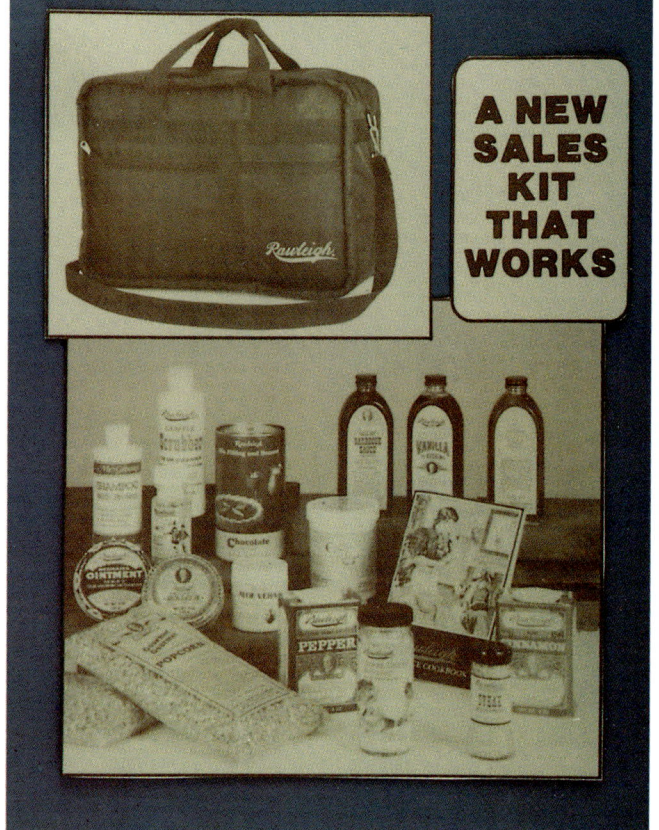

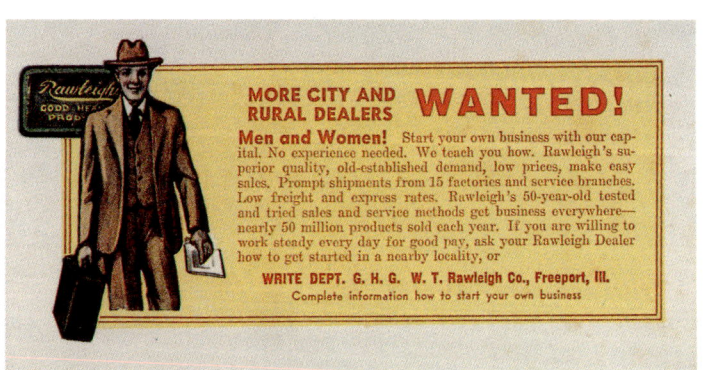

An original "WANTED MORE CITY AND RURAL DEALERS" advertisement from a 1942 Rawleigh's Good Health Guide. $1-$2.

"Rawleigh's Sales Kit," circa 1986. The kit included at least $100 worth of sample products that represented each of the Rawleigh product lines, plus a literature kit. The custom-made carrying case added a degree of professionalism. Rawleigh offered this complete "Sales Kit" to every distributor for the low price of $99.95 (U.S.) and $114.95 (Canada). $100-$125 complete.

Your Recruiting Opportunity

Both Farmers and City Workers Are Now Looking for a Chance to Get Into a Better Business.

"February, March, and April are probably the most unsettled months of the year. Not only is the weather unsettled, but thousands of men, and women too, are unsettled in their business affairs. Farmers who have sold or rented their farms and farm-hands who are out of a job are wondering what they are going to do next. Many business men, clerks and other city and town workers are either dissatisfied or disgusted with their present occupations and are anxious to get into something else. In every community there are scores of good, industrious persons who are seeking ways and means of making a better living in 1926."

"This is doubtless the reason why our records show that more new Customers are started by our old Customers during these three months than at any other season of the year. So now is the opportune time for you to put some extra pep and speed into your recruiting, find out who the dissatisfied and unsettled ones are in your district or location, and then put up the proposition of Rawleigh Retailing to them."

"Tell them from your own experience what you know about the business and assure them that there is no good reason why they should not succeed in it if they will only study and work like the rest of our successful Retailers do. Tell them that if they will give the same good time and attention to Retailing that they probably have to their previous occupations, they not only can reasonably expect to make two or three times as much money as they ever made before, but they will also have the pleasure and satisfaction of owning and conducting their own independent businesses."

"Also tell your Prospects that Spring is the best time of the year to start Retailing because traveling conditions are good and there is a good demand for Products, so it should be possible for them to make unusually large Sales and Profits. Collections are good too, because with the advent of Spring, Consumers seem to part with their money more readily than they do during the cold Winter months. Then tell them that if they will go right ahead and complete all necessary arrangements promptly, there is no good reason why they should not be all ready to start selling by the time the first warm Spring days arrive."

"Now that it will be unusually easy for you to find and interest good prospective new Customers during the next 70 days, we shall expect you to make the most of your opportunity, to look up every possible Prospect in your locality, see that he is fully informed on Rawleigh Retailing and if possible secure his Application. We shall also expect you to send us your Prospects' names and addresses so that we can send them all of our literature. **But don't depend upon us to get your new Customers started.** Remember that your personal interviews with them are worth more than all the letters and Bulletins we could possibly send them. Therefore we shall depend upon you to not only secure your Prospects' Applications, but also see that they get their Contracts or Credit Agreements signed, order their Products, decide upon their Locations or Districts and get started selling without any unnecessary delay." *Rawleigh's Weekly Wednesday, February 17, 1926.*

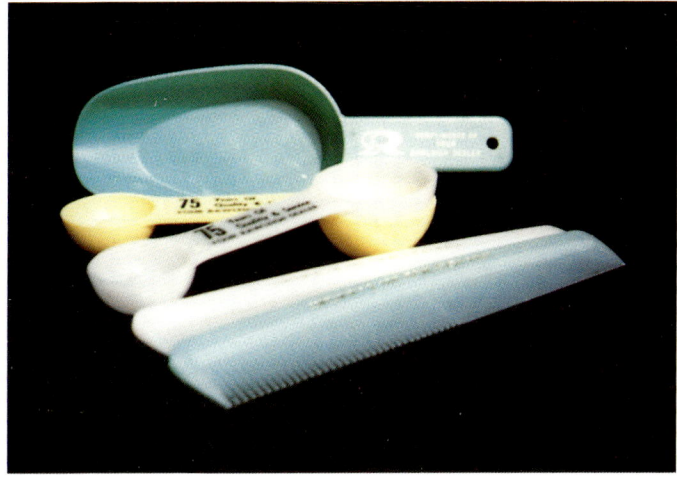

A plastic utility scoop, approximately 6-1/2" in length marked "COMPLIMENTS OF YOUR RAWLEIGH DEALER." Two plastic 5-1/4" long measuring scoops marked "75 Years Of Quality & Service YOUR RAWLEIGH DEALER." Two plastic combs, also marked "COMPLIMENTS OF YOUR RAWLEIGH DEALER." These items may have been "giveaways" to established customers. $10-$15 ea.

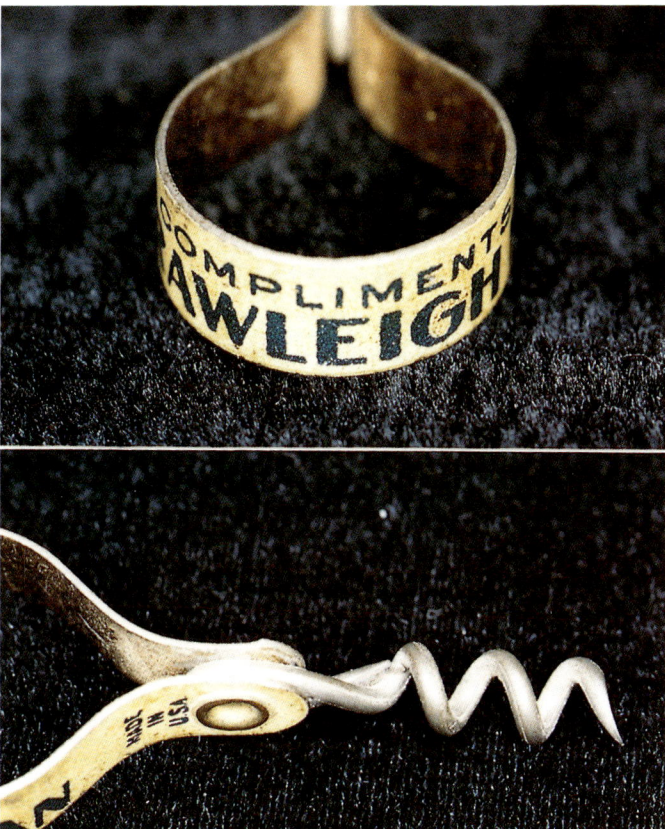

The corkscrew is mark "COMPLIMENTS THE RAWLEIGH MAN" and "MADE IN U.S.A." Approximately 2" in length, this corkscrew was used to pull corks out of bottles. The spiral-shaped pointed head could be folded back into the handle. *Dupler Collection.* $100-$125.

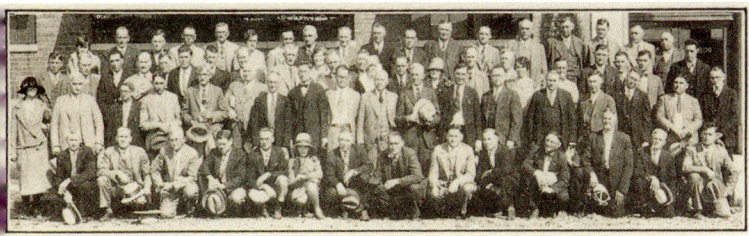

Attending a Annual Conferences to exchange ideas on the improvement of their service to consumers, this group of Rawleigh Dealers posed for a photograph in 1942.

The Rawleigh Foundation

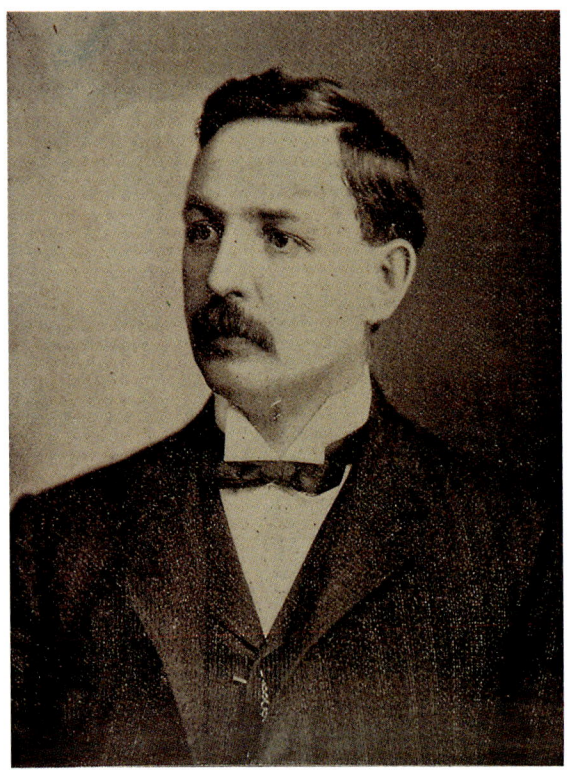

Mr. W.T. Rawleigh, president of the Rawleigh Company and originator of their "Pay After You Are Satisfied Plan."

William Thomas Rawleigh had always shown interest in the social, economic, and political conditions that affect local, state, national, and international affairs. He firmly believed that the proper framework for industry and commerce was based on real service, justice, equal opportunity, the principles of the American Constitution, and true representative government. He also supported the proposition that public service must govern individuals, corporations, and public servants in social, economic, and political life.

W.T. Rawleigh believed and depended on scientific research. He reported the facts as found, and provided aid to the people by supporting legislative action in the interest of the public. His service was expressed through organizations, liberally financed in an effort to render effective public service. The "People's Legislation Service, The Rawleigh Tariff Staff" was located in Madison, Wisconsin, and the "Rawleigh Tariff Bureau" in Washington.

In order to promote a more valuable service, the Rawleigh Foundation was incorporated as a non-profit institution under the laws of the State of Illinois in 1930. This institution was designed to allow Rawleigh to keep their costs down and to keep prices lower for the consumers. The Foundation was headquartered in Freeport, Illinois, with a division office located in Washington, D.C.

In January 1932, the Rawleigh Company observed that about two-hundred million pounds or six thousand six hundred and eleven carloads of incoming and outgoing freight were handled by the Rawleigh industries each year. This freight arrived by river, rail, ocean, and by the Rawleigh motor transport and barge line service.

The ocean freight on raw materials imported annually amounted to approximately $50,000 with import duties paid to the United States Treasury of over $100,000. Freight on vanilla beans totaled $15,000 and on cloves and pepper the annual amount rose to $20,000.

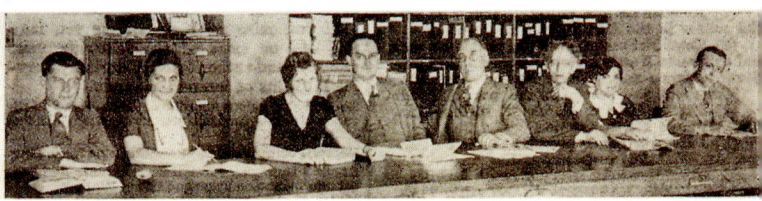

"The Madison Tariff Committee" was under the direction of noted economists J.R. Commons, B.H. Hibbard, and W.A. Morton from the University of Wisconsin. During 1931 - 1932, this committee made an intensive fourteen month study of the tariff on consumers and producers for the Rawleigh Foundation.

The Tariff was studied by B.H. Hibbard and W.A. Morton who had taken a leave of absence from The University of Wisconsin and devoted full time to the 14 months of agricultural tariff schedules. Dr. Commons would join the staff. Their studies of tariff effectiveness and incidence, and various questions of public policy relating to the agricultural duties continued until September 1, 1932.

They would later publish tariff monographs on the following commodities: 1) Sugar 2) Grains 3) Dairy Products 4) Flaxseed 5) Wool 6) Meats and Hides 7) Cotton and 8) Lumber.

Later in 1932, Commons, Hibbard, and Morton's findings were published in several volumes on the various tariff problems.

Taxes, Freight Rates, Anti-Trust Laws, Public Utilities. The Foundation made studies of 1) the effect of higher taxation on rural and urban property; 2) the effect increased freight rates would have on the cost of living; 3) the enforcement of our federal and state anti-trust laws; and 4) the states' efforts to regulate and control utilities.

The outcome of this study could not be located. Rawleigh indicated that the studies would be educational and beneficial to the public and that results would be given to the press, public servants, members of Congress, governors, business men, and laymen in general.

The findings of the Washington and Madison Tariff Bureaus had been widely accepted during the 1931 - 1932 program. So thorough in exposing the inequities of privilege seeking, and potent in stimulating the growing demand for social and economic justice and equality of opportunity was this Bureau that it was decided to develop and carry out a more comprehensive program involving the tariff, taxation, trust legislation, and public utilities. Each problem was studied by a selected research staff of experts.

Golden Pride/Rawleigh, Inc.
Golden Pride International™

In Scottsdale, Arizona, Golden Pride — a privately held corporation that provided people with a unique opportunity to use and market health and beauty products — was incorporated on February 2, 1983. Golden Pride is one of the few remaining family run operations. Tradition will be carried on as the operation passes from father to son and daughter and so on. Continuity is assured.

By August of 1983, Golden Pride had moved its corporate headquarters to Florida and was again incorporated and quickly expanded to all 50 states. In the beginning, only two products were available. However, to meet the changes in American lifestyle, a line of over 70 high quality health food supplements was developed for all ages.

In January 1989, the President and Owner of Golden Pride, Harry W. Hersey, purchased the W.T. Rawleigh Company in the United States and Canada. Rawleigh's 100th Anniversary was held in West Palm Beach, Florida.

In December 1996, Mr. Hersey purchased the Texas based Lady Love Skin Care Company and moved its operation to West Palm Beach, Florida as well. The basic ingredient is aloe vera, which fits perfectly into the Golden Pride and Rawleigh product line.

Golden Pride/Rawleigh's product line, distributor base, and target market has been vastly expanding:

Today's organizational structure retains the underlying separate identity of the founding companies in a way that permits a sharing of the best of the Golden Pride and W.T. Rawleigh traditions and products. Golden Pride International is a management company that was created to coordinate day-to-day administration and business affairs on behalf of the various other companies involved. Those companies, all of which are privately owned are: Golden Pride, Inc. and W.T. Rawleigh Co., Ltd. (of Canada). Collectively, the Company is hereafter referred to as **GPI**.

One of the associations of GPI is the Happy Trails Children's Foundation of which they are pleased to be a part. Providing hope and help for abused children, it is the favorite charity of Roy Rogers and wife, Dale Evans.

"Serving your family with pride" still remains the commitment of GPI.
— *GOLDEN PRIDE INTERNATIONAL HISTORY & FACTUAL INFORMATION.*

As the Golden Pride/Rawleigh products shown here are out-of-date, they are highly collectible. Check your local Yellow Pages for the nearest Golden Pride International™ dealer in your area.

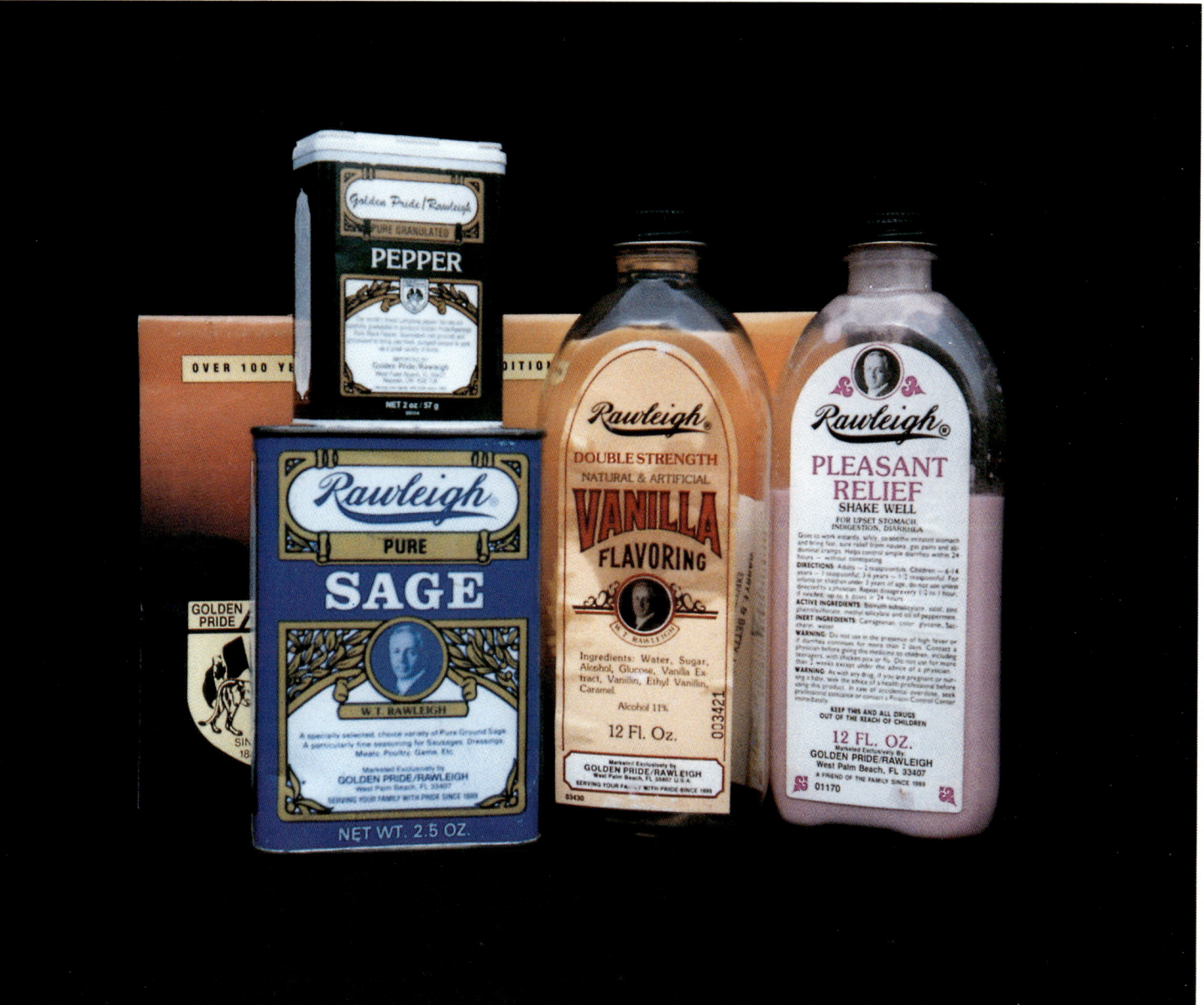

Golden Pride/Rawleigh Pure Granulated PEPPER, Imported By Golden Pride/Rawleigh West Palm Beach, FL 33407 and Nepean, ON K2E 7J6. Rawleigh Pure SAGE 2.5 ounce. Marketed Exclusively by Golden Pride/Rawleigh West Palm Beach, FL 33407 and Rawleigh Natural & Artificial Vanilla Flavoring 12 fluid ounces and 12 fluid ounce Rawleigh Pleasant Relief. Marketed Exclusively by Golden Pride/Rawleigh West Palm Beach, F. 33407 U.S.A. These products are shown with a company publication ©1991, 1990, 1989. $15-$18 ea.

Chapter 2. Rawleigh Method and Health Products

How Rawleigh Used Them

Rawleigh knew their products were of standard and uniform quality because they made them from the raw materials in their own factories, often acquiring additional materials from other countries. Rawleigh's laboratories' tests showed that Rawleigh medicines and other products were not only of superior quality, but the best that years of experience, scientific knowledge, and the most completely equipped factories in American could produce.

The W.T. Rawleigh Company told the public that smaller industries could not be sure of the preparations they sold because they did not make them. Instead they bought ready made compounds, then sold them.

The company went on to reassure the consumer that Rawleigh's, however, had only the highest standards — nothing could be too good. "Everything was made to give the complete satisfaction which every purchaser was entitled to receive."

Why Rawleigh Retailers Served You Best

In 1922, approximately twenty million customers admitted the Rawleigh retailer into their homes. These retailers had established their business directly within their own district or the region within which they resided. Outside their business, they often held public office and became involved in political affairs concerning their community, thus becoming responsible members in their own location.

Rawleigh retailers owned and managed their own business. They purchased their products at wholesale, paid their own freight, selling expenses, and chose their own customers while determining the prices and the terms of sale on their products.

Trading with a Rawleigh retailer was the only link between consumers and this multifaceted international organization. Rawleigh retailers brought these products direct to the consumers' homes and sold them at the lowest prices through the most favorable terms.

Advantages were obtained through patronizing a Rawleigh retailer who was always courteous, obliging, and willing to accommodate their customers by selling at the lowest prices they could make for cash, or allowing consumers to buy "on time" from one trip to another.

Rawleigh retailers could supply all household medicines, spices, extracts, flavors, soaps, toilet articles, food products, veterinary remedies, and poultry supplies. Rawleigh insisted that good health was of the first importance and suggested that customers discuss their needs before the Rawleigh retailer called to learn what was needed for individual members and those required for livestock and poultry. Once those needs were understood, the retailer, having hundreds of customers, would show his entire line of "Good Health Products and Supplies."

Rawleigh suggested to their customers that they accept the advice of their Rawleigh retailer. He was experienced; he knew and understood what the average family needed and what they used most during all the seasons. His advice helped in making the right selection to meet the individual needs of family members and farm livestock.

Becoming acquainted with the Rawleigh retailer made him a friend. When members of the family became sick, copies of Rawleigh's "Good Health Guides" and bulletins were provided in which scientific information was furnished to assist in regaining good health. Rawleigh's Good Health Service was free to all customers using Rawleigh products. However, in 1922 the demand for the bulletins became so large and expensive that it became necessary to restrict their distribution to only those bulletins needed by each family and to charge for part of the printing and postage on bulletins and guides sent by mail. Each of the bulletins and "Good Health Guides" were mailed upon request only if accompanied by stamps to cover the cost of mailing and postage.

Rawleigh provided the most complete and valuable service because they carried the largest number and greatest variety of products and supplied the only scientific and reliable "Good Health Service" available. Ready for distribution in 1922 were the following good health service bulletins. No. 201 - Influenza, LaGrippe, Coughs, Colds, Etc. No. 202 - Health in Spring and Summer. No. 203 - How to Build Good Blood. No. 205 - Constipation, Its Causes and Cure. No. 206 - Intestinal Toxemia and Colitis. No. 207 - Headaches, Their Causes and Prevention. No. 208 - Dyspepsia. No. 209 - Rheumatism, Lumbago and Gout. No. 210 - Neurasthenics, and Nervous Diseases. No. 211 - Care of the Teeth. No. 212 - Your Enemy, The Common House Fly, plus Good Health Guide, Almanac and Cook Book.

These bulletins are becoming highly sought after. However, for the time being, they are readily available at most flea markets, antique shops, and occasionally auctions.

> ☛ Be sure to look for the registered trademark
> *Rawleigh's*
> which appears on all genuine Rawleigh Quality Products
>
> You are warned and cautioned not to be deceived by those who claim their inferior imitations and substitutes are equal to the old, original and reliable Rawleigh Medicines which have been noted for their superiority for nearly 42 years and now have a well earned reputation throughout the United States, Canada and Australia.
> ☛ Don't forget that no so-called sanitary seal can be made to protect the public against the impositions of imitators and others who falsely claim that their medicines are just as good or about the same as Rawleigh's.

Here is the registered trademark that appeared on all genuine Rawleigh products. Rawleigh often cautioned customers not to be deceived.

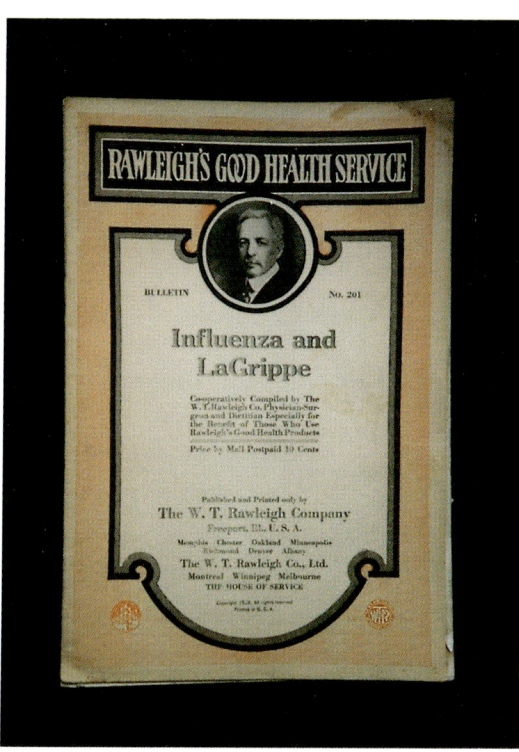

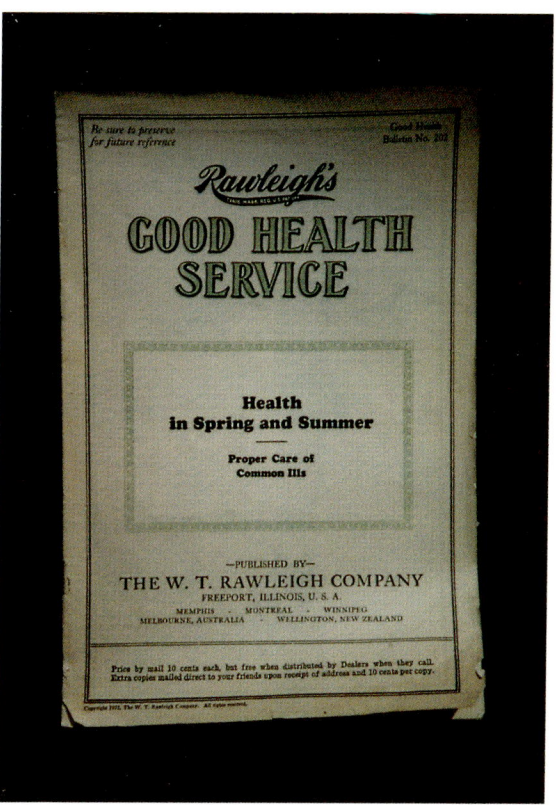

No. 201 Good Health Service bulletin for "Influenza and LaGrippe." This 16 page bulletin was dated ©1928, The W.T. Rawleigh Company. $20-$25.

No. 202 Good Health Service bulletin for "Health in Spring and Summer Proper Care of Common Ills." This 16 page bulletin was marked ©1931, The W.T. Rawleigh Company. $20-$25.

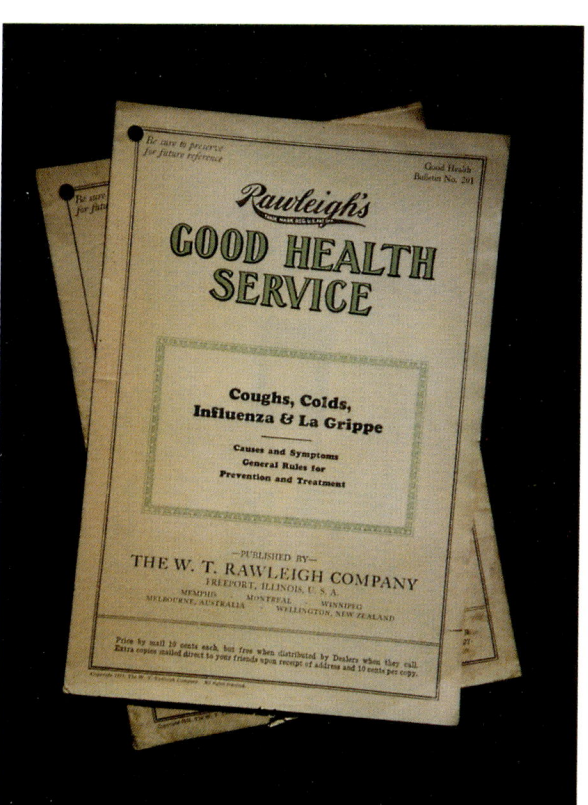

Rawleigh's Good Health Service, which the company claimed to be the only one of its kind in the world, was originated in 1919. Between 1919 and 1922, the company printed over seven million "Good Health Guides" and bulletins at an expense of hundreds of thousands of dollars.

Rawleigh's Good Health Service was no fad; they advocated no abnormal method of diet, fasting, or other impractical, unproven, health measure. It was a simple, scientific explanation of the common diseases and how to prevent or overcome them.

Rawleigh explained the laws of hygiene and good living, various functions of the human body, the importance of right living, need of fresh air, the value of eating the right food, sufficient sleep, exercise, and recreation.

Every bottle and package of Rawleigh's medicine was accompanied by scientific directions explaining the cause of common ailments which caused suffering, sickness, and expenses. In 1953, customers could receive FREE from their dealer a copy of "THE COMMON COLD," an informative publication on what to do for colds. Photograph not available.

No. 201 Good Health Service bulletin for "Coughs, Colds, Influenza & LaGrippe." This 16 page bulletin was dated ©1931, The W.T. Rawleigh Company. $20-$25.

Why Rawleigh Made Their Own Tablets

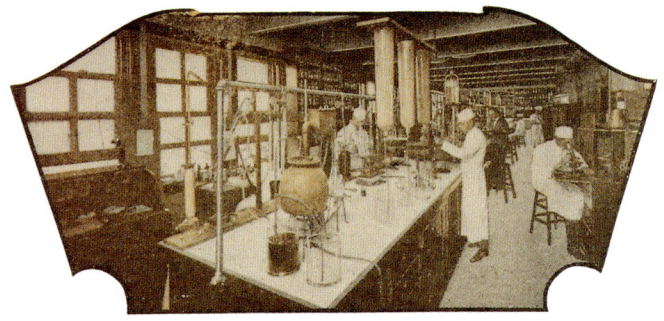

A section of the Rawleigh laboratories where tablets were made and visiting chemists and pharmacists could observe this interesting and fascinating procedure. The photo dates to circa 1922.

Rawleigh laboratories were stocked with thousands of dollars worth of solid and powdered extracts. These extracts were made from roots, barks, leaves, fine chemicals, alkaloids, resins, salts, pepsin, malt diastase, jalap, podophyllin, cinchona bark, ipecac, couch grass, cascara segrada, senna, licorice root, santonin, and numerous other materials used to make Rawleigh's special private formula tablets.

In 1922, Rawleigh was the only manufacturer of proprietary medicines who made all their own tablets. They used no inferior materials; everything used was carefully tested and the most painstaking care was given to every process of manufacturing from beginning to end.

In the mixing room, raw materials were first accurately weighed, then all ingredients thoroughly mixed, chemicals pulverized to a fine powder, and transferred to large mixers which blended the ingredients together thoroughly. The ingredients then moved into a revolving oscillators that granulated the composition into small flakes before going to a big steel oven on hundreds of trays. The composition was thoroughly dried with steam heated air operated by suctions fans.

After sifting, the granulation mass was ready for large steel mixing tanks. Within these tanks, the granulated medicines were prepared for the six automatic tablet compressing machines which had a daily capacity of over 800,000 tablets (annual capacity about 243,000,000). Each tablet was uniform in composition, weight, shape, and color.

After proper seasoning on steel drying racks, the tablets were sent on to the large revolving coating pans where dry air blasts were used in the coating process. They were finished and polished in large, wax-lined revolving pans from which they emerged white, chocolate, pink, or yellow with a smooth, durable coating, and mirror-like polish, ready to be packed and shipped.

The machinery the Rawleigh laboratories used included mixers, breakers, cutting and oscillating machines, pulverizers, automatic rotary presses, coating and polishing pans, steamjacketed copper kettle, heating vat, many electric motors, and a large mill for pulverizing the fine granulated sugar required for making Rawleigh's tablets.

When Rawleigh laboratories made large investments in equipment, it was justified by the immense and steady sales. Rawleigh made uniform, reliable tablets for less than competitive companies were paying to have their tablets produced by manufacturing chemists outside their firms.

Rawleigh further claimed their methods were better because they know exactly what every tablet contained; that the tablets were made right because they were made in Rawleigh's laboratories from the very beginning to the end. Furthermore, "When a customer purchased Rawleigh's tablets they got a carefully compounded, scientifically made pharmaceutical product with exact dosages of ingredients specified in the private formula they were made from and were recognized by medical science as useful in ailments for which the tablet was recommended."

The company warned, however, that Rawleigh's tablets were not recommended for ailments where experience had not proved their usefulness and reliability. They were then quick to reassure that if used according to directions, their tablets were absolutely safe for children and adults.

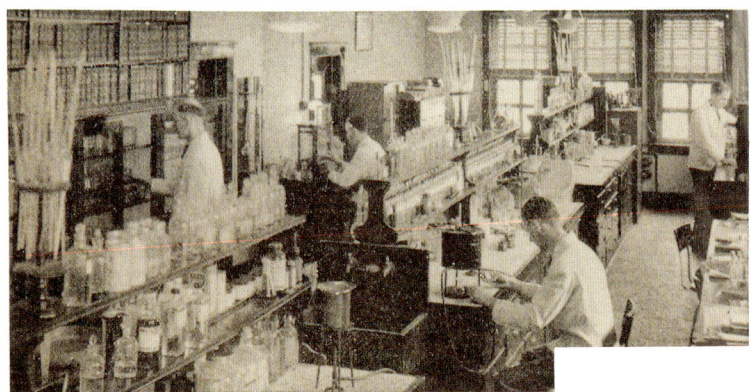

To improve qualities and values of Rawleigh products, only the most extensive scientific equipment was used by Rawleigh chemists, pharmacists, and biologists doing research work. Circa 1939.

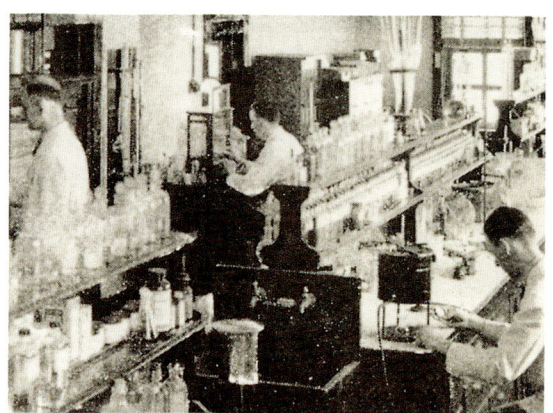

A section of the Freeport laboratories used for testing raw materials and finished products. Chemists controlled all manufacturing processes at all Rawleigh factories. Circa 1941.

Road to Health the Rawleigh Way

In 1922, the public's general ideals regarding health were so low that to most people the expression "to keep well" meant merely to keep out of the sickbed. Rawleigh proclaimed, "Health was and is positive, not negative, and means strength, ability, endurance, magnetism, vitality, vigor, poise, enthusiasm, exuberance of spirit and joy of living." Rawleigh provided the sign posts showing "the road to health" was paved with sanitary surroundings, a sound body, care of the body, and suitable activity.

Rawleigh's "Guide Posts on the Road to Health" were: (1) Clean, simple surroundings; (2) Prevention of infection; (3) Sound body; (4) Cleanliness; (5) Internal cleanliness; (6) Comfortable clothes; (7) Good food and pure water; (8) Good air and sunlight; (9) Good posture and sufficient exercise; (10) Rest and sleep; (11) Work and recreation; (12) The habit of happiness.

Sanitary Surroundings

Rawleigh personnel suggested to customers that their homes should be situated and constructed to admit sun light and air, and to avoid dark, damp places where diseased germs could grow. Plumbing, drainage, heating, and lighting could add, rather than detract from the health of the occupants.

Rawleigh was aware that most people had to adapt themselves to their present houses. However, every person could ventilate his house to get all of the sun light and air possible, and could discard those furnishings which collected dust and dirt, therefore encouraging germs and disease, such as non-washable curtains and draperies, layers of old wall paper, useless ornaments, tacked down carpets, and heavily padded furniture.

Sanitary surroundings involved every person protecting their house from flies, mosquitoes, insects, mice, and rats which carry disease. His duty was to know that the source of water supply, particularly water from private wells, was proof against contamination. Every individual must also be assured that food was properly handled in its manufacture, storage and delivery, and the garbage was disposed of so that it will not cause sickness to the surrounding community.

A Sound Body

In order to have a sound body each person must know the condition of the body. Occasional physical examinations by a doctor and periodic visits to the dentist provided this knowledge. If public schools provide a nurse, parents should cooperate with her and follow her suggestions. Children had a right to the best health. The new idea was to keep well instead of to get well after an illness.

After knowing the physical defects, the next step was to correct them, not to fear them nor accept them blindly. Defects of eyes, nose, ears, and teeth should be corrected, and tonsils and adenoids removed. Feet should be watched for falling arches, and posture, of children especially, supervised so as not to develop bad habits.

Rawleigh pointed out that germs were ever present so each individual's duty to himself and his neighbors was to avoid infection and infecting. A person should not expose himself or his family to crowds during epidemics, nor permit himself or his family to mix with others when ill. Promiscuous spitting, careless coughing and sneezing, the common use of the drinking cup, towel, soap, and dirty hands are the best ways of spreading disease. No article that goes into the mouth or touches the lips should be used by another person or for general service. No article should go into the mouth that is not meant to be eaten. Dirty hands carry germs to the mouth, nose, and eyes, as well as from one person to another. To avoid infection, hands must be absolutely clean and free from cuts, scratches, and ragged hangnails.

Care of the Body

Rawleigh was concerned with the proper care of the body, cleanliness, proper clothing, good food and drink, good bowel habits, good air both night and day, proper posture, care of the eyes, nose, and throat, and sufficient sleep.

Cleanliness involved (1) regular warm baths to get rid of the dirt, sweat, and unpleasant body odors. If possible daily cold baths or sponges to stimulate the blood and nerve systems and to prevent colds were also advisable; (2) thorough washing of hands before eating or handling food and after the use of the toilet, using special care in trimming the nails and hangnails and with proper scissors and not with the teeth or pen knife; (3) liberal use of cold creams for the face and hands to prevent chapping; (4) daily brushing of teeth and the use of dental floss instead of the unsanitary toothpick; (5) regular shampooing and brushing of the hair. Internal cleanliness comes from drinking water — three or four pints a day, eating bulky foods and observing strict and regular bowel habits.

With Rawleigh laundry products clothing were easily cleaned. The selection of proper clothing, suitable to climate and temperature and loose enough to allow freedom for all activities of the body, was of importance.

Deep, slow, regular breathing — always through the nose — feeds the body with air, the most important factor for life. Proper posture keeps the bones and muscles in their natural position, avoiding deformities, and allowing freedom to the lungs. The muscle unused in daily work should be stretched in some regular exercise. The eyes, ears, nose, and throat are delicate organs, not to be strained or injured.

Sleep gives rest and relaxation, both mental and physical. Children especially should not be deprived of sleep in order to do various chores around the house. During the day short periods of relaxation — a vacation between two activities — counteract fatigue and exhaustion. To relax, one should make the body heavy and consciously give up all effort in the body and then the mind.

Activity of Body and Mind

Work is our most important activity. "Overwork" is not too much work, but the wrong way of working and unsanitary living, as is also nervous exhaustion. The habit of relaxing between activities and of stopping worry will counteract these evils. Recreation is half way between work and rest, means "recreating," and should contrast with the daily work. Laughter, games, music, well chosen movies, books, and study can be forms of real recreation.

It is possible to observe all of the preceding points and still miss health. Physically sound people, because of their fault finding and grumbling, can keep themselves and everyone else in an unhappy, unhealthy state of mind which always affects the physical state. To avoid such habits, look beyond the physical and mental troubles and hurt feelings, and see the pleasant and good side of life. Half of the imagined difficulties never come and the actual ones will be entirely forgotten in a few weeks. A healthy mental attitude of happiness, cheer, hope, and serenity causes all of the mental troubles and many physical ones to vanish into thin air. Right habits of living plus right habits of thinking result in good health.

Rawleigh's 1932 Good Health Chart.

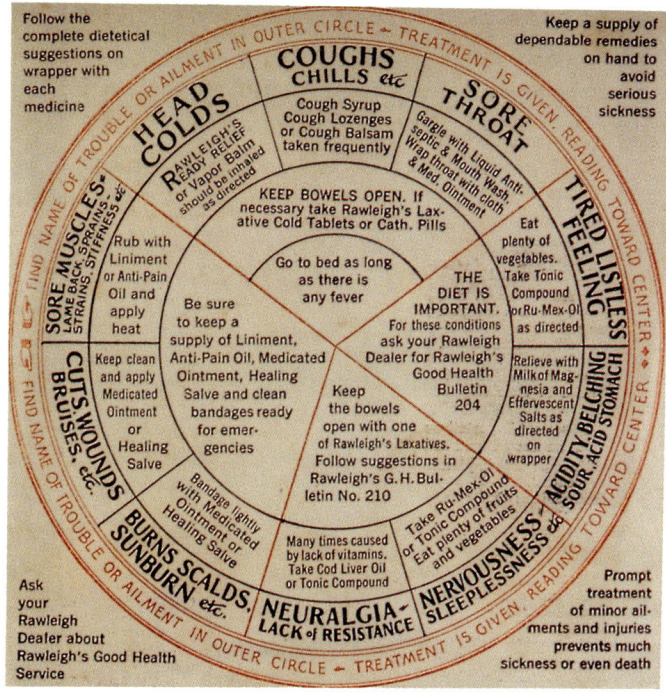

Since the early 1900s, Rawleigh had provided a good health service for consumers consisting of a series of good health bulletins, dietetic directions to accompany important medicines, and other products. In 1932, the cost of this service totaled over a million dollars, with over 50 million bulletins and guides being distributed.

All bulletins published were easily understood. They were scientific, practical, and were written by experienced dietitians, chemists, nurses, and physicians. *See* Chapter 3.

Packing Half a Million Tablets Daily

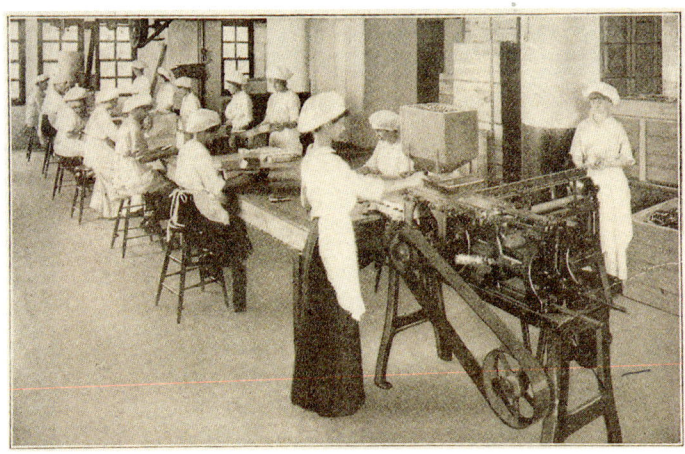

The small machine shown here automatically counted half a million tablets and filled containers daily. This device was invented by Rawleigh's chief chemist, replacing ten girls who had previously done the job.

There is an interesting story connected with the ... picture which again verifies the saying that "Necessity is the Mother of Invention."

The "necessity" was to get Rawleigh tablets packed fast enough to meet the rapidly growing demand for them, and the "invention" which was the result of this necessity is shown in the illustration.

At first not many Rawleigh tablets were sold; one person could easily put them all up by hand, but it now requires in the neighborhood of 75 million tablets to supply the ever-growing demand for those Rawleigh Medicines which are supplied in tablet form. These include Laxative tablets and Wafers, Cold tablets, Kidney tablets, Rheumatic and Digestive tablets, Cathartic and Liver Pills, and Worm Lozenges.

There is no endorsement that so well expresses the satisfaction that users have gotten from using these tablets as the rapid increase in the demand for them in all parts of the United States and Canada. Each is especially prepared for the specific purpose for which it is recommended.

Previous to the invention of the machine ..., the employees were required to put them up, but with the aid of this machine invented by the chief chemist and built by the Rawleigh-Schryer Company, five girls could count, fill, and get ready for shipment approximately half a million tablets per day. This great labor-saving machine not only packed an exact quantity in each package more

An original 1939 advertisement — Rawleigh at various times would emphasize that the medicine cabinet should be full and that "It's better to have them and not need them than to need them and not have them."

accurately than could be done by hand, but it has reduced to the minimum the expense of getting tablets ready for market, another of the many savings which we are able to share with users of Rawleigh Products.

Rawleigh's tablets were made with scientifically correct formulas from the purest drugs of uniform strength; each tablet was exactly the same weight and medicinal strength. When you buy Rawleigh's, you not only get the best but you get a much larger number than sold at the stores — the most, as well as the best, for your money. — *Rawleigh 1916.*

Why Mother Prefer Rawleigh Products

Rawleigh extracted the medicinal properties directly from the drugs they used in making their medicines: lobelia, squill, senega, ipecac, Balm o'Gilead buds, horehound, spikenard, bloodroot, white pine, wild cherry, and sassafras. Thus, Rawleigh was sure of getting the best uniform quality in their medicines.

In manufacturing all of their medicines in their own laboratories, Rawleigh invested over $20,000 in stills, percolators, hydraulic presses, vacuum dryers, evaporating pans, and other equipment used to make all their fluid extracts and tinctures.

The strength and potency of every fluid extract and tincture used in their cough medicines were carefully tested. They insured an exact measure of the active principal of the various drugs and the full therapeutic dose necessary to provide desired results. These methods were necessary to make STANDARD, UNIFORM quality and the most RELIABLE and useful cough medicine.

The Rawleigh Comany assured that in addition to alleviating the cough, Rawleigh's cough medicines assisted in regulating the bowels and increasing the urinary flow, because it was also a mild laxative and diuretic. This helped eliminate poisons from the system and assisted NATURE in restoring the general health.

RAWLEIGH'S COUGH SYRUP was touted as beneficial for coughs, colds, tickling in the throat, hoarseness, and loss of voice due to severe colds. It soothed and healed the irritated membranes of the throat. Rawleigh's cough syrup was recommended for children as it contained no habit-forming drugs and was pleasant to the taste.

RAWLEIGH'S RU-MEX-OL was sold as a helpful preparation of great tonic value, toning the system and assisting in the building of red blood cells. Rawleigh's Ru-Mex-Ol was an old time favorite and in 1922 "was the same dependable preparation that it was when first placed on the market."

See Ru-Mex-Ol in this chapter.

Rawleigh Health Products

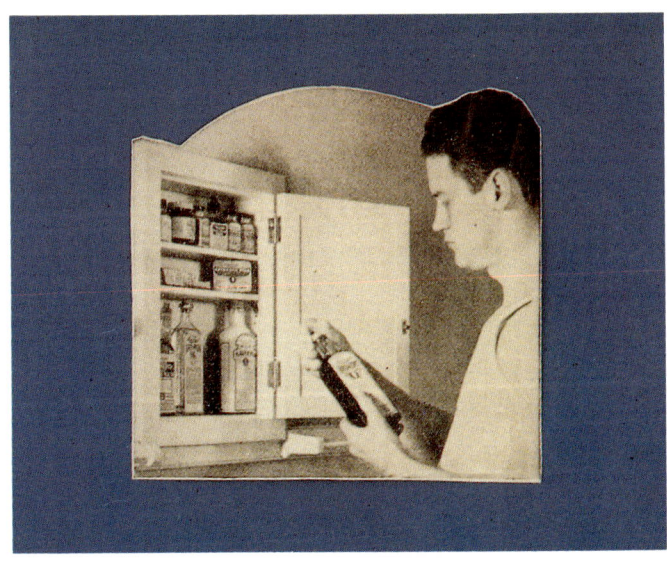

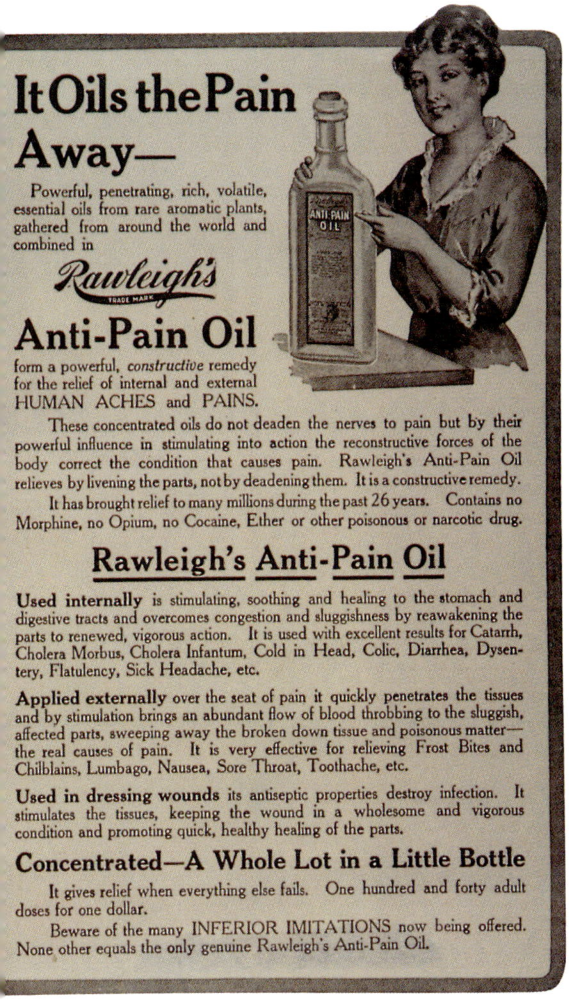

It Oils the Pain Away—
Powerful, penetrating, rich, volatile, essential oils from rare aromatic plants, gathered from around the world and combined in
Rawleigh's
TRADE MARK
Anti-Pain Oil
form a powerful, *constructive* remedy for the relief of internal and external HUMAN ACHES and PAINS.
These concentrated oils do not deaden the nerves to pain but by their powerful influence in stimulating into action the reconstructive forces of the body correct the condition that causes pain. Rawleigh's Anti-Pain Oil relieves by livening the parts, not by deadening them. It is a constructive remedy.
It has brought relief to many millions during the past 26 years. Contains no Morphine, no Opium, no Cocaine, Ether or other poisonous or narcotic drug.
Rawleigh's Anti-Pain Oil
Used internally is stimulating, soothing and healing to the stomach and digestive tracts and overcomes congestion and sluggishness by reawakening the parts to renewed, vigorous action. It is used with excellent results for Catarrh, Cholera Morbus, Cholera Infantum, Cold in Head, Colic, Diarrhea, Dysentery, Flatulency, Sick Headache, etc.
Applied externally over the seat of pain it quickly penetrates the tissues and by stimulation brings an abundant flow of blood throbbing to the sluggish, affected parts, sweeping away the broken down tissue and poisonous matter—the real causes of pain. It is very effective for relieving Frost Bites and Chilblains, Lumbago, Nausea, Sore Throat, Toothache, etc.
Used in dressing wounds its antiseptic properties destroy infection. It stimulates the tissues, keeping the wound in a wholesome and vigorous condition and promoting quick, healthy healing of the parts.
Concentrated—A Whole Lot in a Little Bottle
It gives relief when everything else fails. One hundred and forty adult doses for one dollar.
Beware of the many INFERIOR IMITATIONS now being offered. None other equals the only genuine Rawleigh's Anti-Pain Oil.
ANTI-PAIN OIL

An original Rawleigh's "It Oils the Pain Away - Anti-Pain Oil" advertisement from Rawleigh's 1916 Almanac.

SOME OF THE BIG LEADERS AMONG
Rawleigh's
TRADE MARK
110 QUALITY PRODUCTS
THE LARGEST NUMBER THE GREATEST VARIETY - THE MOST USEFUL AND THE MOST SCIENTIFIC SOLD
FROM FACTORY TO FARM
Rawleigh's COLD TABLETS
Rawleigh LAXATIVE TABLETS
Rawleigh's CAMPHOR BALM
OINTMENT
Rawleigh's ANTI-PAIN OIL
Rawleigh's LINIMENT
Rawleigh's CORDIAL TONIC LAXATIVE
ACUTE OR CHRONIC CONSTIPATION
Rawleigh's RU-MEX-OL COMPOUND
PURIFYING THE BLOOD
Rawleigh's Cough Syrup
SALVE
THE W. T. RAWLEIGH COMPANY
FREEPORT ILL. U.S.A.

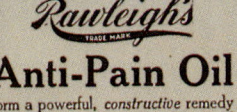

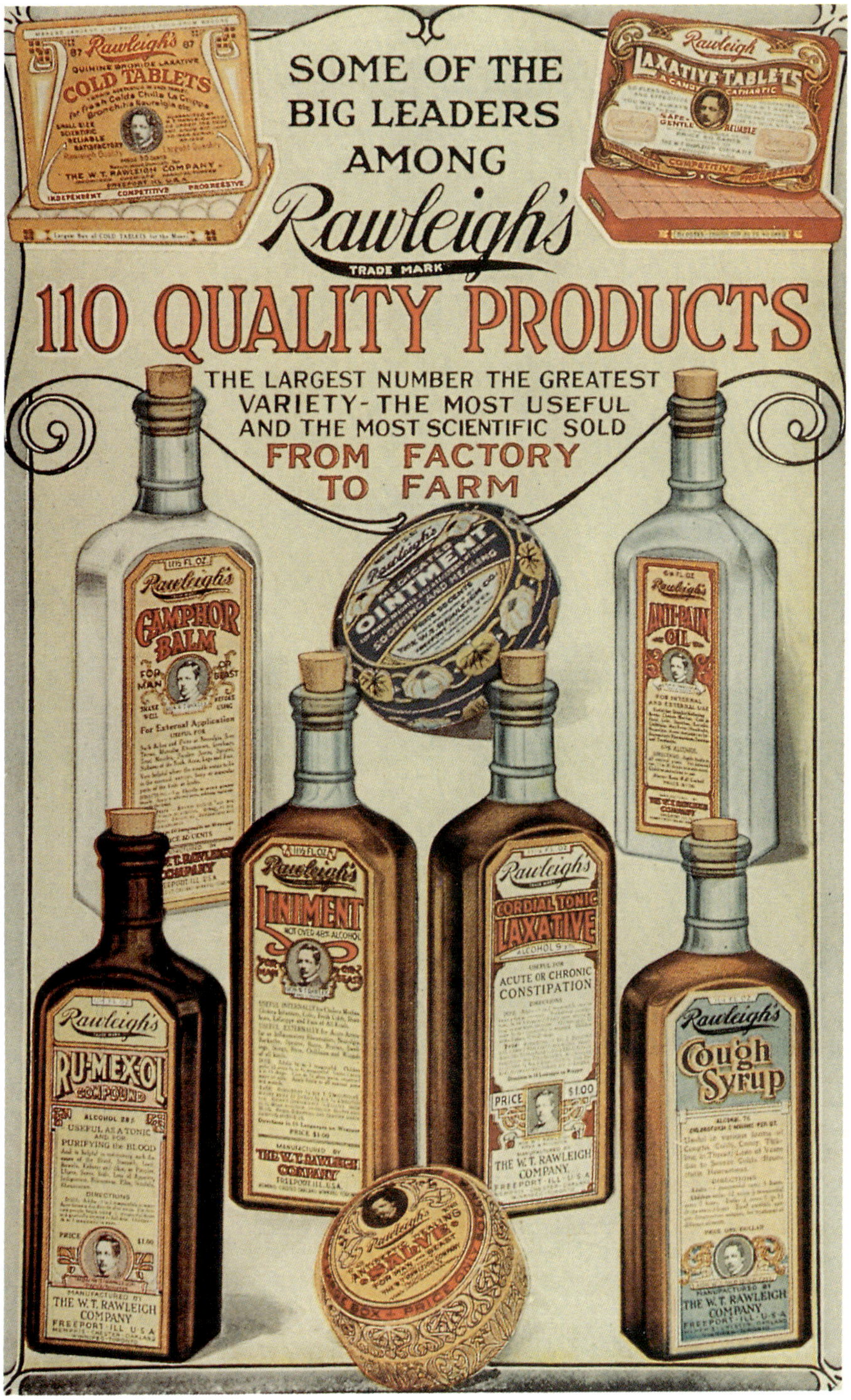

An original advertisement for "Some of the Big Leaders Among Rawleigh's 110 Quality Products." Circa 1917.

In 1932, the W.T. Rawleigh Company announced the following new products which had been developed by the Rawleigh industries during 1931. Each product was scientifically compounded from the best chemicals and other raw materials obtainable. Rawleigh's "Castoria" was made by a scientific process from standardized ingredients which was carefully and properly compounded. Rawleigh's "Castoria" relieved constipation and other ailments of stomach and bowels for babies, children, and adults. Photograph not available.

Rawleigh's "Rectal Ointment" was a soothing application that reduced the irritation and made bowel elimination easier. This ointment was made from a formula of a noted physician specialist who had used it in his successful practice. Photograph not available.

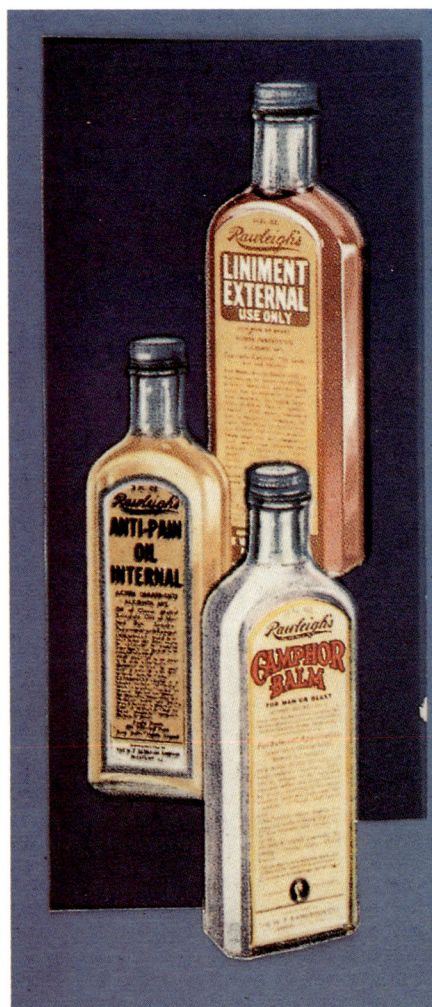

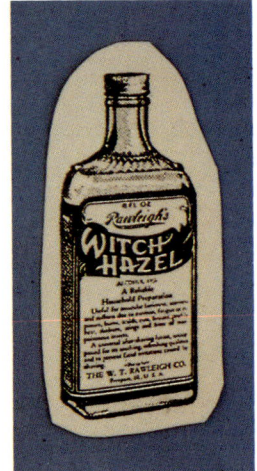

Rawleigh's "Witch Hazel" was a reliable and useful household preparation for muscles, burns, scalds, cuts, bruises, sunburn, stings, non-poisonous insects bites, and also prevented facial irritations caused by shaving. $25-$30.

Rawleigh's "Liniment" — both internal and external — had "provided continuous satisfaction in 1951 to millions for over 62 years." Rawleigh's Liniment External Use Only, Anti-Pain Oil Internal, and Rawleigh's Camphor Balm had proved their value in millions of homes for aches, pains, stiffness, lameness, neuralgia, and for sore muscles.

Many farmers kept one bottle of Liniment in the house for the family and another in the barn for their livestock.

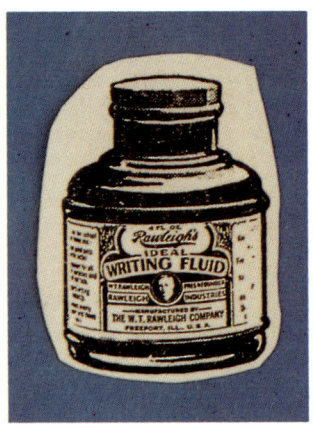

Rawleigh's "Ideal Writing Fluid," a 4 ounce high grade of serviceable writing fluid that flowed freely. It dried quickly and did not fade. This 1932 product was excellent for fountain pens. $35-$40.

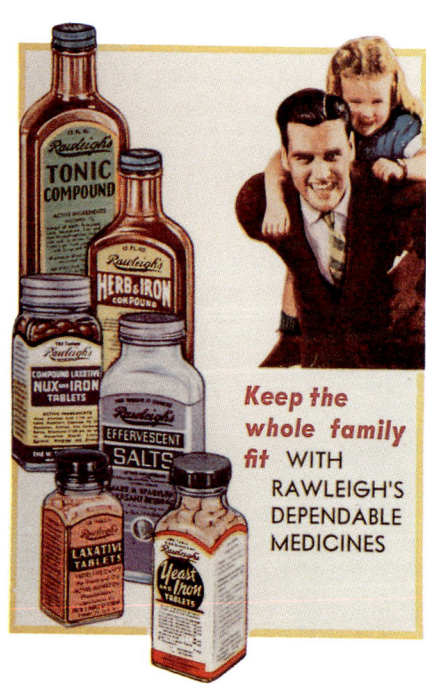

Rawleigh's "Silver Polish" was also announced in 1932 as, "A practical, economical necessity for cleaning, polishing and brightening silverware, cutlery, and nickel plating." It was supposed to polish quickly and easily with less effort and not to scratch or mar the finish. Photograph not available.

Rawleigh's Starch-Aid, which made ironing easier, is shown elsewhere in this publication as is the new 1932 Rawleigh's Fruit Pectin and Celery Salt. Not shown is a new 1932 hand soap that was a specially prepared cleaner that easily removed dirt, grease, grime, ink stains, paint, and oil while leaving the hands clean, smooth, and soft. This new hand soap was economical and better than most other soaps.

In 1951 Rawleigh promoted their Tonic Compound, Herb & Iron Compound, Nux-Iron Tablets, Effervescent Salts, Laxative Tablets, Yeast and Iron Tablets, as a way to "Keep the whole family fit."

Rawleigh often warned customers to "Always be sure to follow the directions on the label of each laxative."

It is estimated nearly five-hundred carloads of cans and bottles were required yearly for Rawleigh packaging and one hundred thirty eight tank cars of oils were used annually for soaps, insecticides, and disinfectants.

In 1932, Rawleigh announced "MORE FOR THE MONEY, Bigger Bottles and Better Values" when they introduced a new 12 ounce bottle for: cough syrup, thyme cough compound, cough balsam, Ru-Mex-Oil, tonic compound, cod liver oil, and pure cod liver oil. With Rawleigh's bigger bottles customers got more medicine for the same amount of money, because the new bottles contained about 10% more than the old bottles with no increase in prices.

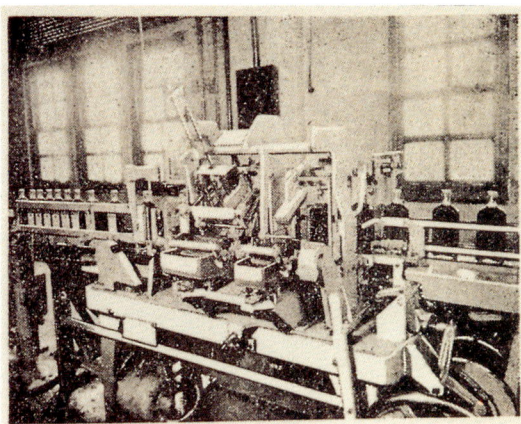

This machine automatically labeled bottles at the rate of 70 per minute in 1932.

In 1981, the Rawleigh tradition was emphasized by the reintroduction of authentic containers originally created eighty years ago for Rawleigh's "Medicated Ointment and Antiseptic Salve." These two products were big sellers for almost the entire history of the Rawleigh Company. The reintroduced ointment and salve were once again made with natural ingredients from the early formula.

Rawleigh's 16 ounce "Antiseptic Solution" that killed germs on contract and contained a bacteria fighting ingredient. This solution was an effective mouthwash recommended for family use and appeared in a ©July 1986 brochure. Manufactured by The W.T. Rawleigh Company, Freeport, Illinois 61032 U.S.A. $10-$15.

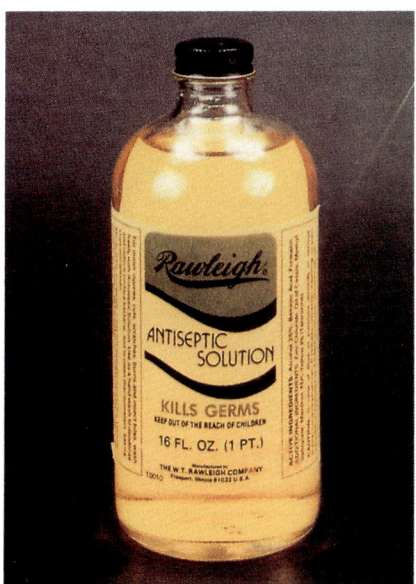

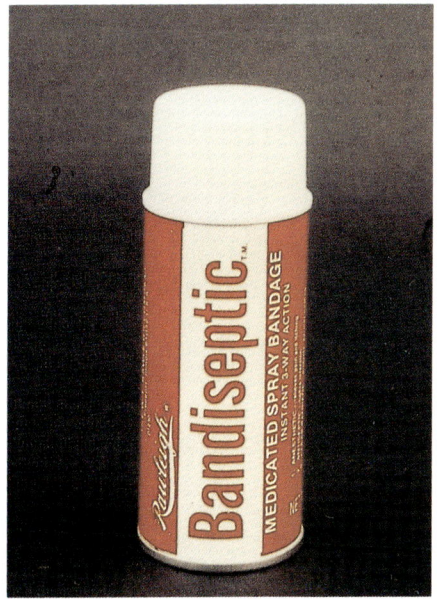

Rawleigh's 4.5 ounce "Bandiseptic" was a medicated aerosol spray bandage that gave a three-way action. Ingredients included Benzocaine, "a local anesthetic for relieving discomforts of minor injuries." Bandiseptic appeared in a © July 1986 brochure. $5-$10.

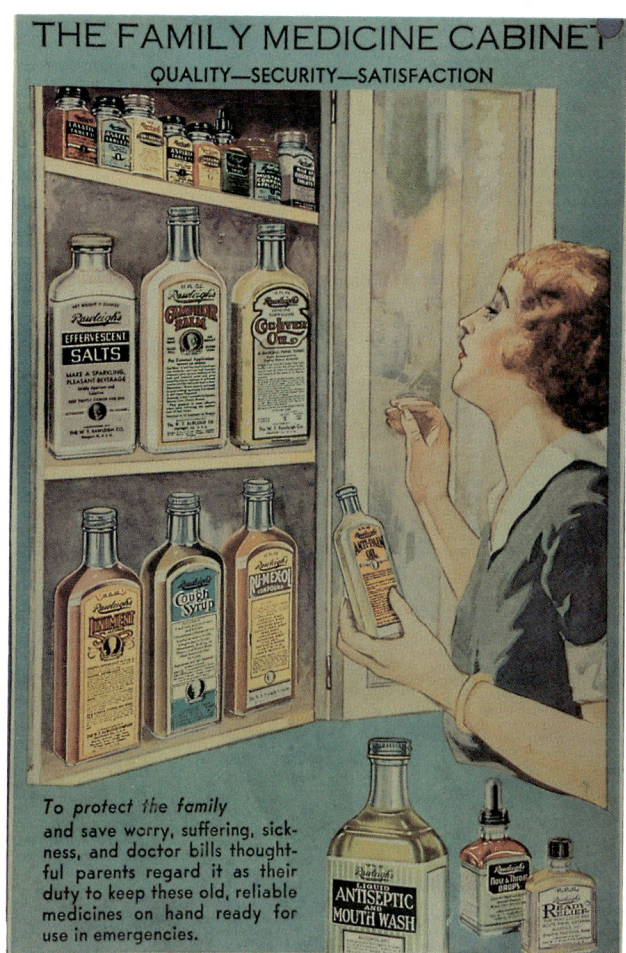

An original 1939 advertisement, "The Family Medicine Cabinet". Ready for any emergencies, the family medicine cabinet was stocked with reliable medicines.

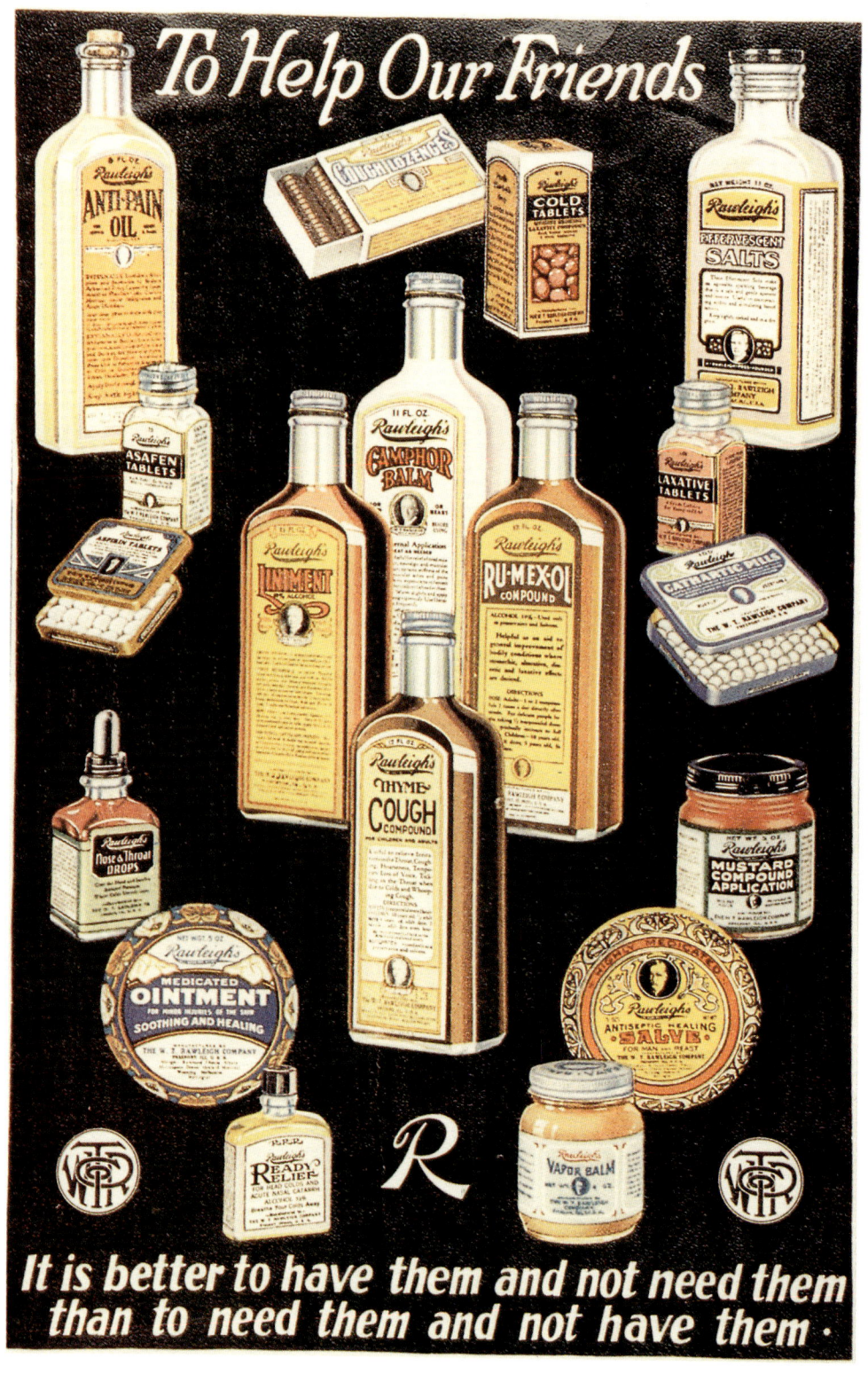

An original 1935 advertisement, "To Help Our Friends". Note the "WTRCo" marking near the bottom; this is the same marking that appears on the lid to Rawleigh's "Effervescent Salts" shown later in this chapter. Original advertisements can help date many Rawleigh products.

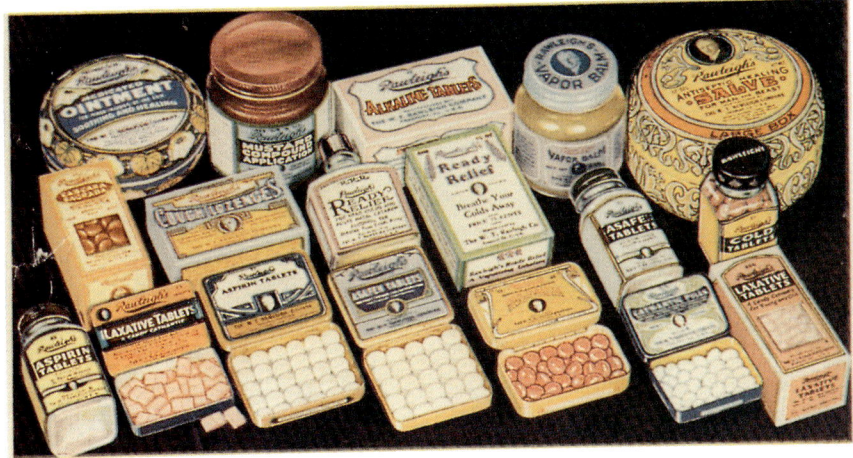

A selection of Rawleigh's tablets and other "NECESSITIES NEEDED IN EVERY HOME." Many of these products are shown elsewhere in this publication. Circa 1939.

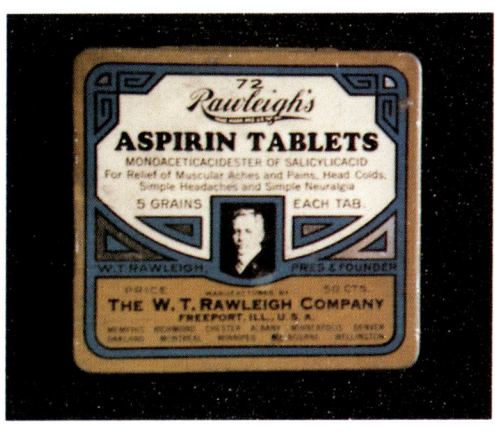

Rawleigh's Aspirin tablets. For relief of simple headaches and neuralgia, muscular aches and pains, head colds, and as a gargle for relief of minor throat irritations. *Dupler Collection.* $10-$15.

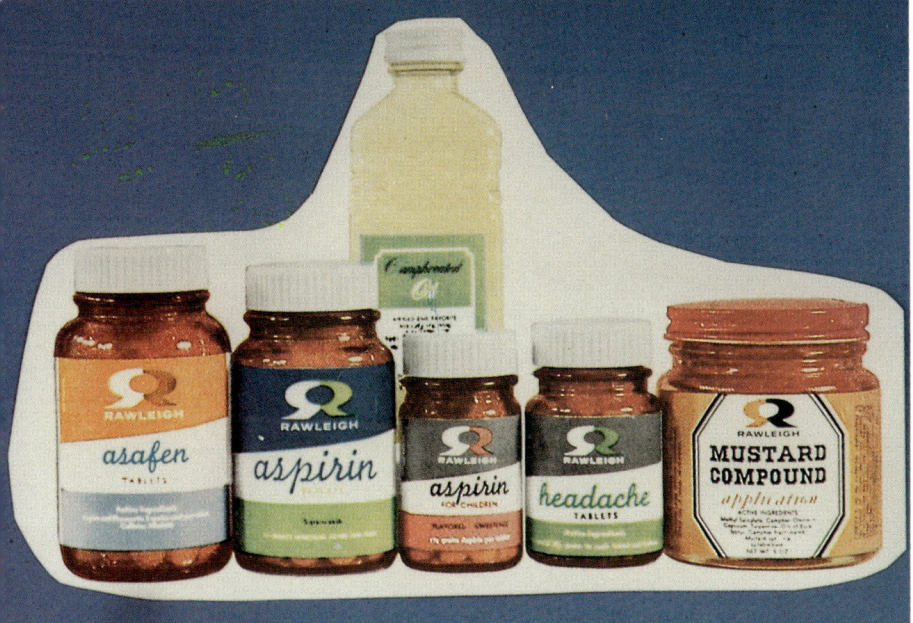

A 1960s selection of Rawleigh's Asafen, Aspirin, Aspirin for children, Headache Tablets, Mustard Compound, and Camphorated Oil. Rawleigh Asafen was a reliable compound for headaches, neuralgic pains, muscular pains and to relieve symptoms of the common head colds. Aspirin for Children was a widely used medicine to relieve the discomfort of the common cold among children. Headache tablets reduced the pain of ordinary headaches. Mustard Compound helped relieve aching, painful muscles and Camphorated Oil was an old time favorite for sore muscles, coughs, minor throat irritations, sprains, bruises, and cold sores.

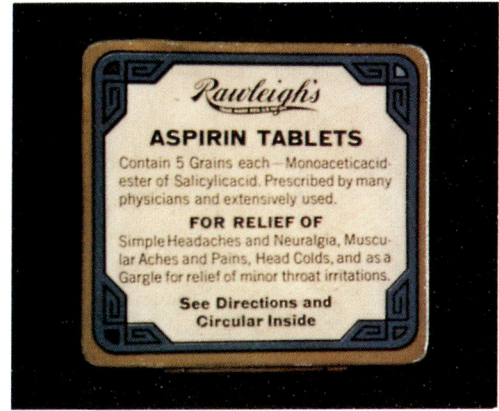

The reverse side of Rawleigh's Aspirin Tablets. Directions and a circular were provide inside. Flat rectangular hinged lid tin. Manufactured by THE W.T. RAWLEIGH COMPANY FREEPORT, ILL., U.S.A. Memphis - Richmond - Chester - Albany - Minneapolis - Denver - Oakland - Montreal - Winnipeg - Melbourne - Wellington. Circa 1930s. *Dupler Collection.* $10-$15.

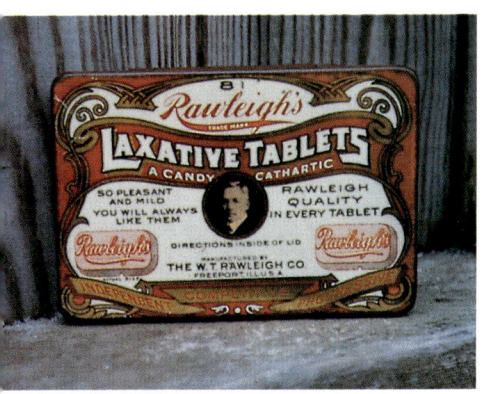

Rawleigh's Laxative tablets, a candy cathartic. Enough for thirty to forty days or eighty-one doses. Flat rectangular hinged lid tin. Manufactured by THE W.T. RAWLEIGH COMPANY, FREEPORT, ILL., U.S.A. $10-$15.

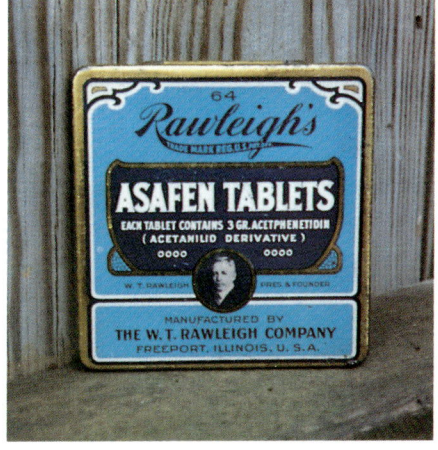

Rawleigh's Asafen Tablets, one of the safest and most useful general pain-relieving preparations for reducing pains, aches, colds, and La Grippe. Manufactured By The W.T. Rawleigh Company Freeport, Illinois, U.S.A. *Dupler Collection.* $10-$15.

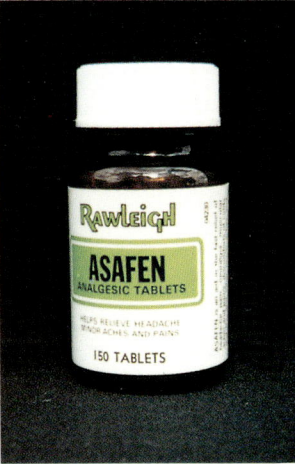

Rawleigh Asafen Analgesic Tablets. Distributed By The W.T. Rawleigh Company Freeport, Illinois 61032. *Dupler Collection.* $10-$15.

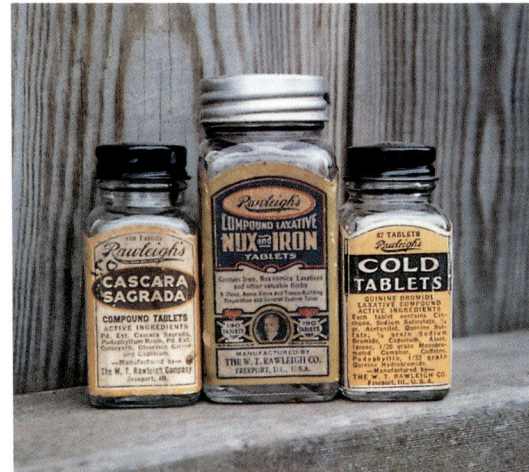

Rawleigh's Cascara Sagrada Compound Tablets, Rawleigh's Nux & Iron Tablets, and Rawleigh's Cold Tablets. *Dupler Collection.* $10-$15 ea.

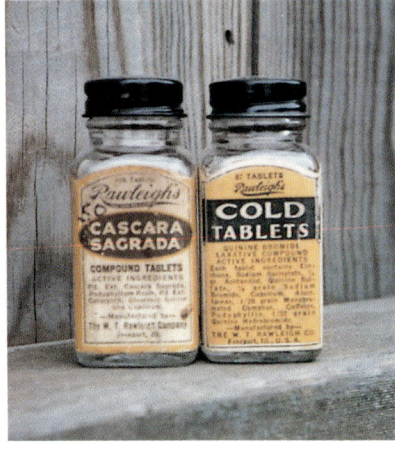

Rawleigh's Cascara Sagrada Compound Tablets and Rawleigh's Cold Tablets. Manufactured by THE W.T. RAWLEIGH COMPANY FREEPORT, ILL., U.S.A. Top of Cold Tablets lid is marked "Rawleigh's Trade Mark Reg. U.S. Pat. Off." *Dupler Collection.* $10-$15.

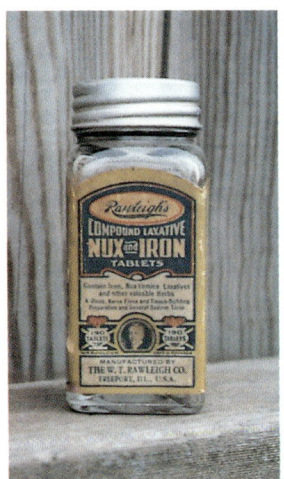

Rawleigh's Compound Laxative Nux and Iron Tablets. Manufactured By The W.T. Rawleigh Co. Freeport, Ill., U.S.A. Both lid and glass bottle is embossed with the Rawleigh name. *Dupler Collection.* $10-$15.

An original 1954 advertisement for Rawleigh's Cold tablets and Rawleigh's Ready Relief (RRR). Rawleigh believed everyone should "Be prepared to fight colds at the first symptom."

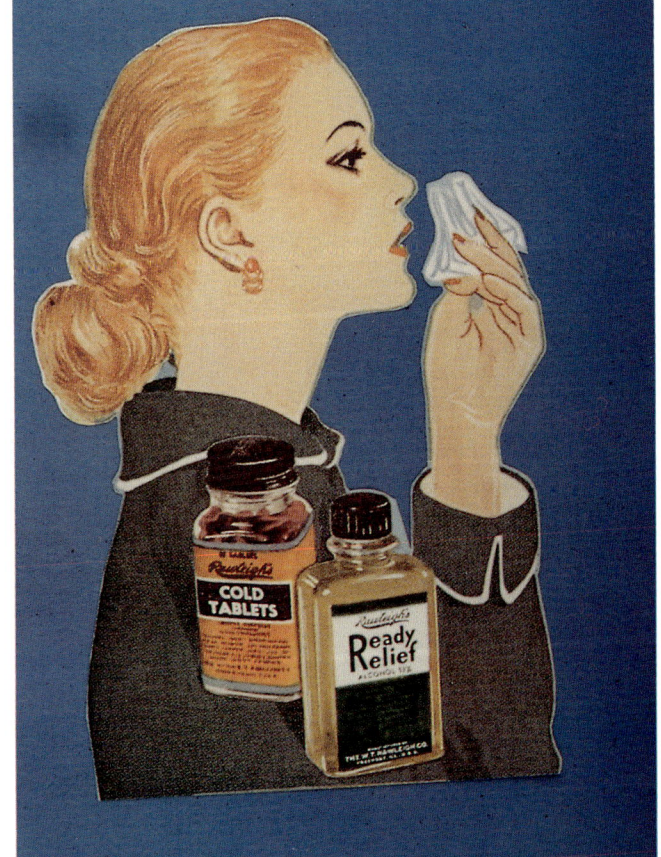

In 1932, Rawleigh's Ready Relief (RRR) had sold particularly well that year — since first introduced — because it brought quick relief. Rawleigh imported the volatile ingredients ("which, when breathed, reach all the nasal cavities and the seat of infection") from France, Spain, Italy, and Japan.

From the very beginning, the Rawleigh Industries had produced a larger bottle and a product (Rawleigh's Ready Relief) that was stated to be over "100% stronger in actual medicinal power, it provided consumers by far the best values and satisfaction."

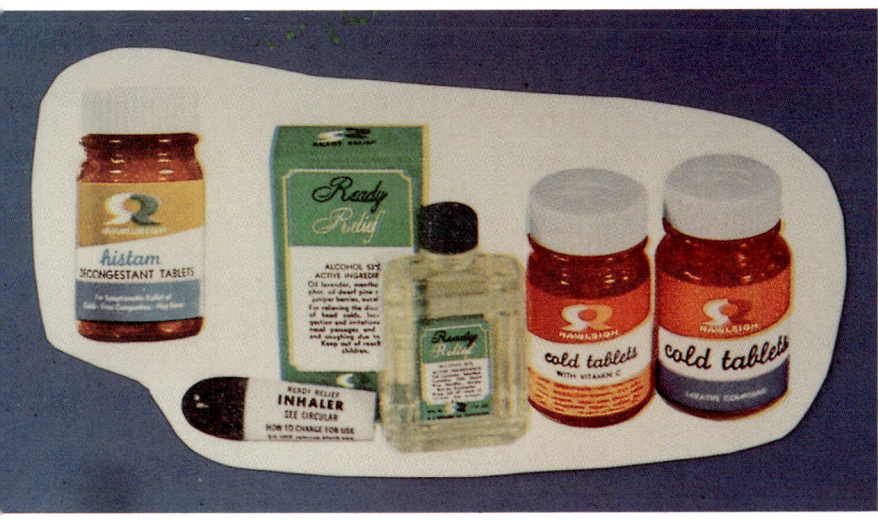

An original 1960s advertisement, "Be Ready when colds come." NEW Histam Decongestant tablets relieved the symptoms of colds, sinus congestion, and hay fever. Ready Relief, when applied to a handkerchief, made breathing easier. The Inhaler was offered empty. Rawleigh's Cold tablets with vitamin C helped to relieve pain and supplied vitamin C; this product was also offered without vitamin C.

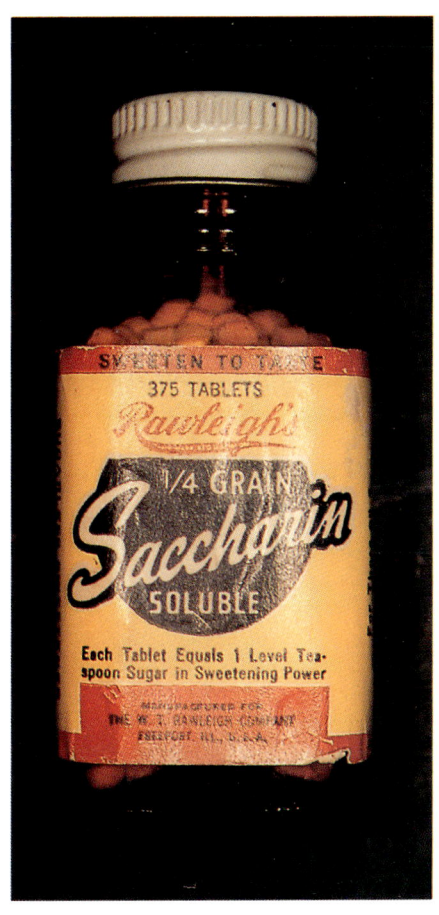

Rawleigh's 1/4 Grain Saccharin Soluble Tablets. Manufactured For THE W.T. RAWLEIGH COMPANY FREEPORT, ILL., U.S.A. Glass bottle with metal screw on lid, paper label. 375 Tablets. *Dupler Collection.* $10-$15.

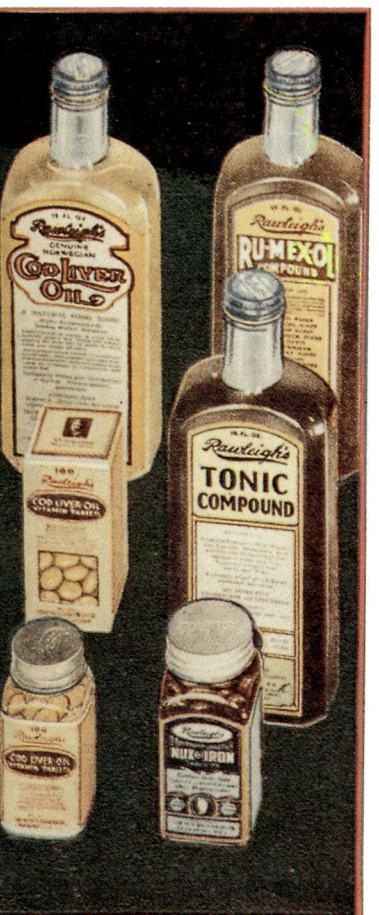

An original 1939 advertisement for Rawleigh's Cod Liver Oil, Ru-Mex-Ol Compound, Cod Liver Oil Tablets, Tonic Compound, and Nux & Iron Tablets.

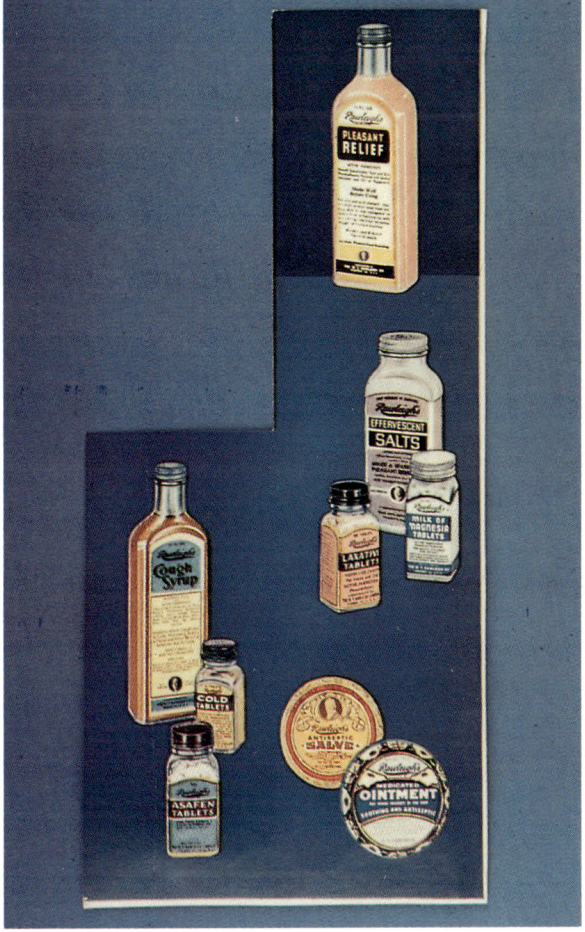

An original 1951 advertisement for reliable medicines. Note the similarities of the 1951 packaging when compared to those of the 1930s shown elsewhere in this publication.

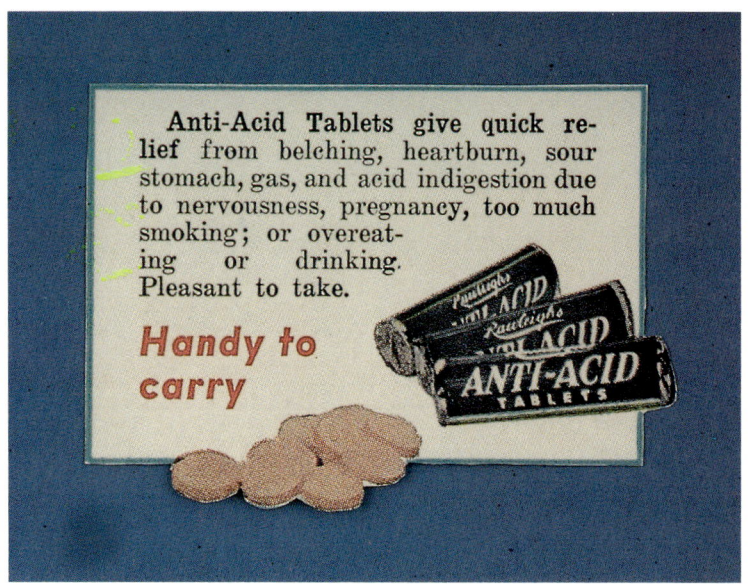

The original advertisement for Rawleigh's ANTI-ACID tablets. This advertisement appeared in a 1953 publication.

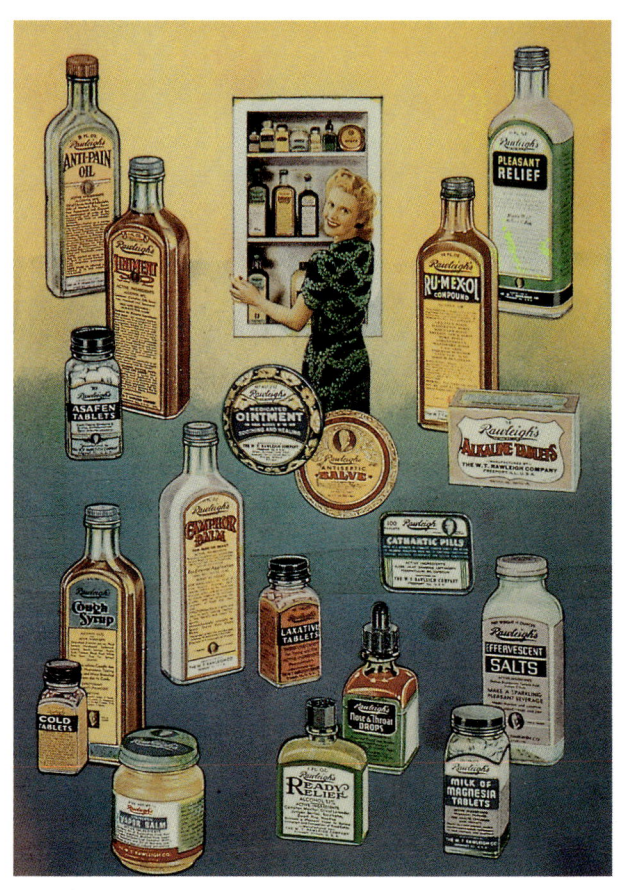

In 1946, was *your* cabinet full of Rawleigh medicine? To relieve aches, pains, and colds, this Rawleigh advertisement promoted reliable Rawleigh medicines, tablets, and ointments.

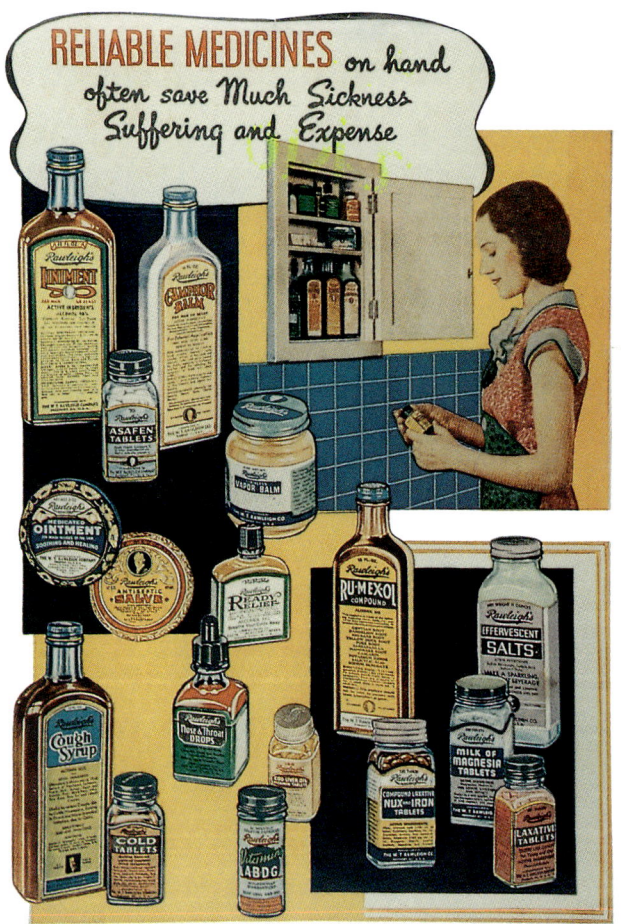

The Reliable Medicines advertisement appeared in a 1942 Rawleigh's Good Health Guide Almanac Cook Book. Note asafen, cold tablets, cod liver oil, laxative, Milk of Magnesia, nux and iron tablets, medicated ointment, salva, Ready Relief, drops, vitamins, and various other products. Many of these products appear throughout this publication.

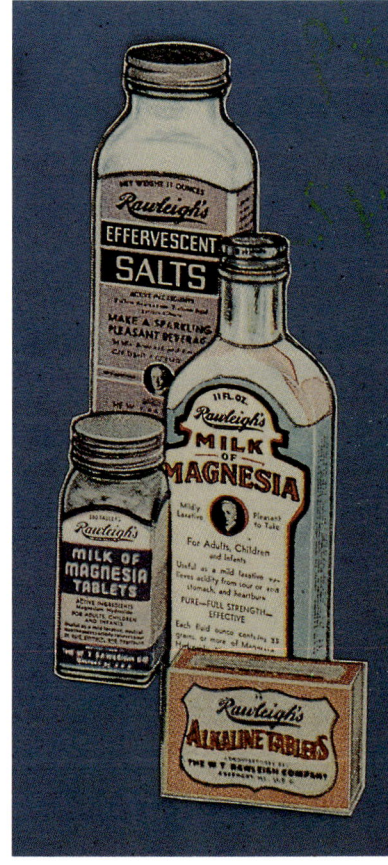

An original 1946 Rawleigh advertisement for Rawleigh's Effervescent Salts, Milk of Magnesia in either liquid or mint-flavored tablets, and Alkaline tablets.

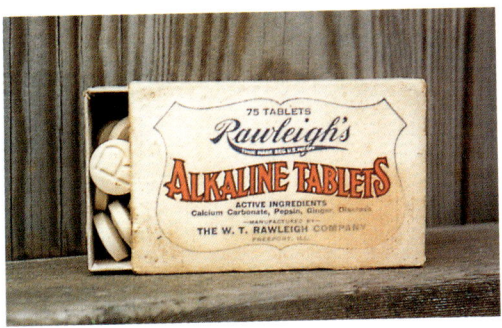

A full carton of Rawleigh's Alkaline Tablets. Manufactured By The W.T. Rawleigh Company Freeport, Ill. *Bushue Collection.* $15-$20.

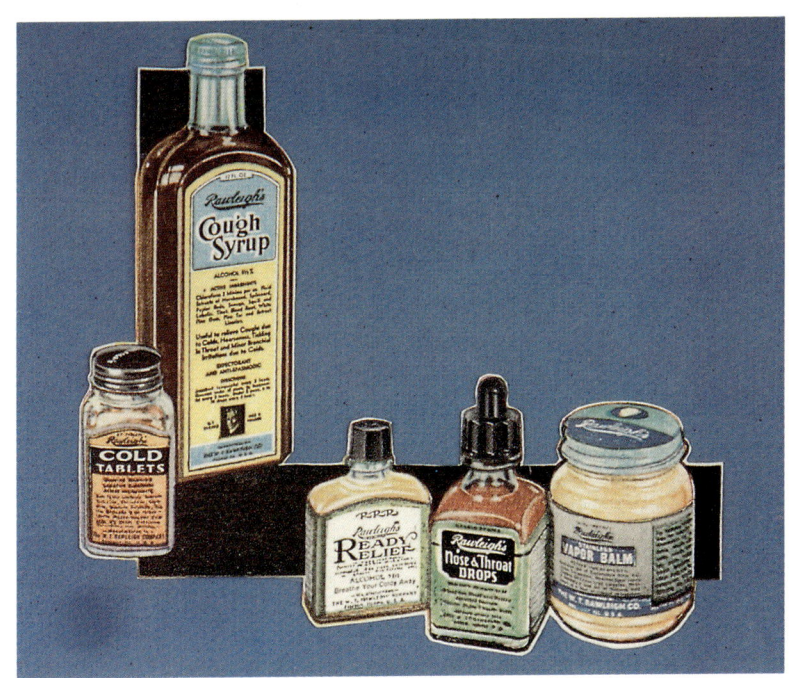

An original 1946 "Coughs and Colds" advertisement for Rawleigh's Cold tablets, Cough Syrup, Ready Relief, Nose and Throat drops, and Vapor Balm. Rawleigh reminded customers to keep these medicines handy.

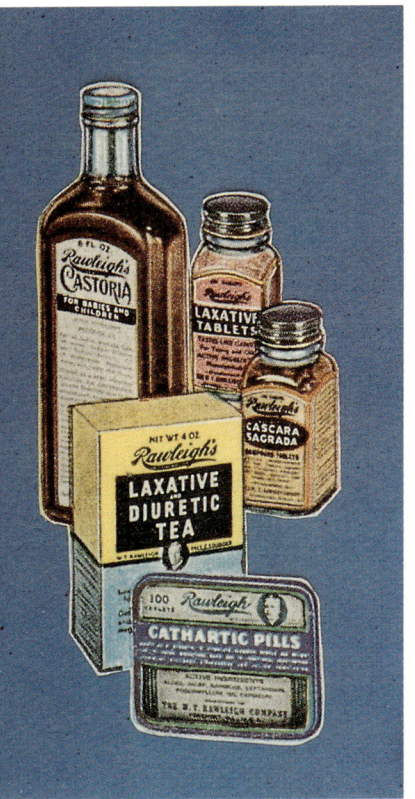

Rawleigh's Castoria, Laxative tablets, Cascara Sagrade, Laxative Diuretic tea, and Cathartic pills. Circa 1946.

Two variations of "Rawleigh's Ready Relief" with an original cardboard carton. Both Mfg. by The W.T. Rawleigh Company Freeport, Illinois. One bottle has a zip code which indicates a date of manufacture after 1959 and the other does not. The five digit zip code number was introduced by the U.S. Post Office in 1959. Directions were provided with "Rawleigh's Ready Relief" inside the packaging. This liquid compound relieved the discomfort of head colds, congestion, and irritation of nasal passages and throat, and coughing due to colds. Manufactured by The W.T. Rawleigh Co., Freeport, Ill., U.S.A. *Shepard Collection.* $10-$15 ea.

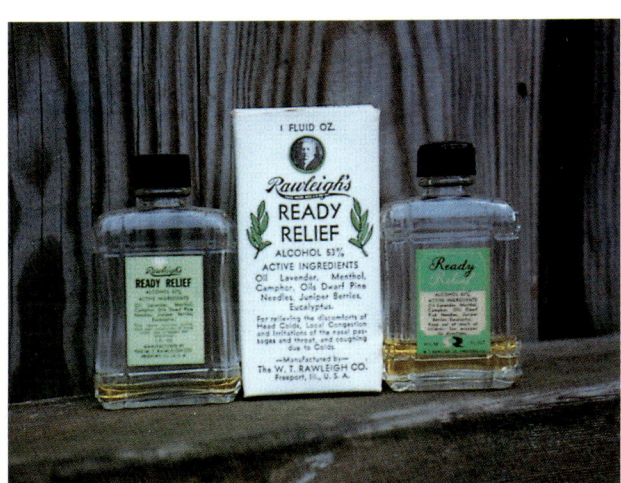

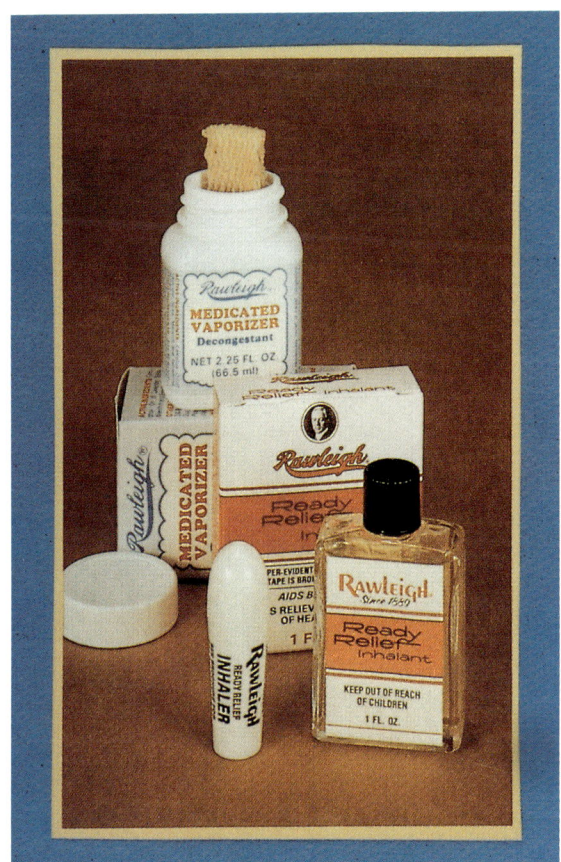

Rawleigh Medicated Vapor Decongestant 2.25 ounce and Rawleigh Ready Relief with 1 ounce inhaler. Circa 1986.

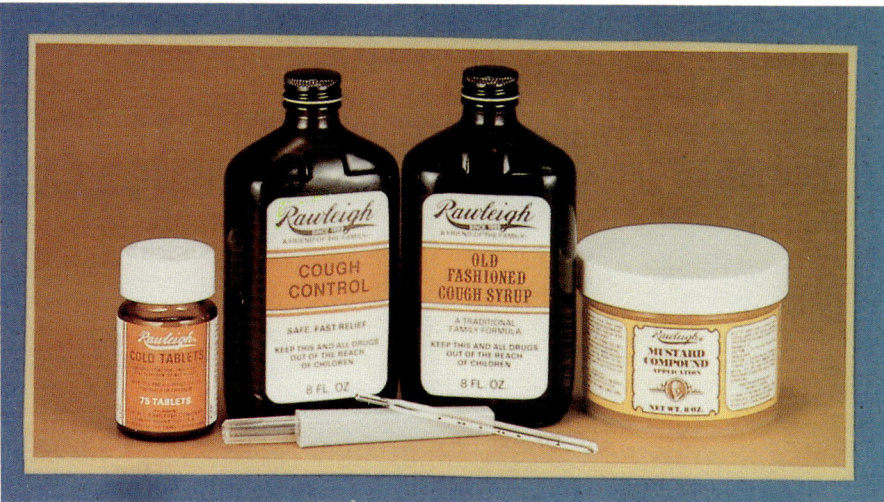

Rawleigh's Cold tablets, Cough Control, Old Fashioned Cough Syrup, and Mustard Compound. Circa 1986.

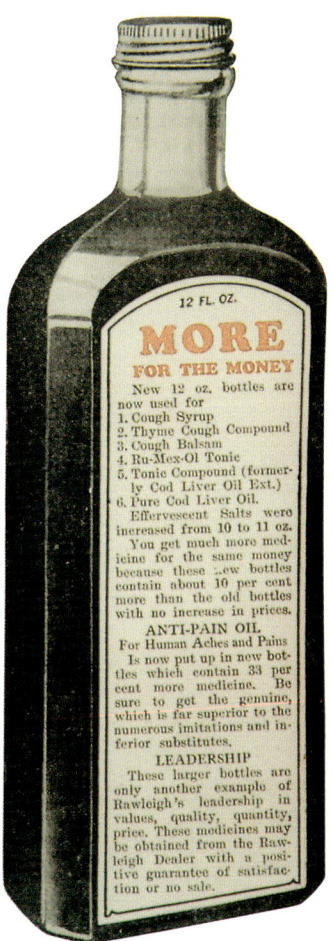

In 1932, Rawleigh promoted the new 12 ounce bottle being used for Cough Syrup, Thyme Cough Compound, Cough Balsam, Ru-Mex-Ol Tonic, Tonic Compound (formerly Cod Liver Oil), and Pure Cod Liver Oil. Effervescent Salts were increased from 10 ounce to 11 ounce. These bottles were advertised as "Bigger Bottles — Better Values — No increase in Price."

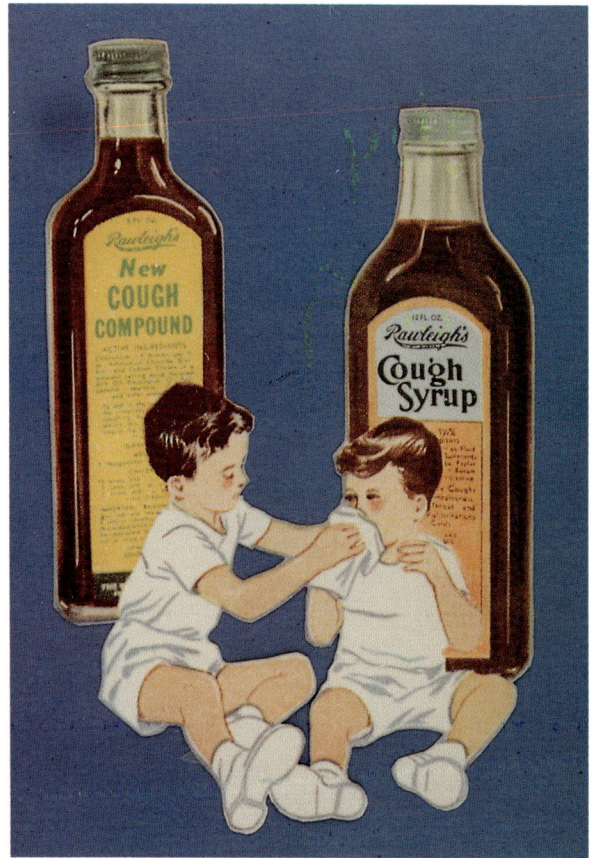

When Rawleigh promoted its Rawleigh's New Cough Compound and Cough Syrup in 1954, Rawleigh's medicines had "given wonderful satisfaction for 65 years."

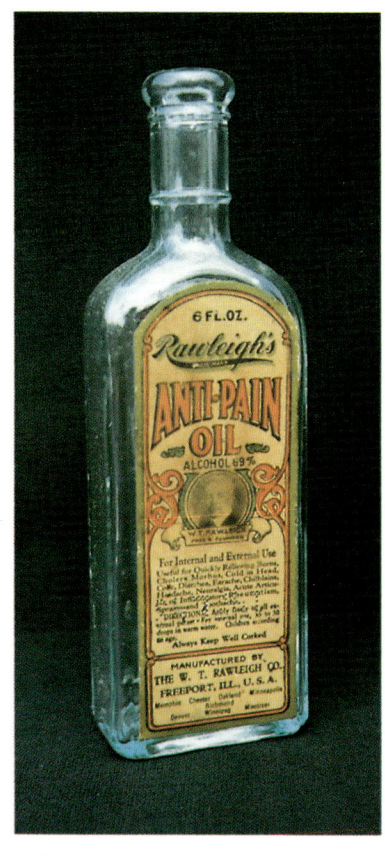

Rawleigh's 6-oz. "Anti-Pain Oil", for internal and external used. Glass bottle with paper label and cork cap. Manufactured by The W.T. Rawleigh Co. Freeport, Ill., U.S.A. Memphis - Chester - Oakland - Minneapolis - Richmond - Denver - Winnipeg - Montreal. Refer to Chapter One of this publication, where each Rawleigh plant opening has been discussed. This should provide you with some idea as to the date of production when locations are referred to on the packaging. *Dupler Collection.* $15-$20.

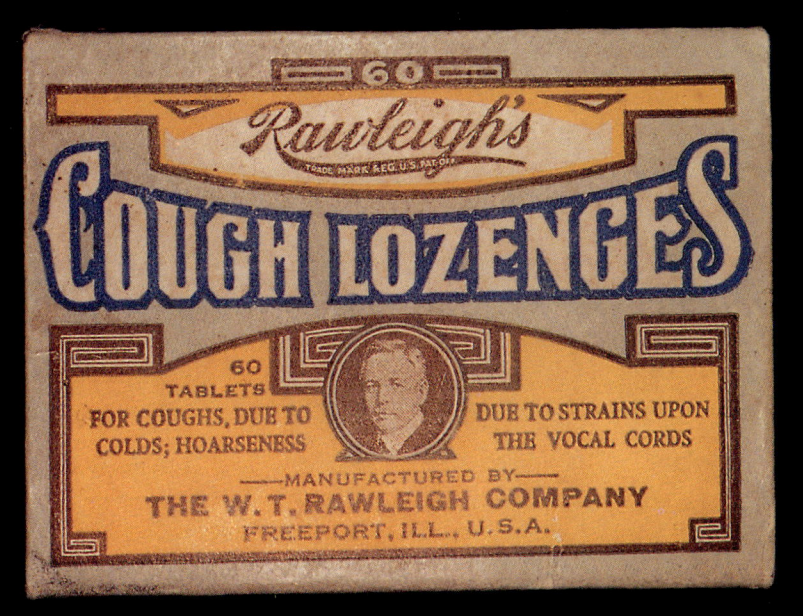

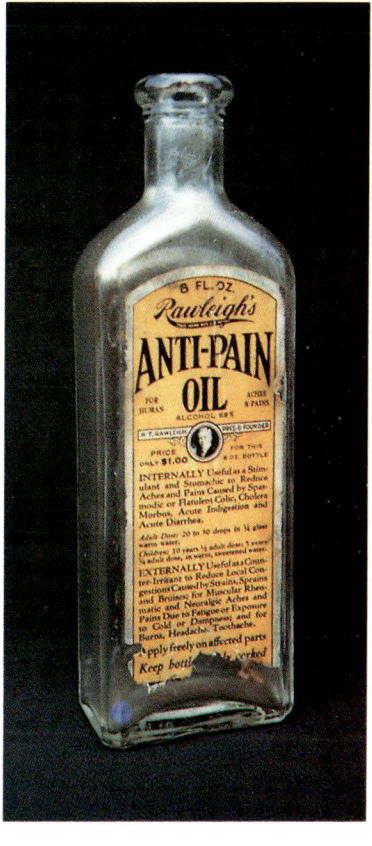

Rawleigh's 8 ounce "Anti-Pain Oil", for internal and external use. Glass bottle with paper label, and cork cap. A small section of the label is missing; this lowers the price. *Dupler Collection.* $15-$20.

The front and reverse of a cardboard container for Rawleigh Cough Lozenges. Manufactured By The W.T. Rawleigh Company Freeport, Ill., U.S.A. *Dupler Collection.* $25-$30.

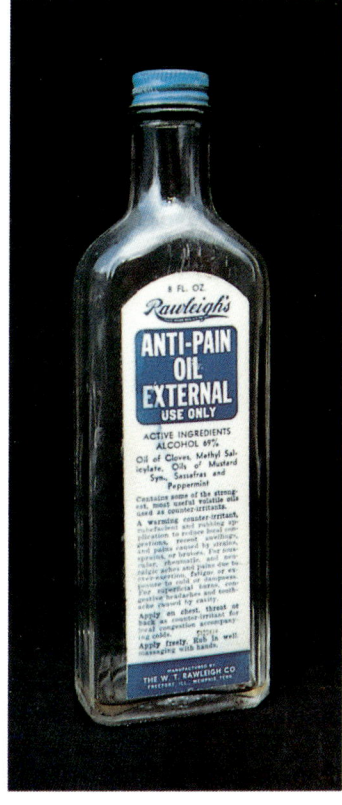

Rawleigh 8 ounce "Anti-Pain Oil External Use Only." Manufactured by The W.T. Rawleigh Co. Freeport, Ill., Memphis, Tenn. Contained some of the strongest, most useful volatile oils used as counter-irritants. *Dupler Collection.* $15-$20.

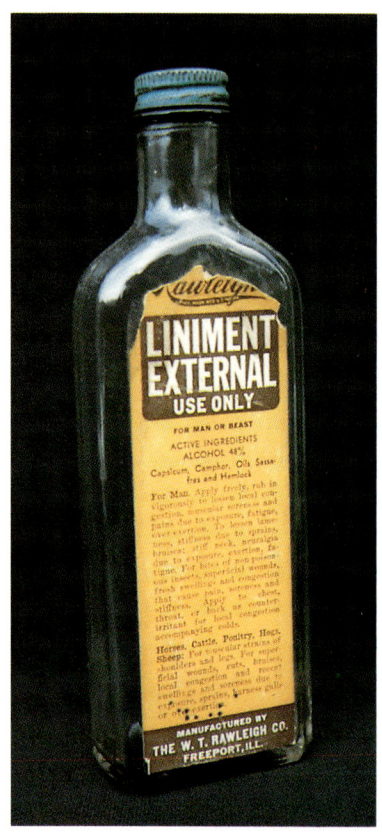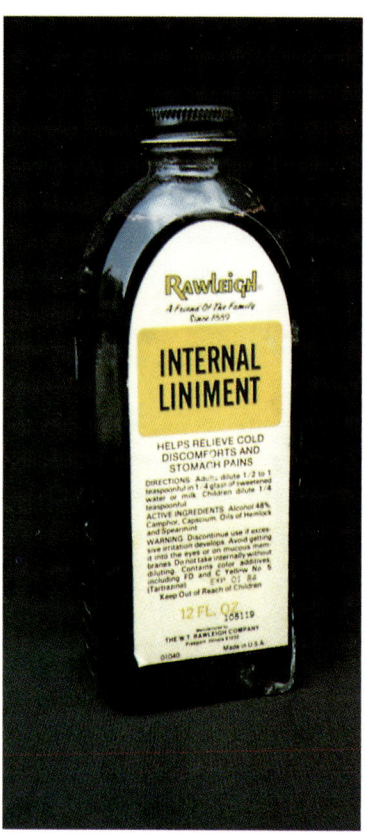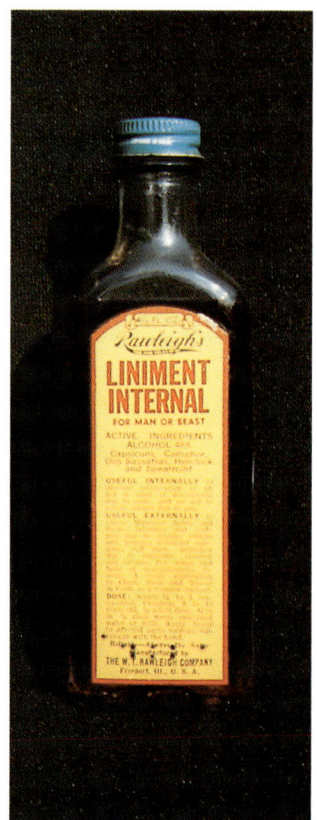

Rawleigh's 4-1/2 ounce "Liniment Internal For Man or Beast." Manufactured by The W.T. Rawleigh Company Freeport, Ill., U.S.A. *Dupler Collection.* $15-$20.

Rawleigh's "Liniment External Use Only. For Man or Beast." Manufactured by The W.T. Rawleigh Co. Freeport, Ill. A small section of the paper label is missing; this hinders the selling price. *Dupler Collection.* $15-$20.

A full 12 ounce glass container of Rawleigh "Internal Liniment." Helps relieve cold discomforts and stomach pains. Manufactured by The W.T. Rawleigh Company Freeport, Illinois 61032. *Dupler Collection.* $15-$20.

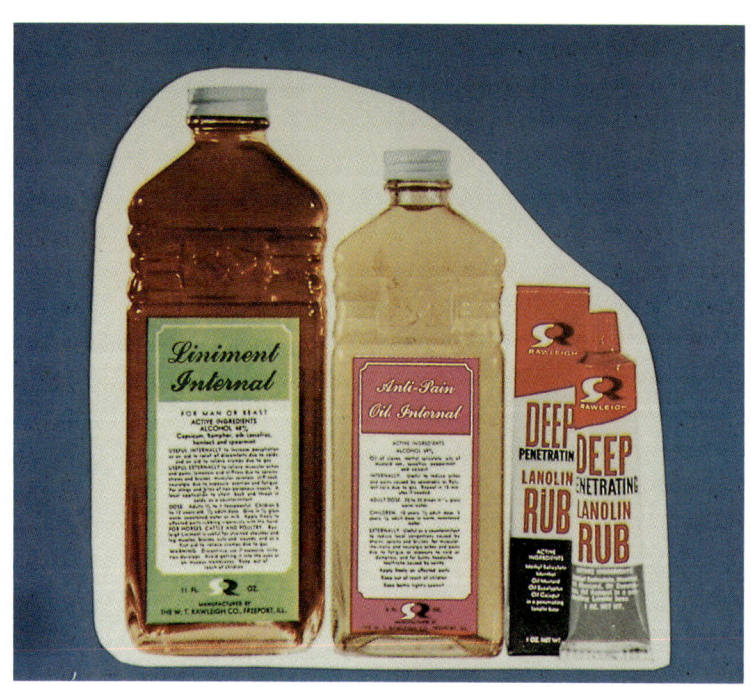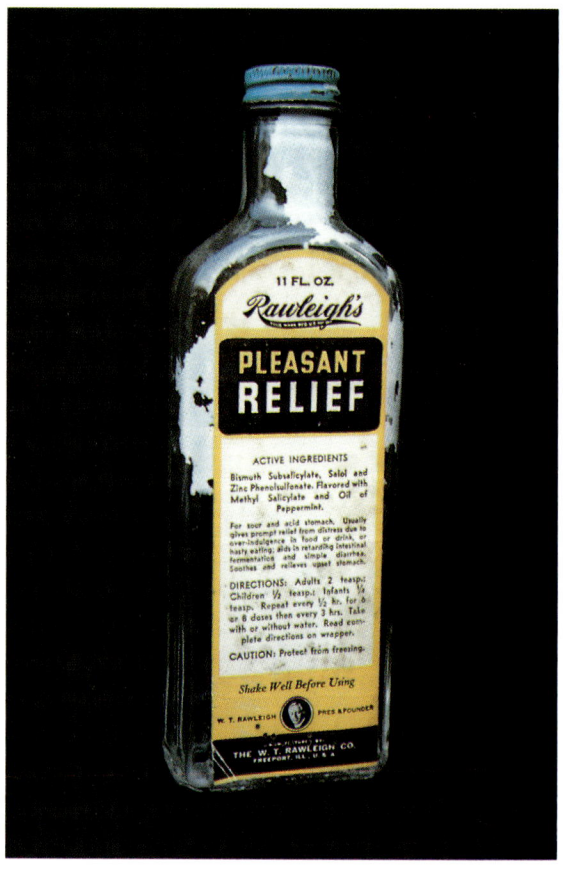

Rawleigh 11 ounce Liniment Internal. For over 50 years Rawleigh red Liniment Internal had been a favorite to relieve discomfort of colds, aching muscles, sprains, bruises, fatigue. Rawleigh 8 ounce Anti-Pain Oil Internal and Deep Penetrating Lanolin Rub. Circa 1960s. $15-$20.

Rawleigh's 11 ounce "Pleasant Relief." Glass bottle with screw on lid and paper label. Manufactured by The W.T. Rawleigh Co. Freeport, Ill., U.S.A. *Dupler Collection.* $15-$20.

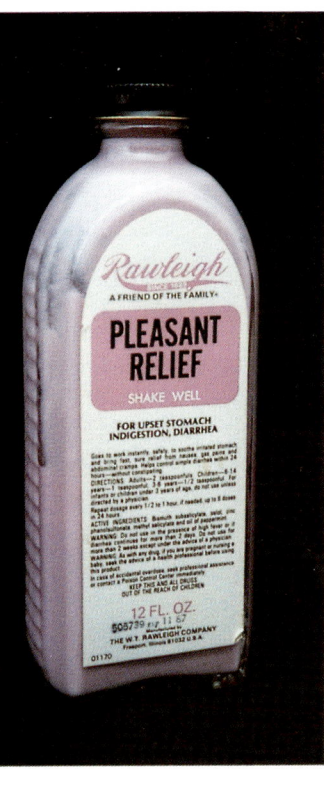

A partially full 12 ounce glass bottle, screw on lid, and paper label. Rawleigh's "Pleasant Relief" was Manufactured by The W.T. Rawleigh Company Freeport, Illinois 61032 U.S.A. *Dupler Collection.* $15-$20.

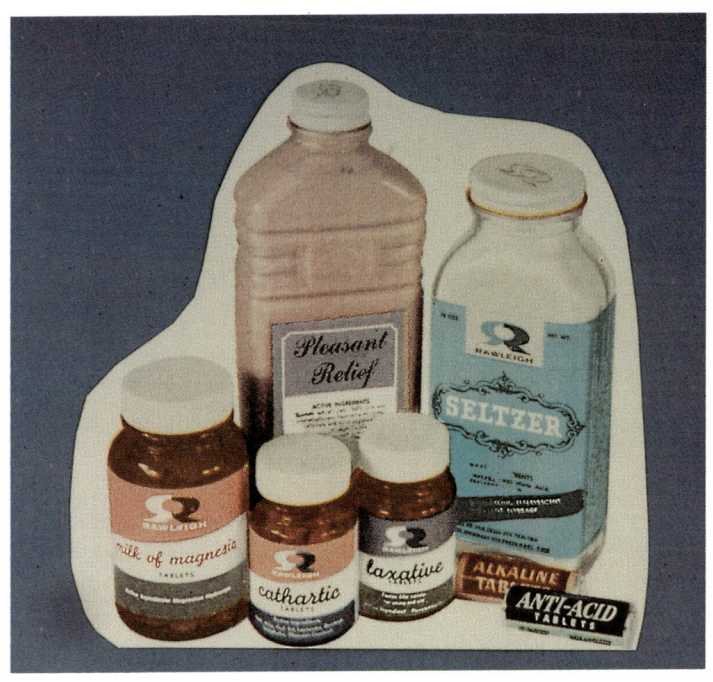

Rawleigh 11 ounce "Pleasant Relief Seltzer" was promoted in 1960 with Rawleigh's Anti-Acid tablets, Alkaline tablets, Laxative, and Cathartic tablets, Milk of Magnesia, and Pleasant Relief. $20-$25.

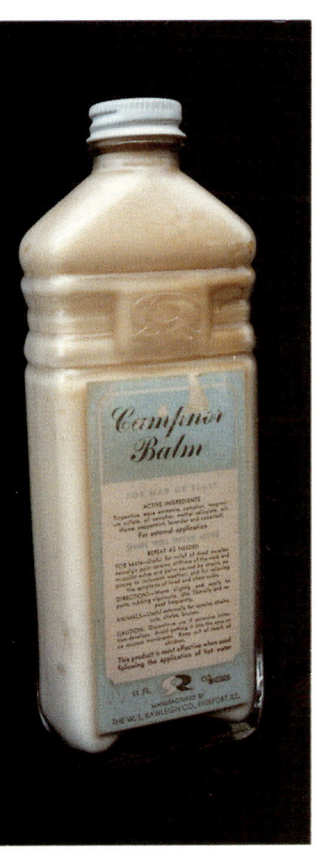

A full 11 ounce "Camphor Balm" For Man or Beast. Manufactured by The W.T. Rawleigh Co., Freeport, Ill. *Dupler Collection.* $15-$20.

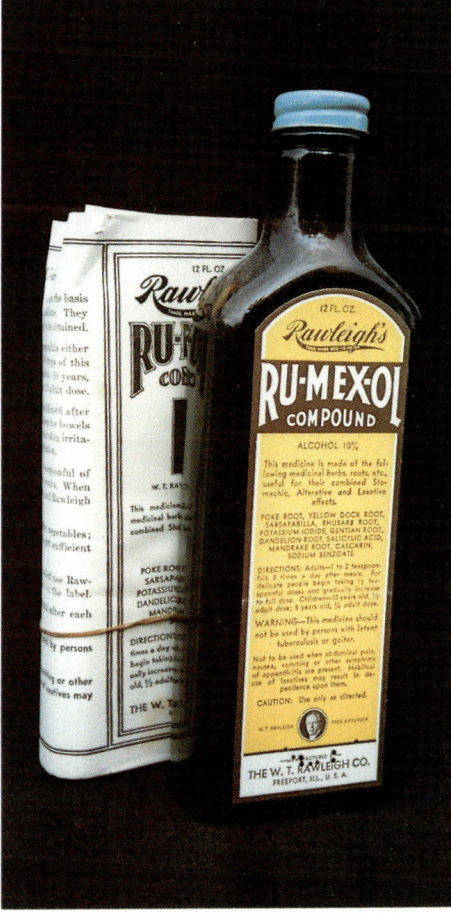

A full 12 ounce glass container of Rawleigh's "Ru-Mex-Ol Compound" with directions. Manufactured by The W.T. Rawleigh Company Freeport, Ill., U.S.A. *Dupler Collection.* $45-$50.

The original directions surround the bottle of Rawleigh's "Ru-Mex-Ol Compound." Directions for using, value, and brief descriptions of some of the many useful and dependable Rawleigh products needed in every home. *Dupler Collection.* $45-$50.

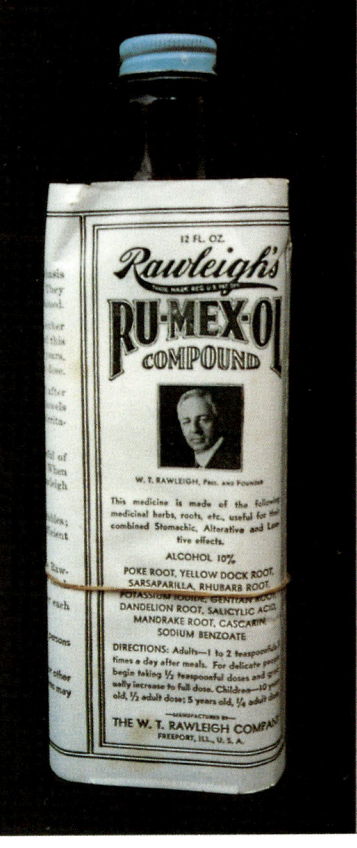

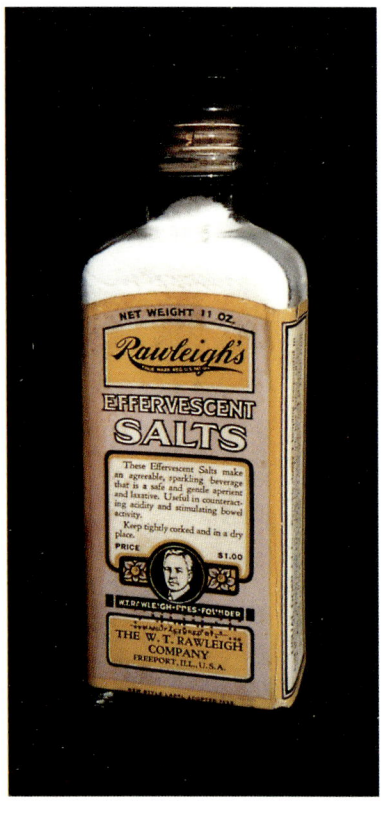

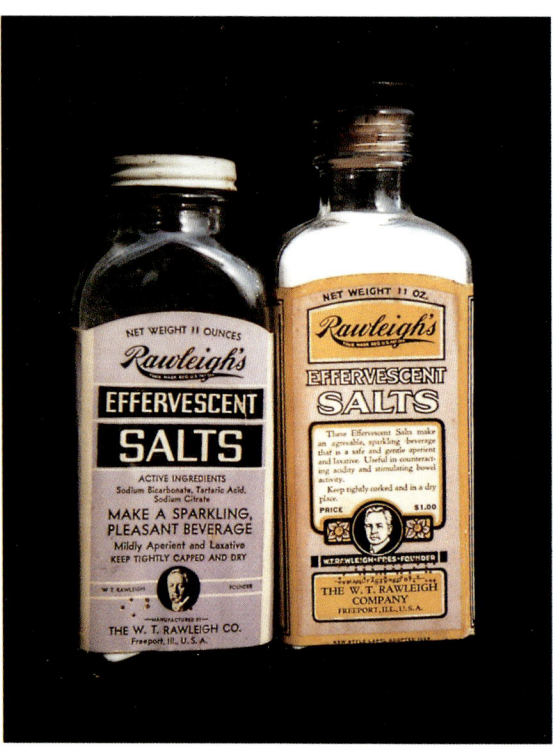

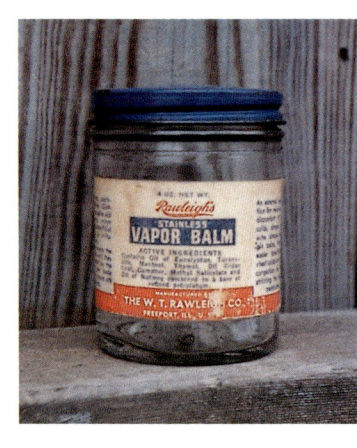

Rawleigh's "Vapor Balm" 4 ounce glass jar with paper label and screw on lid. Manufactured by The W.T. Rawleigh Co., Freeport, Ill. *Dupler Collection.* $10-$15.

A full 11 ounce glass bottle with paper label of Rawleigh's "Effervescent Salts." The initial "WTRCo" is embossed on the cap/lid. Manufactured by The W.T. Rawleigh Company Freeport, Ill., U.S.A. Also marked "New Style Label Adopted 1925." *Dupler Collection.* $35-$40.

Two variations of Rawleigh's "Effervescent Salts." *Shepard Collection.* $35-$40 ea.

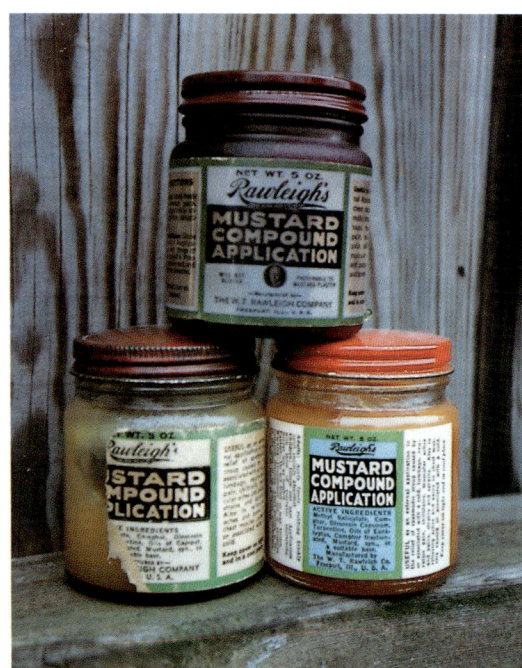

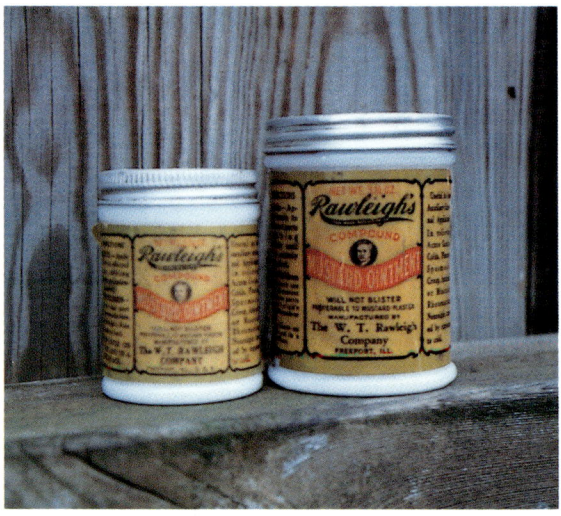

Two milk glass containers of "Rawleigh's Mustard Ointment." Manufactured by The W.T. Rawleigh Company Freeport, Ill. The smaller container held 1-1/4 ounces and the larger 3-1/2 ounces. *Dupler Collection.* $10-$15 ea.

Three different 5 ounce containers of Rawleigh's "Mustard Compound Application." Manufactured by The W.T. Rawleigh Co. Freeport, Ill., U.S.A. Missing paper sections hinders the selling price. *Dupler Collection.* $10-$15 ea.

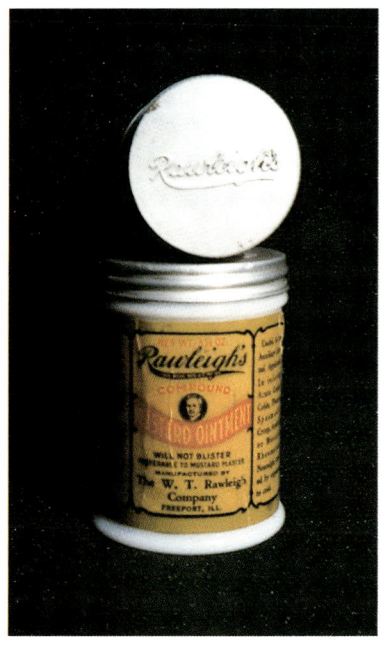

"Rawleigh's Mustard Ointment", each lid is embossed "Rawleigh's." *Dupler Collection.* $10-$15.

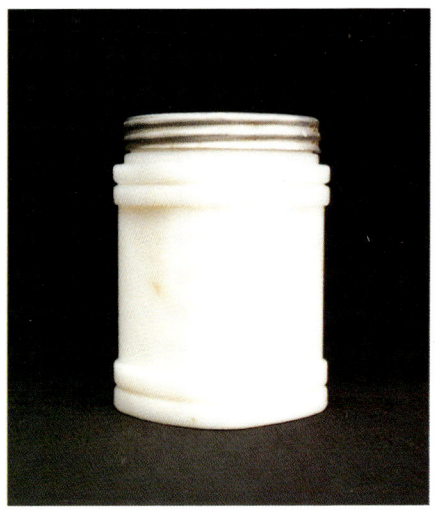

A milk glass Rawleigh container. The content is unknown. The lid is embossed "Rawleigh's." *Shepard Collection.* $5-$10.

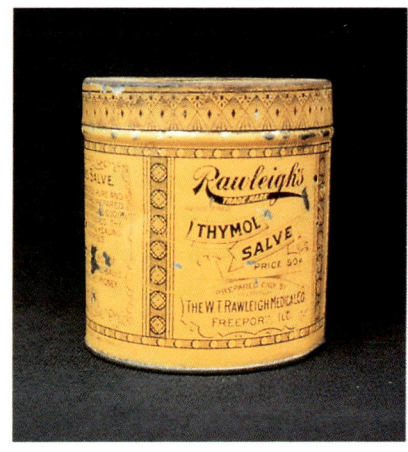

Rawleigh's "Thymol Salve", found in a metal container, was "Prepared Only By The W.T. Rawleigh Medical Co. Freeport, Ill." Original price 50 cents. Containers marked "The W.T. Rawleigh Medical Co." have escalated in both price and demand. *Dupler Collection.* $50-$60.

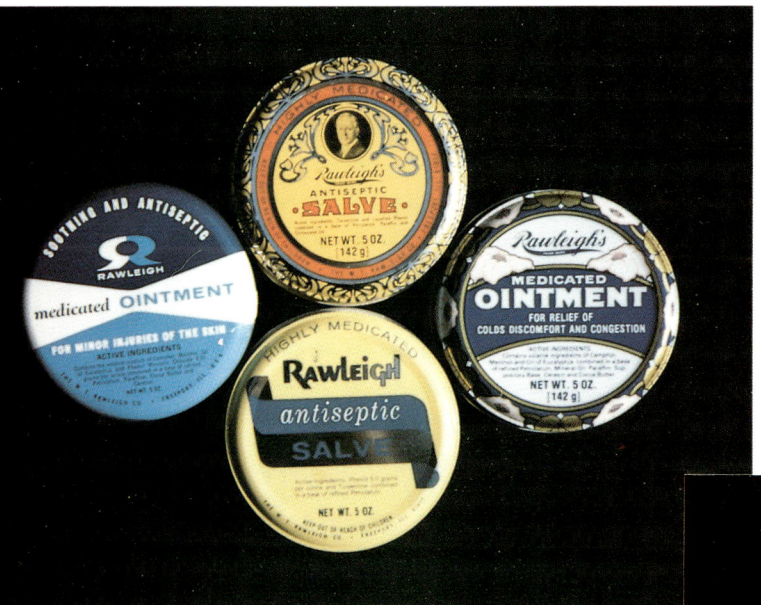

A selection of Rawleigh Antiseptic Salve and Medicated Ointment tins. These round containers are readily available to collectors and are moderately inexpensive. *Dupler Collection.* $10-$15 ea.

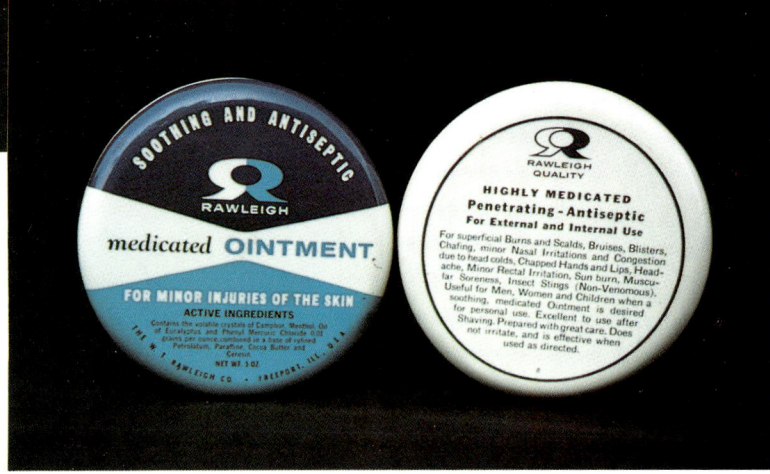

The front and reverse side of Rawleigh "Medicated Ointment." The W.T. Rawleigh Co. Freeport, Ill. U.S.A. Each container held 5 ounces and is slightly different but the contents remain the same. *Dupler Collection.* $10-$15 ea.

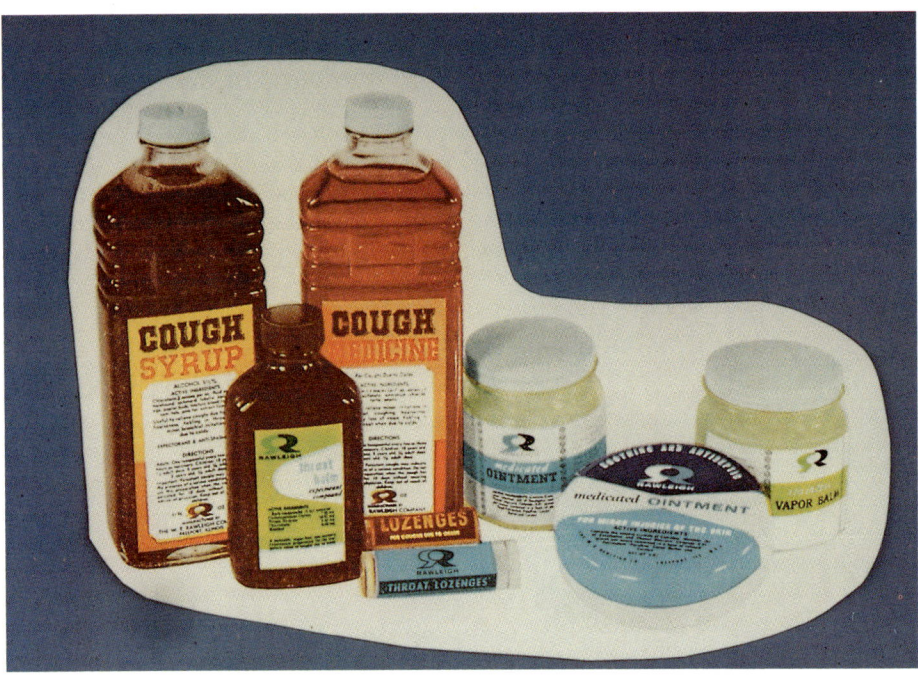

An original 1960s advertisement for Rawleigh 11 ounce Cough Syrup that had been a favorite since 1892. Rawleigh 4 ounce Throat Balm and Cherry flavor Cough medicine, 11 ounce. Rawleigh Lozenges relieved hoarseness, throat irritations, and coughs due to common colds. Rawleigh offered their famous medicated ointment in either 5 ounce cans, 5 ounce jars or in a 2 ounce can. Vapor Balm worked two ways: when rubbed on the chest, it acted as a counter irritant; however, it also released volatile oils that helped make breathing easier.

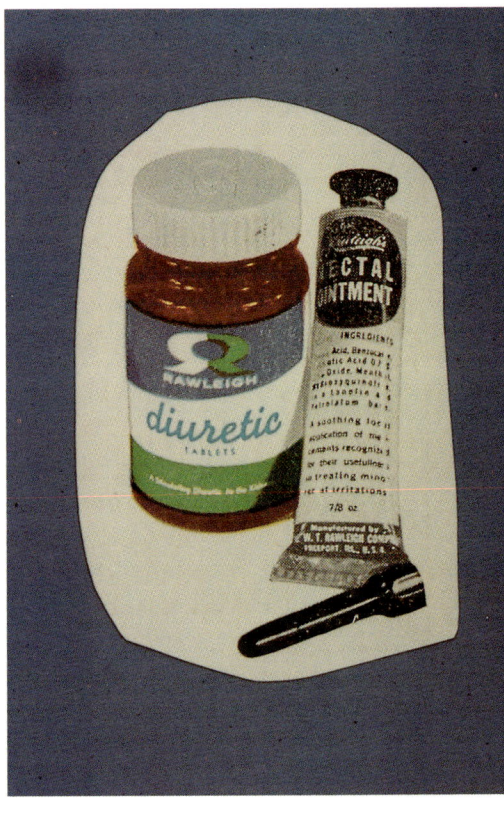

Rawleigh Diuretic tablets and Rawleigh's Rectal Ointment. Circa 1960s. $10-$15 ea.

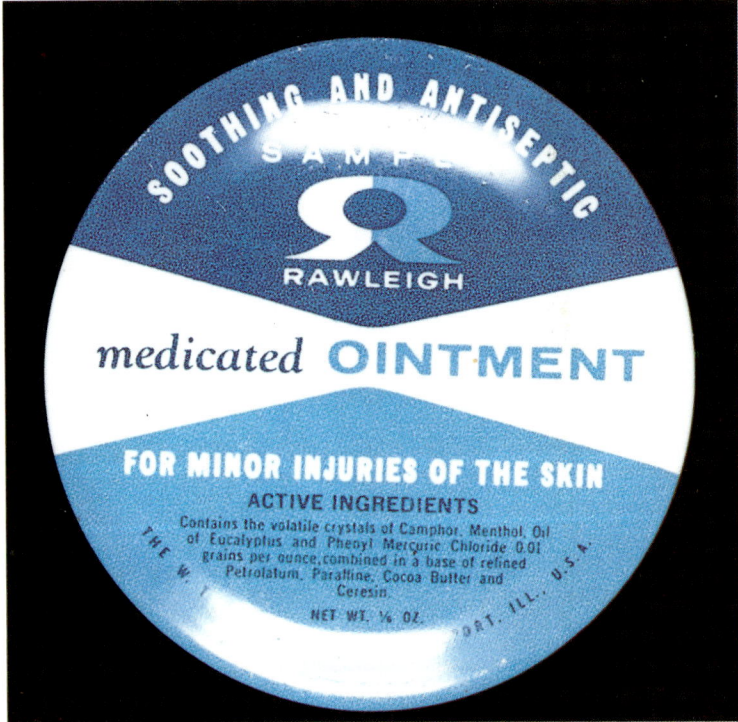

The front and the reverse sections of "Rawleigh's Medicated Ointment." The W.T. Rawleigh Company Freeport, IL. This is a highly collectible SAMPLE and has become expensive. *Dupler Collection.* $25-$30.

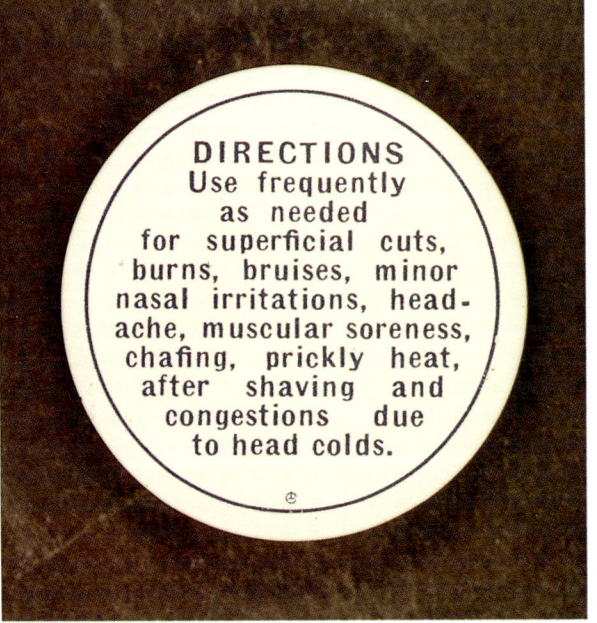

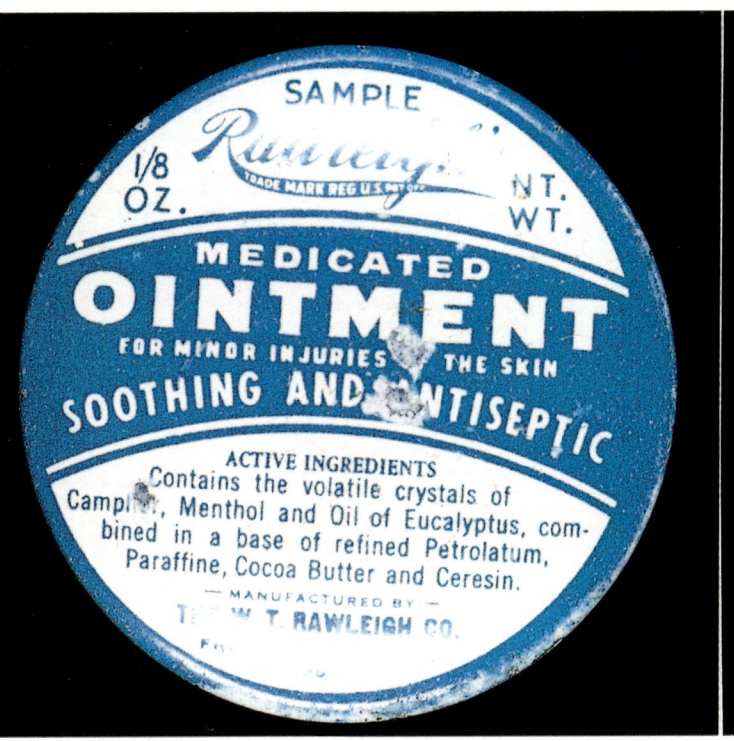 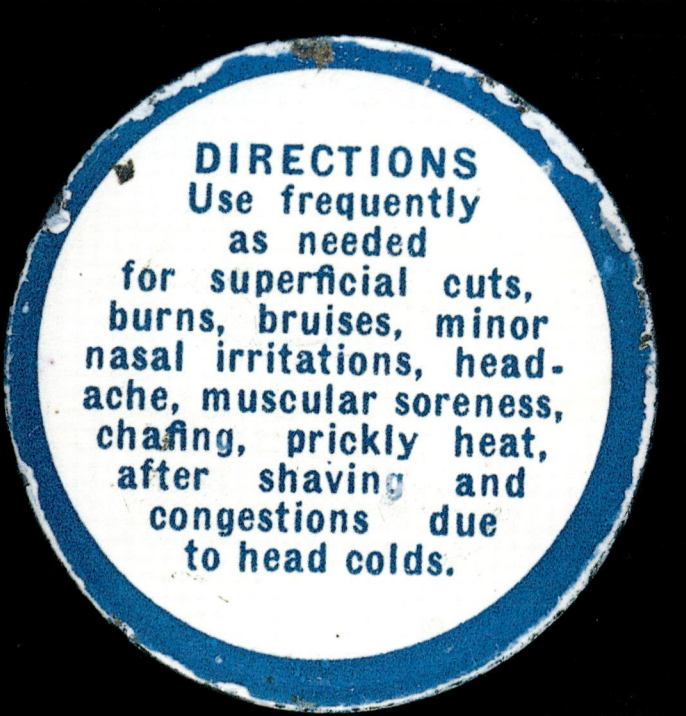

Shown here, the front and the reverse sections of another SAMPLE variation of "Rawleigh's Medicated Ointment." This SAMPLE held 1/8 ounce and was manufactured by The W.T. Rawleigh Company Freeport, IL. *Dupler Collection.* $25-$30.

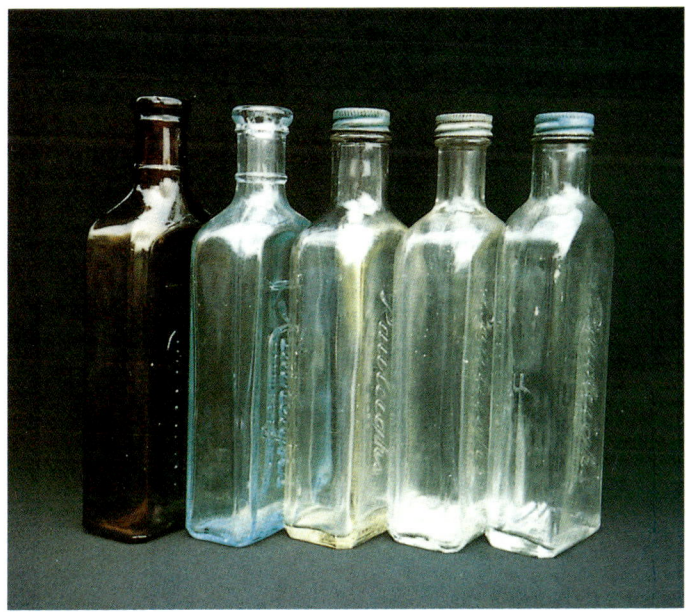

A selection of empty Rawleigh bottle. Each bottle is embossed with the "Rawleigh's Trademark." Two bottles require cork stoppers and three have metal screw on lids. Missing labels hinders the selling price. Contents unknown. *Dupler Collection.* $15-$20 ea.

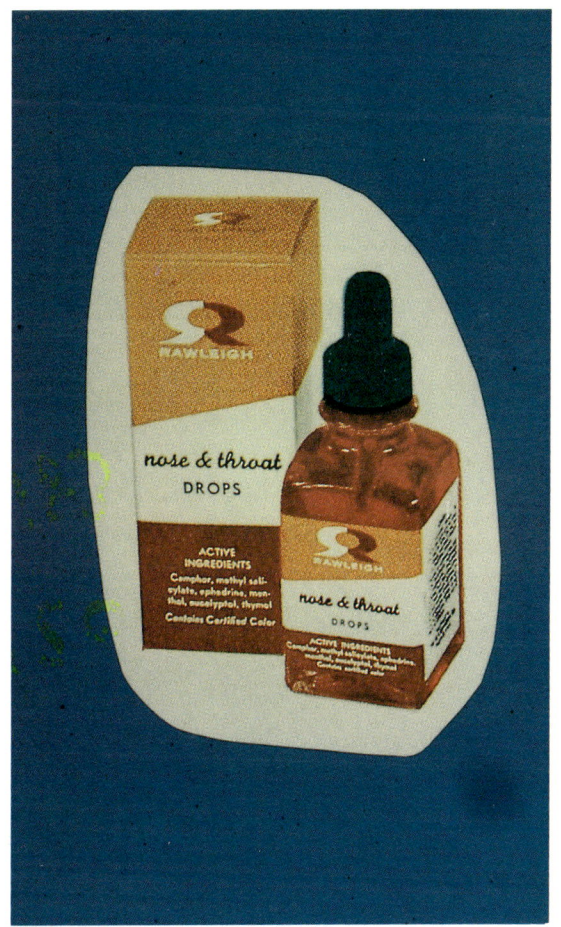

An original 1960s promotion for Rawleigh 2 ounce Nose and Throat Drops. These drops soothed irritated passages where colds often started. $10-$15 ea.

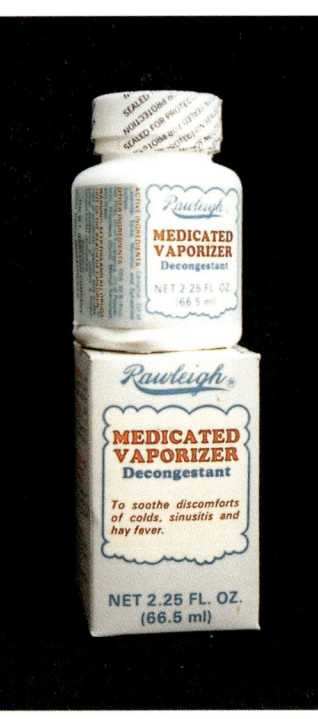

Rawleigh® Medicated Vaporizer Decongestant. To soothe discomforts of colds, sinusitis, and hay fever. Distributed by The W.T. Rawleigh Company Freeport, Illinois 61032 U.S.A. An expiration date of 12/86 appears on a side panel of the original carton and the plastic bottle. The bottle is full and the original seal is intact. *Bushue Collection.* $10-$15.

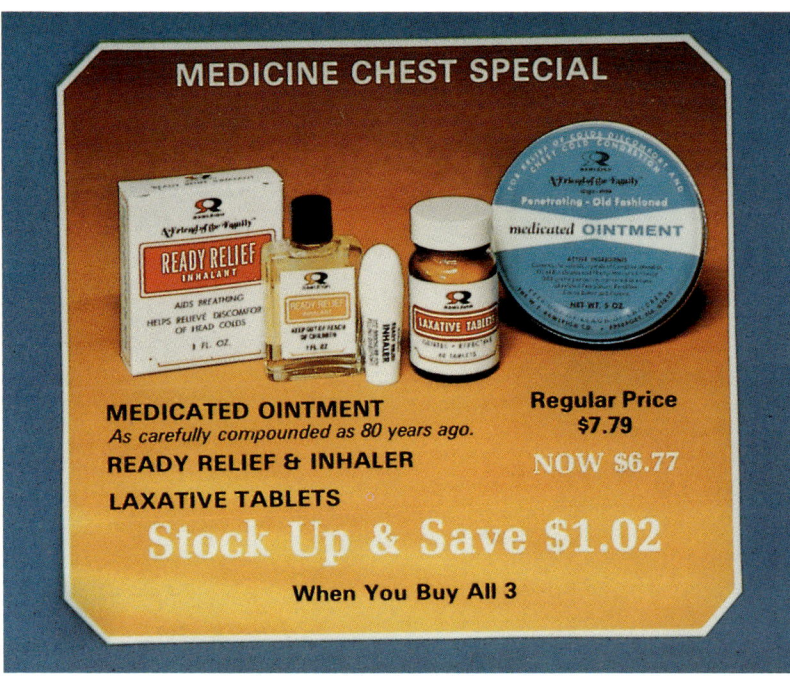

In 1976, Rawleigh promoted this "Medicine Chest Special."

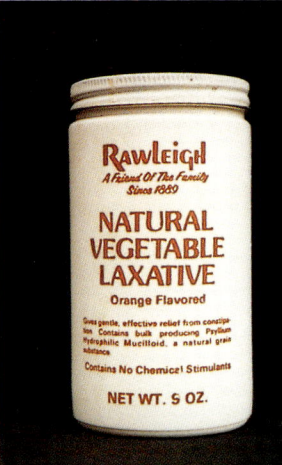

Rawleigh Natural Vegetable Laxative. Manufactured by The W.T. Rawleigh Company Freeport, Illinois 61032. An expiration date of 12/63 appears on a side panel. *Bushue Collection.* $10-$15.

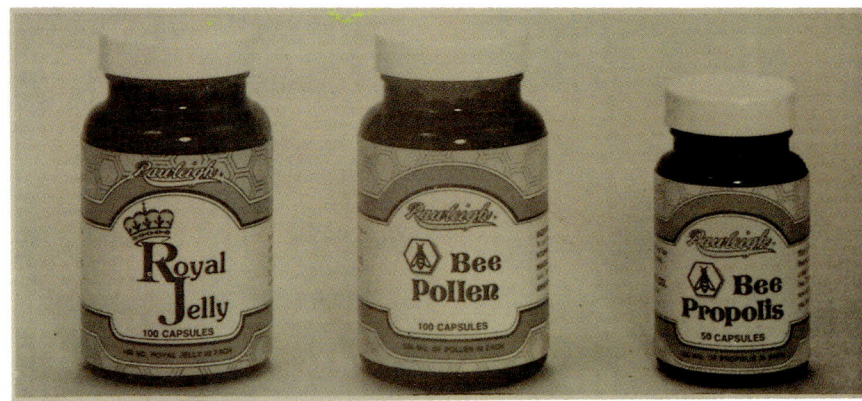

"Nature's Most Perfect Foods." The W.T. Rawleigh Company was proud to introduce these new products during the 1980s. Appearing across the country during their introduction was "Rawleigh Royal Jelly, Bee Pollen, and Bee Propolis." Royal Jelly was helpful in slowing the aging process and increasing longevity. Bee Pollen increased energy, stamina and good health. Bee Propolis was a natural enemy of harmful germs, bacteria, and viruses. *Dupler Collection.* $10-$15 ea.

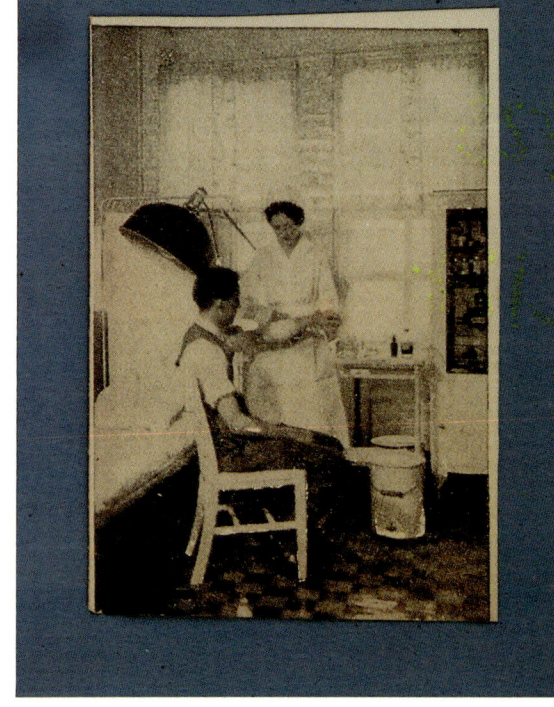

A section of the first aid facility at Rawleigh's Freeport factories. Circa 1939.

Chapter 3. Rawleigh's Paper Memorabilia

Paper Care

Many collectors of historical paper products — issues of Rawleigh's Good Health Guide Almanac & Cookbooks, calendars, catalogues, pamphlets, and brochures — do not realize that their paper collectibles could be in danger. Collectors of such items should become aware of the "enemies of paper." Seek professional advice in preserving your Rawleigh paper memorabilia.

Paper documents should be stored completely flat in acid free boxes. It is not wise to place valuable paper items in plastic storage bags purchased from your local grocery store. If moisture develops inside the bag, your valuable paper item may become worthless.

Never subject paper collectibles to direct sunlight which will cause fading. Acid burn can occur from wood, wood pulp mats, backings, and cardboard. Ultraviolet light causes colors and inks to fade. Infrared light accelerates aging, causing brittleness and discoloration.

Permanent mounts (including dry mounting, wet mounting, and most glues and tapes) cause permanent and irreversible damage. Improper framing actually causes and encourages all of the above. No matter how good your framed piece looks, what matters most is out of sight, inside the frame.

The greatest danger to your paper items comes from insects that like to feed on them. The older the paper, the greater the risk.

Paper collectibles retain their greatest value in pristine condition. Anything that happens to change the condition of the item reduces its value. It is wise to consult a professional in paper to retain the value of such items. Be prepared; this can be quite costly.

When choosing a paper professional, be sure to consult only those who use the finest materials and methods — methods and materials which are used or endorsed by all conservation authorities, such as the Library of Congress, the National Archives, the American Institute of Conservation, and the Professional Picture Framers' Association. Protect your investment, and avoid the enemies of paper.

Rawleigh's Printing Department

In 1915, it was estimated that the 2,000 men who distributed Rawleigh products visited approximately 20,000 customers daily. The company did no expensive newspaper or magazine advertising which would add nothing to the value of its products. Instead, it relied entirely upon the intrinsic merits of its preparations and the value, the fairness, and liberality of its business methods to introduce its goods, and upon satisfied patrons to extend their business.

Practically the only money spent for advertising was for useful booklets which were distributed by salesmen while supplying their customers' needs. The enormous volume of business done by Rawleigh in these booklets also enabled the company to buy the paper it used first hand by carload lots.

All Rawleigh documents were printed entirely by the Rawleigh company; no outside organization was used. This saved time and expense as Rawleigh had its own printing and book-binding machinery. In fact, Rawleigh maintained one of the largest private printing plants in the country. The company explained that this provided, "a large savings because each machine was kept busy producing its own work."

Millions of copies of Rawleigh's Almanac, Cook Book and Medical Guide, Salesmen's Advance Notice Catalogs, and Stock and Poultry Preparations booklets were required annually. During the early years, the most important of these were printed in four languages (English, French, Norwegian, and German). Later on, directions were printed in nine different languages for using various Rawleigh's products.

These booklets were produced in such enormous quantities that it required six large presses, four equipped with automatic feeders, to handle the load. One press was an enormous Perfecting Press, printing on both sides of the sheet with one operation.

Approximately 16,000 pounds of paper (the equivalent of 121,000 sheets) were required for a nine hour day run. Four large folding machines with automatic feeders had a daily capacity to create 110,000 thirty-two page booklet. Another machine stitched, wired, and looped 50,000 booklets a day. With one of the latest typesetting machines used by the largest newspapers, and modern cutting, book-trimming, and other equipment, Rawleigh had an annual capacity estimated at 45 million almanacs, booklets, labels, wrappers, and other paper products.

Rawleigh's Printing Department required over 20,000 feet of floor space and employed between 30 and 50 people. During the busiest seasons, it was necessary to keep the machinery operating night and day to supply the demand.

In 1921, seventy million pieces of printed material were produced. To educate consumers about the reliability and every day practical usefulness and benefits obtainable from Rawleigh's Good Health Service, over seven million guides and bulletins were printed at a cost of over $100,000 for paper and labor.

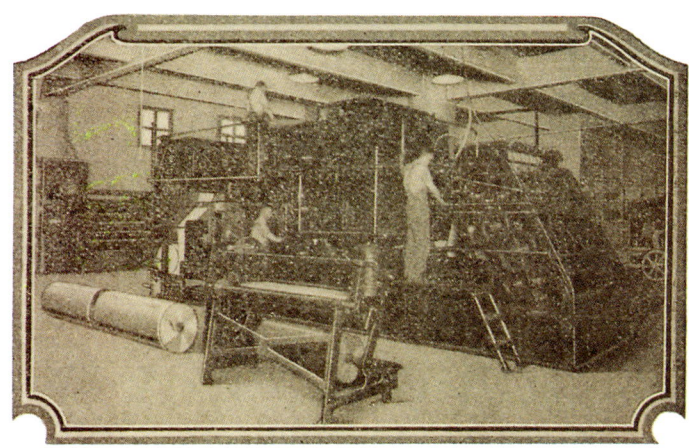

In 1921, Rawleigh drew attention to their 36-ton press, built especially for printing Rawleigh's "Good Health Guide" and other advertising matter. It was an immense and expensive machine of great capacity, using 7 tons of paper daily. This press printed in two colors, cut, folded, and delivered ready for binding (all in one operation) 30,000 64- or 96-page guides, or similar books, per day.

Over 300 different kinds of paper were kept in stock. Millions of labels were printed in different languages providing directions for medicines. Rawleigh's weekly magazine, salesmanship literature, booklets, bulletins, pamphlets, and circulars were printed every month in one, two, three, and four colors, requiring tons of ink in all colors.

Rawleigh had a large investment in the Rawleigh Printers, but by making all their boxes and cartons, printing all their labels, advertising material, literature, stationary, and other supplies, the company's costs were reduced to the minimum and large savings proved effective.

A 1922 general view of Rawleigh's Printing Department in Freeport, Illinois.

The Year 1906

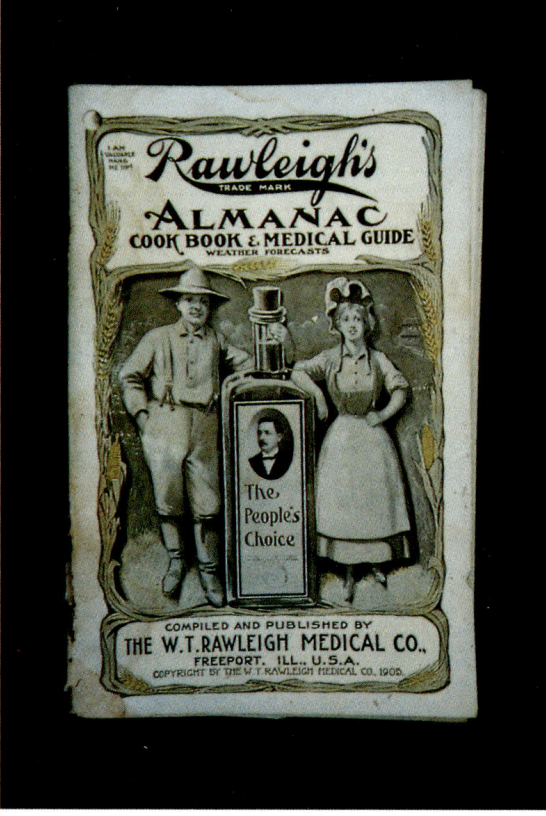

Rawleigh's 128 page 1906 Almanac Cook Book & Medical Guide. Compiled and Published By THE W.T. RAWLEIGH MEDICAL CO., FREEPORT, ILL., U.S.A. ©1905. $20-$25.

Good Health Guide and Almanac

Beginning each year, Rawleigh "renewed its determination to serve everyone concerned with confidence that the new year would bring them better health, greater happiness, and prosperity and that Rawleigh would continue to serve them faithfully and to the best of their ability." In each issue of the yearly almanac, Rawleigh provided high points of each year, promoted new and improved old products, tested recipes, provided medical information, and shared with the consumer the continued growth of the Rawleigh organization.

An "Introduction" often appeared in the front, written by W.T. Rawleigh and/or another administrator after his death. Rawleigh's Almanac Cook Book and Medical Guide was published once a year and given free to customers. Today, these publications are moderately priced when found at local flea markets, antique shops, and paper shows.

Whenever possible, I have provided verbatim the personal messages as they appeared in the yearly Almanac Cook Book and Medical Guide. All Rawleigh's Almanac Cook Books and Medical Guides were not available for this research. If you should have those that are missing, I would appreciate hearing from you.

"In issuing this, the tenth edition of our Almanac, Cook Book and Medical Guide, we feel that a word ought to be said about *The Man* and *The Plan* that have made possible this continued and increasing success."

"A little over ten years ago — notice the ten — Mr. Rawleigh organized his Company. It then had but $25,000 Capital — 1,200 feet of floor space — the right ideas and a good constitution. It started to grow and has never stopped since."

"Results: Capital of $1,000,000.00 — Floor Space Measured by Acres — Millions of Cures — Millions of Friends and Customers, and Mr. Rawleigh, the greatest medical manufacturer in the world, all in ten year — not 40, but 10. Remarkable progress, unequaled growth, wonderful achievement."

"Reasons: Ability and Character of Mr. Rawleigh, high quality, purity and great efficiency of his preparations, the generous honesty of his "Pay After You Are Satisfied Plan.""

"Proof: The largest and best equipped medical laboratory, the longest list of satisfied customers, the greatest number of cures, the largest and most valuable Almanac of any similar institution on the Globe."

"Wouldn't it be nice if there were a store where you could buy your shoes on six months' trial — "satisfaction or no pay?" But you can't. The fellows who sell you footwear, headwear and backwear don't make their stuff and they don't know how it is made. They'd trust you if they could trust their good — but they can't."

"We believe in our preparations; we make them, we know them — we're not afraid they'll go back on us — THEY WONT! We are spreading the gospel of good health on Rawleigh's now famous **"Pay After You Are Satisfied Plan."**

"It's fair; it's honest; it's generous. It inspires confidence because there is no chance for deception — the preparations must stand the test or they cost you nothing. 10,000,000 packages sold, used and paid for each year prove the superior quality of our preparations."

"To the millions who have tested our plan — our friends and customers — to the millions who will test it in the coming year — our future friends and customers, we dedicate this valuable Almanac, Cook Book and Medical Guide." *Rawleigh's Almanac Cook Book & Medical Guide © The W.T. Rawleigh Medical Co., Freeport, IL., U.S.A. ©1905.*

The Year 1907

Not Available.

The Year 1908

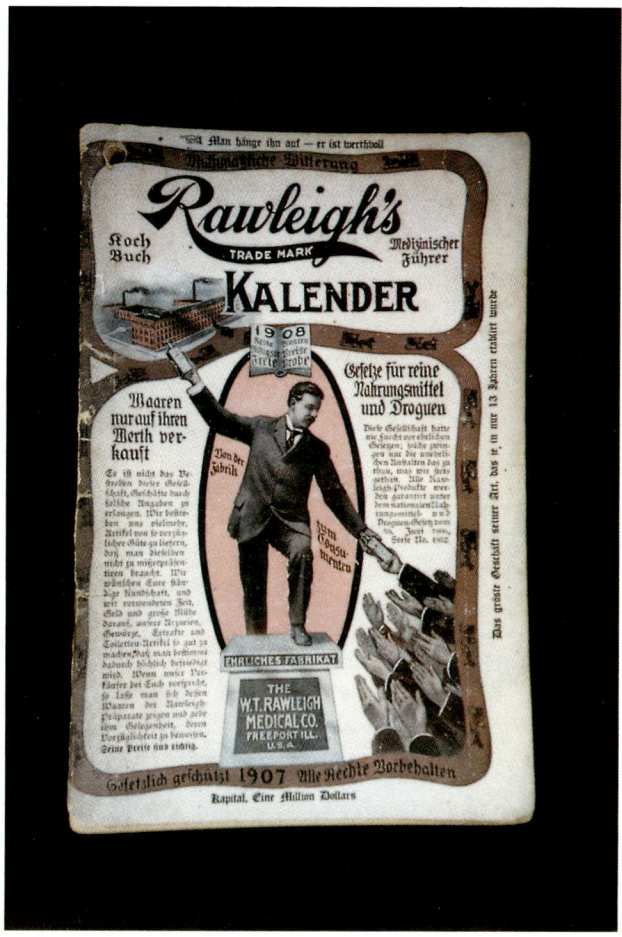

Rawleigh's 1908 Kalender. The W.T. Rawleigh Medical Co. Freeport Ill. U.S.A. 95 pages printed in German, ©1907. $20-$25.

The Years 1909 - 1912

Issues not available.

The Year 1913

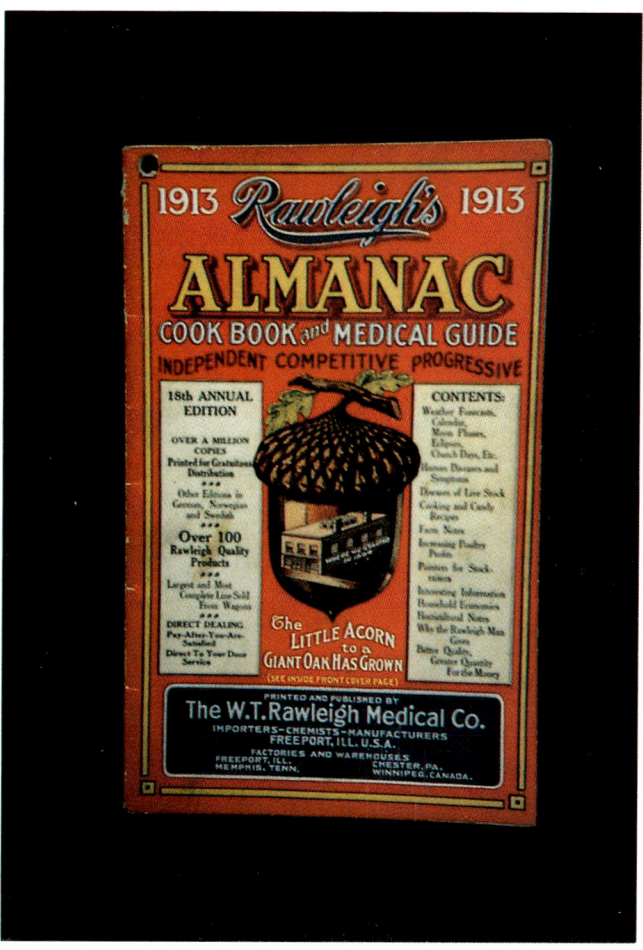

Rawleigh's 1913 Almanac Cook Book and Medical Guide. Published by The W.T. Rawleigh Medical Co. Importers - Chemists - Manufacturers Freeport, Ill. U.S.A. $20-$25.

"The W.T. Rawleigh Medical Company was organized and began business with a small line of products 18 years ago. Its business has grown and spread each succeeding year until now it has become one of the greatest buying, manufacturing and selling organizations of its kind in the world."

"During All These Years the policy of the Rawleigh Company has been one of absolute independence, aggressively competitive, and always progressive. It has at no time during its history been a part of any combine, trust or organization in restraint of trade or to increase, regulate, or control prices or sales. On the contrary, its policy has always been to give consumers better values in quality, quantity and price than they can obtain from others." *The W.T. Rawleigh Medical Company Importers - Chemists - Manufacturers 1913.*

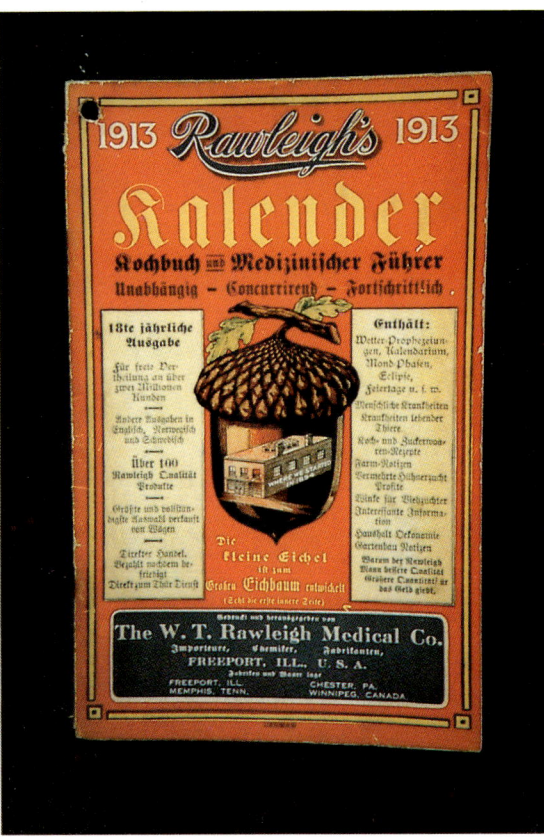

Rawleigh's 1913 Kalender. The W.T. Rawleigh Medical Co. Freeport Ill. U.S.A. 64 pages printed in German. $20-$25.

"When we organized way back in 1895 we recognized that correct, economic and business principles were absolutely essential for success, so the first year we went STRAIGHT to the farmer. We PASSED BY the jobber and the dealer. We took the SHORTEST route to the GREATEST market. We were among the first pioneer manufacturers to offer a free trial and guarantee absolute satisfaction or no sales."

"When we began manufacturing in the little building our aim was to make Rawleigh's Medicines and other Products good and reliable so that users who depended upon them might obtain the best possible results. No pains or reasonable expense has since been spared to give the best values, unsurpassed service, and the fairest and most liberal terms made possibly by our enormous capital and resources. We have spent the best part of our lives in a persistent and earnest effort to make a reputation for reliable and superior quality Products."

"While the hundreds of thousands of dollars we have invested in great factories and modern machinery are all valuable and necessary for the success, extension and perpetuation of the business, we know that the most valuable business asset we now have is our millions of satisfied customers whose good will, loyalty, confidence and patronage we treasure more highly than the miser can treasure his gold."

"For years we have been manufacturing and selling the largest and most complete line sold from wagons."

"Our policy has always been absolutely independent and so aggressively competitive and progressive that we are now recognized among the foremost, most successful, responsible and reliable companies in existence."

The Year 1915

The Year 1914

Rawleigh's 96 page 1914 Almanac Cook Book and Medical Guide. Published by THE W.T. RAWLEIGH MEDICAL CO. FREEPORT, ILL. U.S.A. $20-$25.

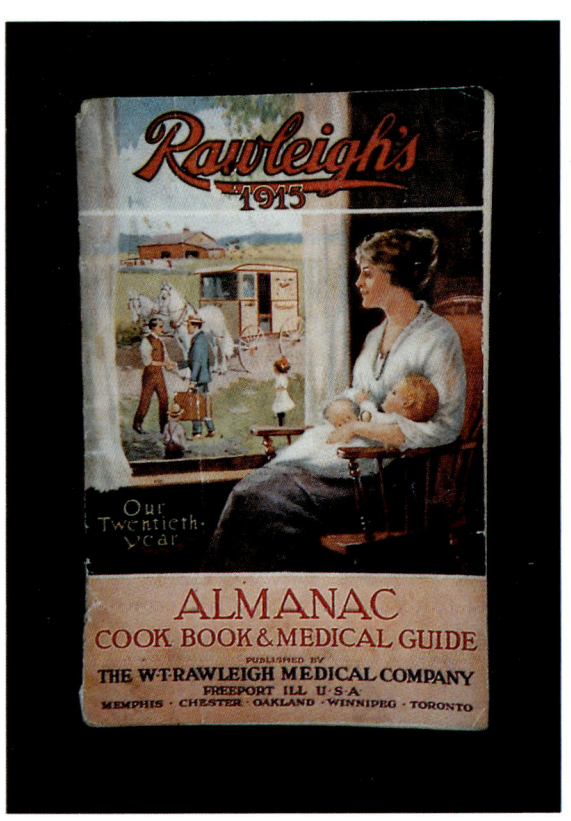

Rawleigh's Twentieth year 100 page 1915 Almanac Cook Book & Medical Guide. Compiled and Published By THE W.T. RAWLEIGH MEDICAL CO., FREEPORT, ILL., U.S.A. $20-$25.

The Year 1916

Issue not available.

The Year 1917

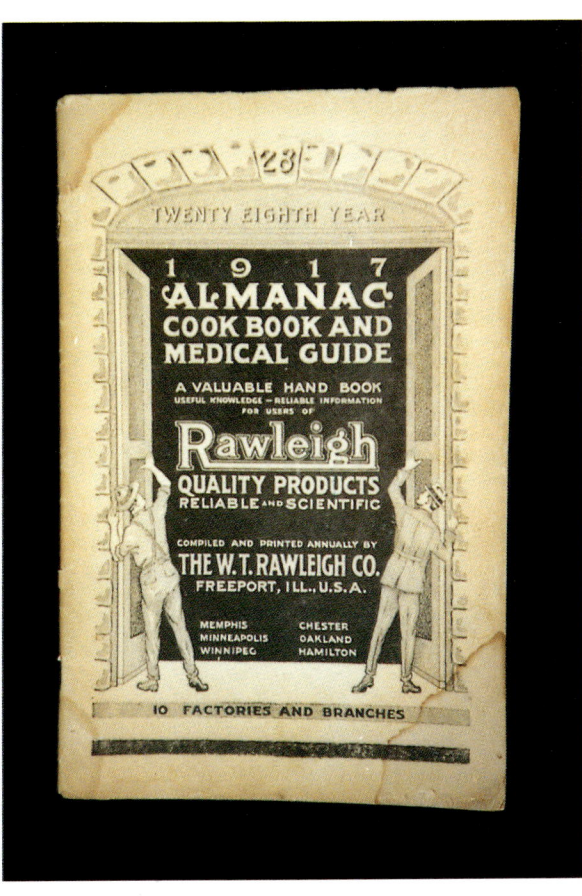

Rawleigh Twenty-Eight Year 104 page 1917 Almanac Cook Book and Medical Guide. Original cover is missing and no introduction was provided, the following did appear in this issue. $20-$25 complete.

"The leadership of the Rawleigh line in 1917 was more pronounced than ever before; it consisted of 140 separate and distinct products, in 238 sizes. This figure included the 140 new products of 1917."

"31 Medicines, 15 Extracts and Flavors, 10 Spices, 9 Toilet Soaps, 25 Toilet Articles, 16 Stock and Poultry Preparations, 8 Miscellaneous Products, 15 Power Supplies and 11 new Products which included Temperance Drinks, Toilet Waters, Concentrated Flavors, Vanilla, Lemon and Orange."

The Years 1918 - 1919

Issues not available.

The Year 1920

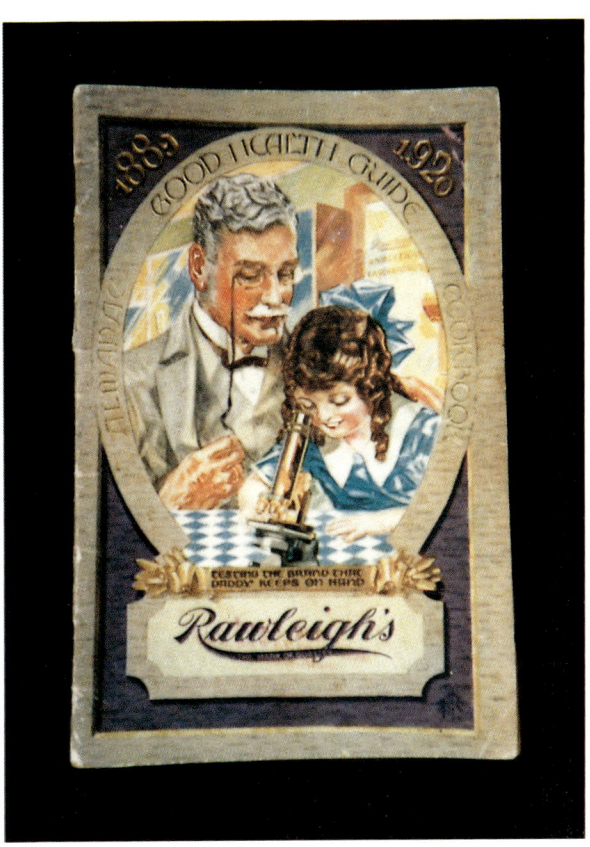

Rawleigh's Good Health Guide Almanac & Cook Book 1920. Published by The W.T. RAWLEIGH CO. FREEPORT, ILL. U.S.A. $20-$25.

"THE HOUSE OF RAWLEIGH is now over a quarter of a century old. Beginning practically without capital only thirty years ago in competition with well established businesses, The W.T. Rawleigh Company has developed and enlarged amidst keen competition until now over 130 Good Health Products are delivered through Rawleigh Retailers to the homes of millions of people throughout North America."

"When W.T. Rawleigh made his first sales and laid the foundation for the international organization that now bears his name, he made **Service** the fundamental principle in his business structure. With a comprehensive knowledge of the needs of the people he had aimed to give his customers the largest and best line of Good Health Products obtainable anywhere. Faithful devotion to this ideal, steadfast adherence to correct business methods, together with superior laboratories, centrally located factories, modern manufacturing facilities, large resources and conservative management have made The W.T. Rawleigh Company one of the foremost of its kind."

"Rawleigh's were the first manufacturers of their kind to establish analytical laboratories. Their methods of analysis and manufacture are similar to the most approved practices of noted American and European laboratories, and their line of products includes not only reliable medicines, but foods, food flavors, spices, extracts, soaps, toilet accessories, washing compounds, cleansers, polishes, insecticides, veterinary remedies and stock and poultry preparations."

"In addition to this, the House of Rawleigh supplies the latest scientific information upon healthful living and disease prevention, so that those using the products of the Rawleigh laboratories may be benefited in the greatest degree possible from such service." *Rawleigh's Good Health Guide Almanac & Cook Book 1920.*

The Year 1921

Issue not available.

The Year 1922

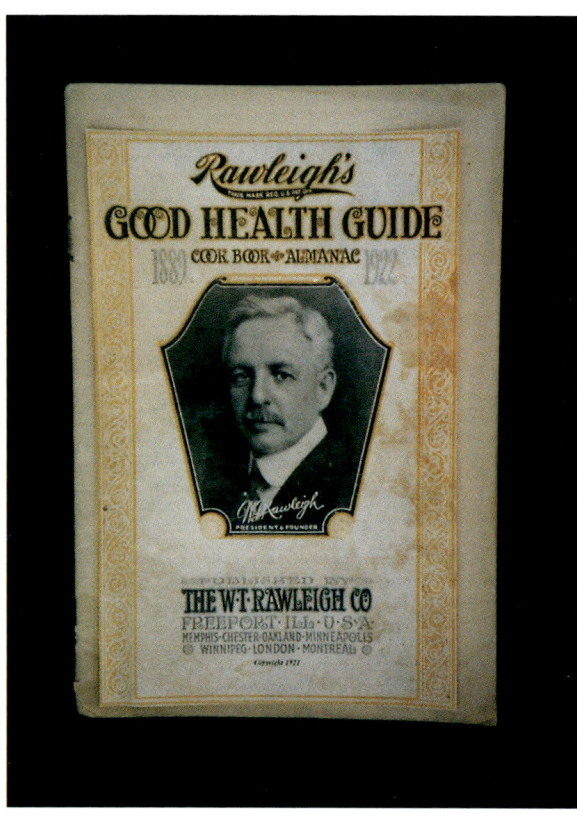

The inside cover of Rawleigh's Good Health Guide Almanac & Cook Book 1922. The original cover is missing which affects the selling price of paper documents. Published by The W.T. RAWLEIGH CO. FREEPORT, ILL. U.S.A. ©1921. $20-$25.

"During the past year the Company paid more than Three Quarters of a Million Dollars in land and ocean freight charges. Over 1300 full carloads raw materials and freight were received and shipped. There were 650 carloads equalizing 16 train loads, of over 40 cars each, of Rawleigh's Products shipped from Rawleigh's Factories and Branches during the year." *Rawleigh's Good Health Guide 1922* ©1921

The Year 1923

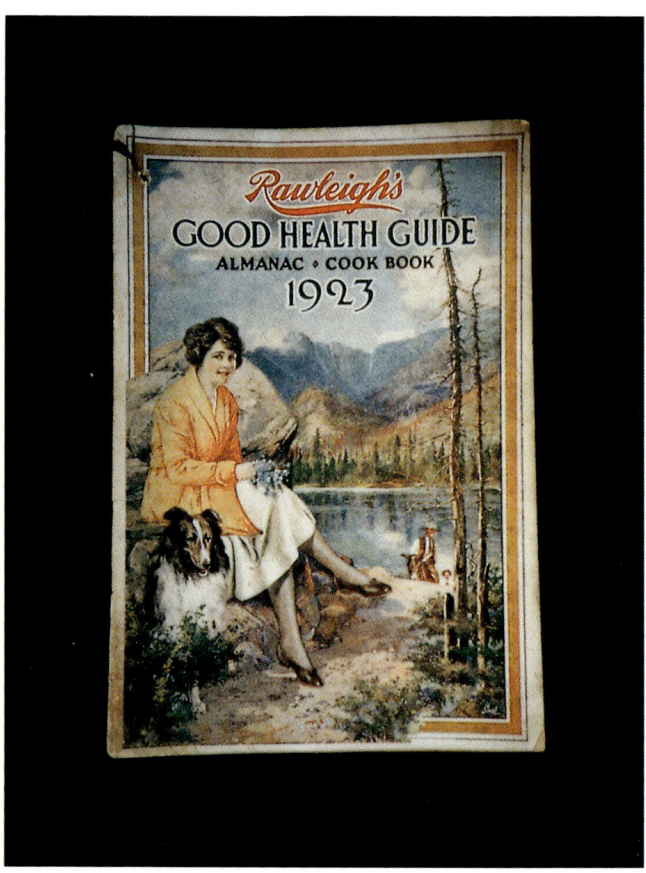

Rawleigh's Good Health Guide Almanac & Cook Book 1923. Published by The W.T. RAWLEIGH CO. FREEPORT, ILL. U.S.A. ©1922. $20-$25.

"Throughout all America The W.T. Rawleigh Company has become popularly known as the "House of Service." Through 34 years of unprecedented growth and success, SERVICE has constantly been its keynote. To give something more — something better, to make it easier to supply a need, to give more complete satisfaction, to render everyone a superior and more reliable service than is obtainable from any other similar industry in the world, is Rawleigh's constant ideal, aim and conscienticus endeavor."

"There is no greater SERVICE that can be rendered to a person or to society than the SERVICE that helps to restore, to maintain and to preserve health, to prevent disease and sickness and suffering, and to promote that strength, beauty, comfort and happiness which are the accompaniments of health. This is the field in which Rawleigh's chose to serve." *Rawleigh's Good Health Guide Almanac & Cook Book 1923.*

The Year 1924

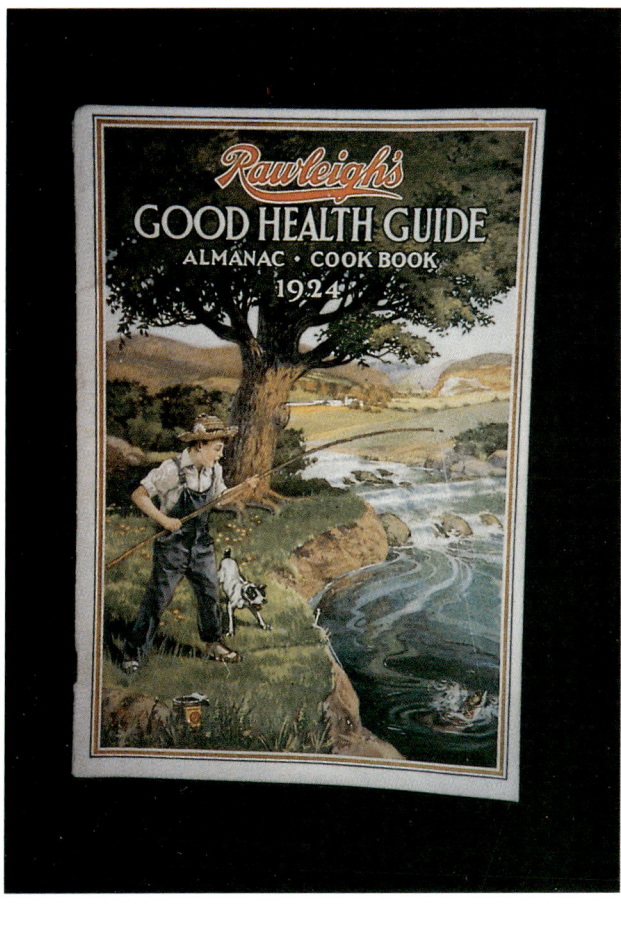

Rawleigh's 64 page Good Health Guide Almanac & Cook Book 1924. Published by The W.T. RAWLEIGH CO. FREEPORT, ILL. U.S.A. ©1923. $20-$25.

The Year 1926

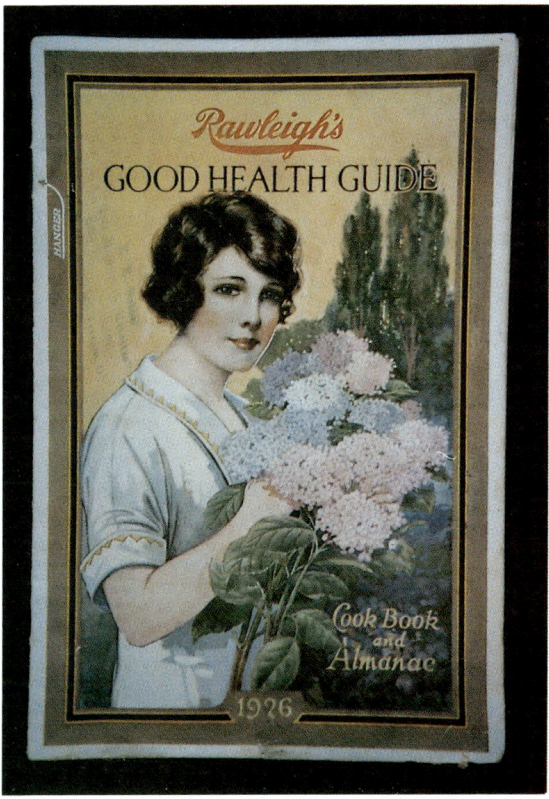

Rawleigh's 32 page Good Health Guide Cook Book 1927 and Almanac. Published by The W.T. RAWLEIGH CO. FREEPORT, ILL. U.S.A. ©1925. $20-$25.

The Year 1925

"The name "Rawleigh's" is a symbol and a guaranty of highest merit, of intrinsic value, of good faith, of highest integrity, and of a genuine service."

"The power to satisfy human wants is utility. Rawleigh's is an institution of great and unusual utility with an enviable record, worthy of your confidence, deserving of your patronage, capable of giving you the most complete service and satisfaction, conscious of the responsibilities of Leadership and with a future whose limits only time and a continued faithful devotion in service can discover." *Rawleigh's Good Health Guide Almanac & Cook Book 1925.*

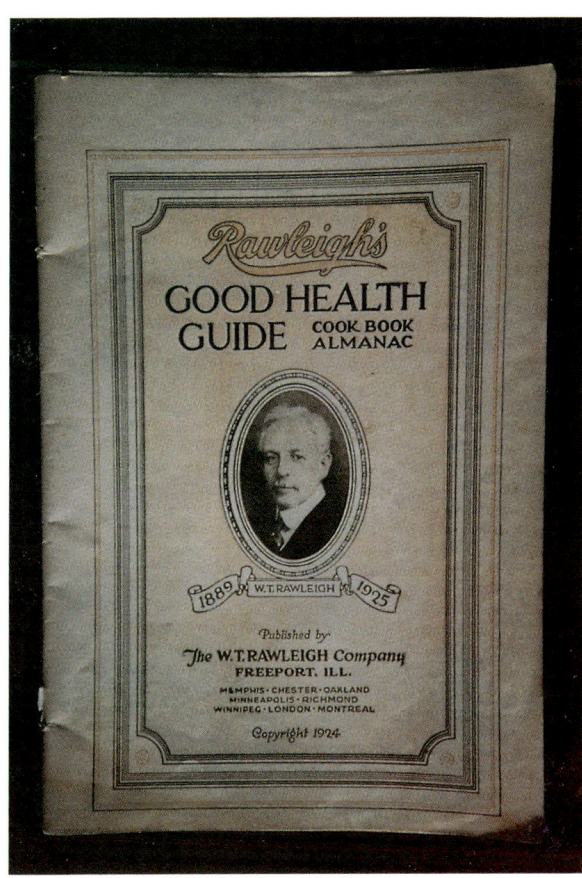

Rawleigh's Good Health Guide Almanac & Cook Book 1925. The original cover is missing. Published by The W.T. RAWLEIGH CO. FREEPORT, ILL. U.S.A. ©1924. $20-$25 mint.

The Year 1927

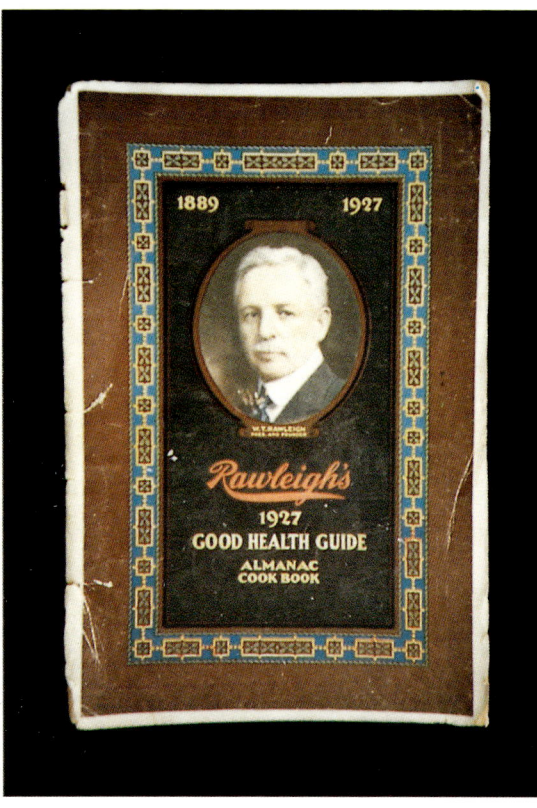

Rawleigh's Good Health Guide Almanac & Cook Book 1927. Published by The W.T. RAWLEIGH CO. FREEPORT, ILL. U.S.A. ©1926. $20-$25.

"Back in 1889 there was only one Rawleigh Retailer — the founder of Rawleigh Retailing — selling a few products to farmers in Northern Illinois. Then in 1895 came the first little factory. There were only three employees, a small number of Products and about a dozen Retailers selling to Consumers."

"Now there are thousands of Rawleigh Retailers regularly selling about 150 Products to more than six million families in practically every community in every state and province of the United States and Canada. Now there are many big factories, numerous branches, warehouses, offices, farms, foreign plantations, branches, and curing establishments and hundreds of employees, specialists in many trades and professions and speaking many different languages in the Unites States, Canada and many foreign countries."

"Most of the compounded earnings of a fast growing business, have been used to build factories and equipment, secure stocks and extend, increase and improve its service. More than fifteen million dollars ($15,000,000.00) in active resources without any indebtedness and the policy of paying cash for everything make Rawleigh's financially the strongest organization of its kind."

"From its small beginning, the Rawleigh business has steadily grown to a great international industry which grows, prepares and buys its raw materials in many lands, makes practically everything it sells directly from raw materials completely within its own factories and sells its Products by direct to the home methods, which give Consumers the best values and service obtainable." *Rawleigh Good Health Guide 1927 ©1926.*

The Year 1928

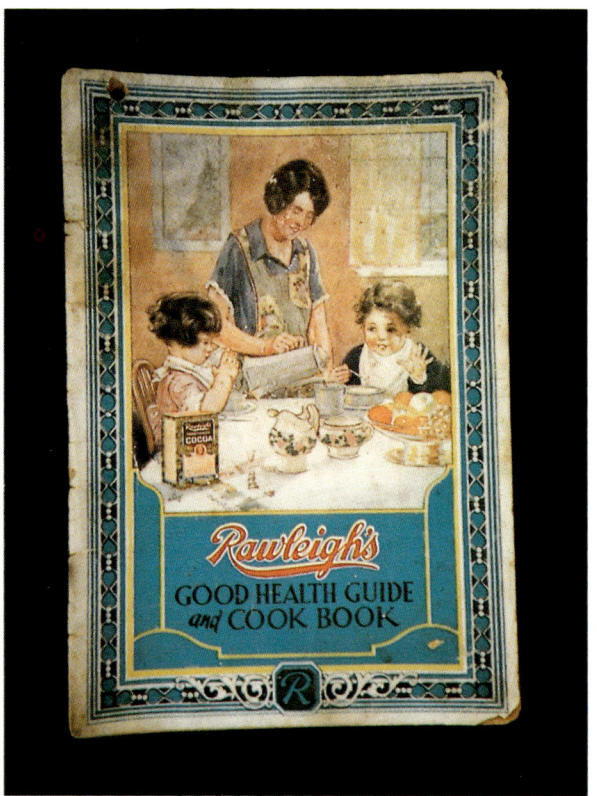

Rawleigh's 1928, 32 page Good Health Guide and Cook Book. The W.T. RAWLEIGH COMPANY FREEPORT, ILLINOIS ©1927. $20-$25.

"To be sure everything is right, it is a Rawleigh policy to make its Products in its own Factories, to get the best materials from producers and in its chemical laboratories to test materials, and standardize finished Products. It does everything necessary to protect Consumers of its Products fully and makes improvements whenever practical to do so."

"Some of its cork sealed medicines are not put up in bottles with a metal screw cap. This makes a better package and it is more convenient to open the bottle and close it secure from spilling. In many cases where Products could not be improved, packages were improved or provided with cartons and new labels."

"New Products include Sweet Milk Chocolate, Pie Fillings, Black Walnut Flavor, Raspberry Fruit Drink, Poultry Worm Capsules, Cholera tablets, Double Strength Extract of Vanilla and the La Jaynees distinctive toilet articles, Body Powder, Talcum, Perfume, Toilet Water, Face Powder, etc."

"Over 105 million pieces of printing including 20 carloads of Good Health Guides, 12 carloads of Calendars, 6-1/2 million Advance Notices, 1-1/2 million Good Health Bulletins and 12 carloads of Ideal Farming books were completed."

"Two million samples of Rawleigh Products, including Effervescent Salts, Medicated Ointment, Baking Powder and Cocoa were distributed in 1927."

"With increased experience and training in Rawleigh Methods the organization has greater capacity and more determination than ever before to give Consumers the most needed and practically useful Products and the most complete service and satisfaction from producers to Consumers." *Rawleigh's Good Health Guide 1928 ©1927.*

The Year 1929

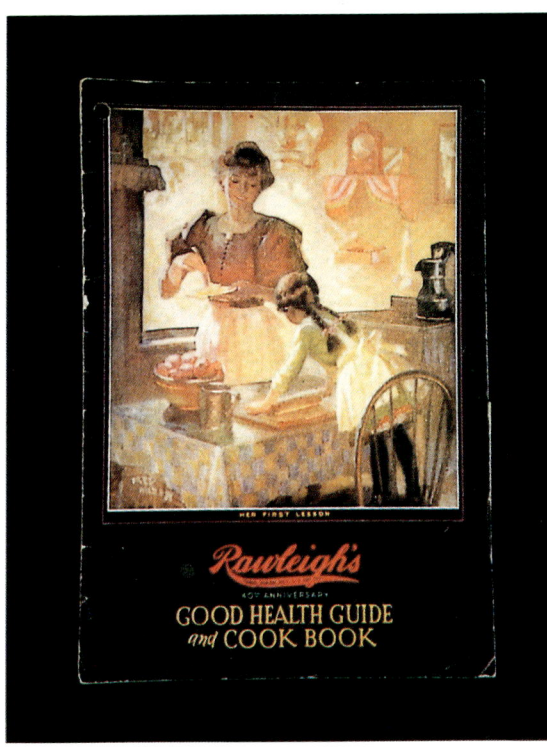

Rawleigh's 1929 40th Anniversary Good Health Guide and Cook Book. Published by THE W.T. RAWLEIGH CO. FREEPORT, ILL., U.S.A. ©1928. Cover painting titled "Her First Lesson." $20-$25.

"In 1895 a rented factory started with three employees. Within a year 30 men were retailing its products and factory space was doubled. In 1898 a factory was built and in 1904 the first building on the present location. In 1909 the first branch was started and in 1912 a Canadian factory opened. A three year million dollar building program closed in 1927 and early in 1928 Rawleigh's became established in Australia. Later in the year another Branch was opened at Albany, New York which gives a quicker, more economical and improved service to Retailers and Consumers in New England and New York in response to the fast growing demand for Good Health Products and Service." *Rawleigh's Good Health Guide and Cook Book 1929, ©1928.*

The Year 1930

Issue not available.

The following appeared in Rawleigh's 1931 Good Health Guide issue:

"NOTWITHSTANDING world-wide depression in nearly all lines of industry, trade and commerce the year 1930 has been one of the busiest and most successful in the entire 42 years history of the Rawleigh Industries."

"During and after the World War the cost of the four prime necessities of life — food, clothing, shelter and medicines, and the farmers' and home owners' taxes became so burdensome that the people generally rebelled at the high cost of everything, began complaining about hard times and demanding lower prices, and the false and fictitious prosperity caused by the war was deflated and the foundations laid for a new and more substantial and enduring prosperity."

"There never had been such a thing as hard times with the Rawleigh Industries. Sales have increased each and every year because during peace times and war times they have adhered strictly to their old fundamental policy of always producing the best qualities and values by keeping costs and wholesale and retail prices as low as possible."

"At the beginning of the year 1930 the Rawleigh Industries made tremendous reductions in their wholesale prices, which not only enabled Dealers to give consumers better values but the result was that more of Rawleigh's Good Health Products were made and sold during 1930 than ever before."

"While other industries have been complaining about hard times and there has been much unemployment and agricultural depression all Rawleigh factories have worked full time every day, week and month throughout the year, new branches have been established, offices and warehouses enlarged and service extended to hundreds of thousands of new families in the United States, Canada and Australia."

Improvements and Extensions

"Among the most important improvements and extensions made by the Rawleigh Industries during the year 1930 may be mentioned in the following:"

"In the Far East we began manufacturing in a new modern equipped factory in Melbourne, Australia."

"In the Dutch East Indies new offices and warehouses were opened at Telok-Betong to buy pepper, cinnamon, oil of citronella and other raw materials which are used in large quantities by all Rawleigh factories."

"In Japan offices were opened to buy menthol, camphor and pyrethrum flowers which are imported in large quantities for use in making powdered and liquid insecticides."

"In France larger offices and warehouses were secured at Marseilles to provide enlarged facilities for handling vanilla beans and other raw materials that are bought from first hands in France, Spain, Italy and Northern Africa for making extracts, flavors, toilet preparations and other Products."

"In Madagascar new offices and warehouses were completed to give enlarged facilities for buying vanilla beans, cloves, ylang ylang and other raw materials produced in the French Colonies in Madagascar, the Comore and Reunion Islands."

"Never before have the Rawleigh Industries bought so many different kinds of raw materials at their source as they now buy from first hands. This world-wide buying policy has resulted in securing better qualities at lower costs which means lower wholesale and retail prices and better values to consumers."

"In the Rawleigh Laboratories much research work was done in 1930 to improve qualities and reduce costs and studies were made to increase production and lessen the cost of transportation. Many important investigations were made to learn more about stocks, crops and conditions under which raw materials are grown, produced and marketed. These investigations extended into Northern and Western Africa, Jugo-Slavia and in the Far East into Japan, Java and other remote places."

"Never before in their history have the Rawleigh Industries had as much of everything necessary to give consumers the best values, service and satisfaction. Therefore, at the beginning of the new year we again renew our determination to serve everyone concerned with confidence that the new year will bring better health, greater happiness and prosperity to everyone we have always tried to serve faithfully and to the best of our ability." *Rawleigh's 1931 Good Health Guide.*

The Year 1931

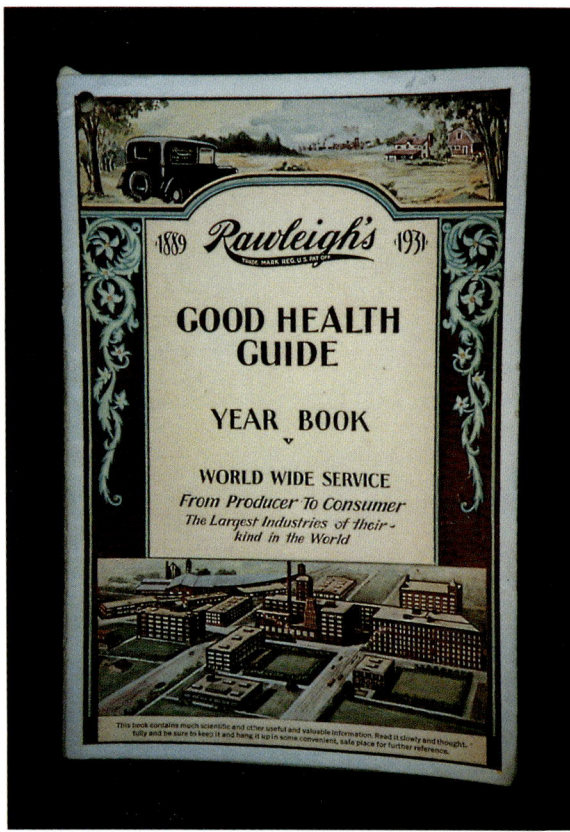

Rawleigh's 1931, Good Health Guide Year Book. "This publication contains much scientific and other useful and valuable information. Read it slowly and thoughtfully and be sure to keep it and hang it up in some convenient, safe place for further reference." The W.T. Rawleigh Company Freeport, Illinois, U.S.A. $20-$25.

"In presenting Rawleigh's Good Health Guide and Year Book for 1931, we desire to express our sincere appreciation for the good will and steadfast patronage of those millions of consumers in the United States, Canada, Australia and other countries whose continuous patronage during the last 42 years has enabled the Rawleigh Industries to do more research work to improve the quality, usefulness and reliability of its products, to build new factories and branches, increase production, enlarge distribution and extend its "Good Health Service" to many millions of new consumers throughout many countries."

"A Fundamental Rawleigh policy is to give consumers everywhere superior quality, the best values, the most and best of everything, on the most fibril terms, frequent, regular and dependable service, and a positive guarantee of satisfaction or no sale."

"Upon these fundamental policies, principles and methods the sale of Rawleigh Products have increased each and every year for 42 years and now the Rawleigh Industries buy more raw materials, make and sell more household medicines, insecticides, disinfectants, veterinary remedies, stock and poultry raisers' supplies and other home and farm necessities than all other similar industries combined."

Rawleigh's Good Health Guide
"With new engineering and research work, the enlargement of the Freeport and Melbourne factories, opening new offices in France and a new factory in New Zealand, the enlargement of the glass furnace and extension of transport service, the installation of much new machinery and equipment to increase production and lessen costs, and all factories working full time, the year 1931 was one of the busiest of the 43 years of continuous progress of the Rawleigh Industries."

Research Work
"Much important research work was done in our Laboratories during the year to improve processes, lessen costs and increase values. Some 5000 chemical analyses were made in standardizing materials. Other research work to improve the qualities and usefulness of products included studies of citrus oils; making aspirin; biological tests of liquid insecticides; feeding experiments and veterinary studies at Rawleigh's Ideal Farms; development of new Products; and producing insecticides about 25 per cent stronger, yet at lower costs than can be obtained by other methods."

New Machinery
"Immense sums were invested in new manufacturing equipment, including dryers, mills, stills, many large glass-lined storage and aging tanks, typesetting machines, printing presses, cutters, etc., and hydraulic, toggle and stamping presses, trimmers, beaders, thread rollers, slitters, for making products and all of our sprayers."

The Rawleigh Glass Factory
"The most important 1931 improvement at the Rawleigh Glass Factory was the enlargement of the furnace, and increasing the capacity nearly 50 percent by the addition of new and improved annealing ovens or lehrs, pyrometers to record automatically tremendous temperatures in the furnace, centrifuge vacuum pumps, air compressors, potentiometer recorders and conveyors. A new warehouse 440 ft. by 60 ft., for carrying reserve stocks of some 12 million bottles, increased the bottle storage area to nearly two acres."

Larger Bottles
"Consumers' attention is especially called to the larger bottles which give 33 per cent more Anti-Pain Oil and about 10 per cent more Effervescent Salts, Cough Syrup, Thyme Cough Compound, Cough Balsam, Ru-Mex-Ol Tonic and Tonic Compound (formerly Cod Liver Oil Extract). There has been no change in the Rawleigh quality of these medicines and no increase in price, consequently the result is much larger values than ever before."

Brushes, Mops and Dusters
"One of the most important improvements made in the manufacture of Rawleigh's Brushes was the installation of new automatic machinery to make all our own tooth brushes at lower cost. But many other additions and improvements were also made to the Rawleigh Line of Brushes, Mops and Dusters."

The Rawleigh Transport Service
"In 1931 the Rawleigh Transport Service was also enlarged until it now carries shipments between Freeport, Minneapolis, Chicago, Rockford and Memphis, also connecting with the Rawleigh River Transport Service. New tractor transports also bring bottles from the Glass Factory to the main Freeport Factories."

Europe and the Far East
"At Marseilles, France, large offices and warehouses were opened where Rawleigh's receive, inspect, and re ship vanilla from Madagascar and the Islands, and purchase perfume-making materials, essential oils and other raw materials from France, Spain, Italy, Algeria and elsewhere in Europe, Asia, Africa and South America. In the Far East, Branches were opened at Batavia, Java, and Kobe, Japan."

New Factories
"A new factory for the manufacture of Rawleigh Good Health Products was opened at Wellington, New Zealand to give the people of those islands Good Health Service. New and larger factories at Melbourne were also opened to provide for the great increase in Australian sales."

Better Service, Qualities, Values
"Everything considered, substantial progress was made during the year, not only at the main factories in the United States,

but in France, the Far East, New Zealand and Australia, which has resulted in improved qualities, lower costs, better values, lower wholesale prices to Dealers and lower retail prices to Consumers." *Rawleigh's Good Health Guide 1932.*

The Year 1932

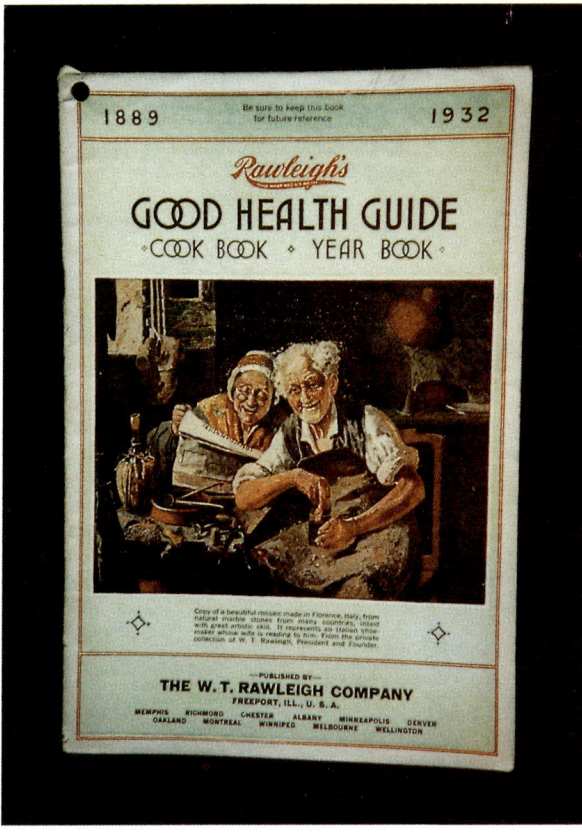

Rawleigh's Good Health Guide Cook Book Year Book 1932. Published By THE W.T. RAWLEIGH COMPANY FREEPORT, ILL., U.S.A. © 1931. The W.T. Rawleigh Company. $20-$25.

The Year 1933

"Our 1932 world-wide activities besides the opening of new factories at Wellington, New Zealand have been concentrated upon (1) savings and extensions in buying the best raw materials, (2) improvements in quality and usefulness of products, and (3) delivery of the best values, service and satisfaction to the homes of an increased number of Consumers." *Rawleigh's Good Health Guide 1933.*

Rawleigh's Good Health Guide Cook Book Year Book 1933. Published By THE W.T. RAWLEIGH COMPANY FREEPORT, ILL., U.S.A. ©1932. The W.T. Rawleigh Company. $20-$25.

The Year 1934

Issue not available.

The Year 1935

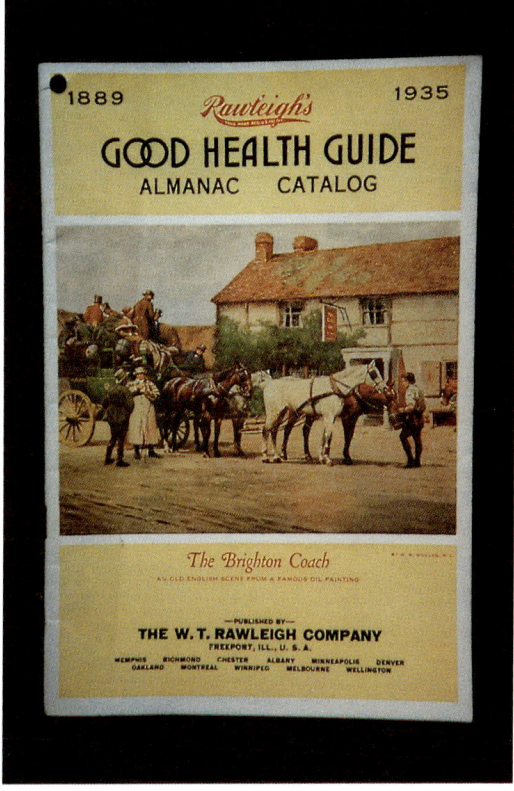

Rawleigh Good Health Guide Almanac Catalog 1935. Published by THE W.T. RAWLEIGH COMPANY FREEPORT, ILL., U.S.A. ©1934 The W.T. Rawleigh Company. $20-$25.

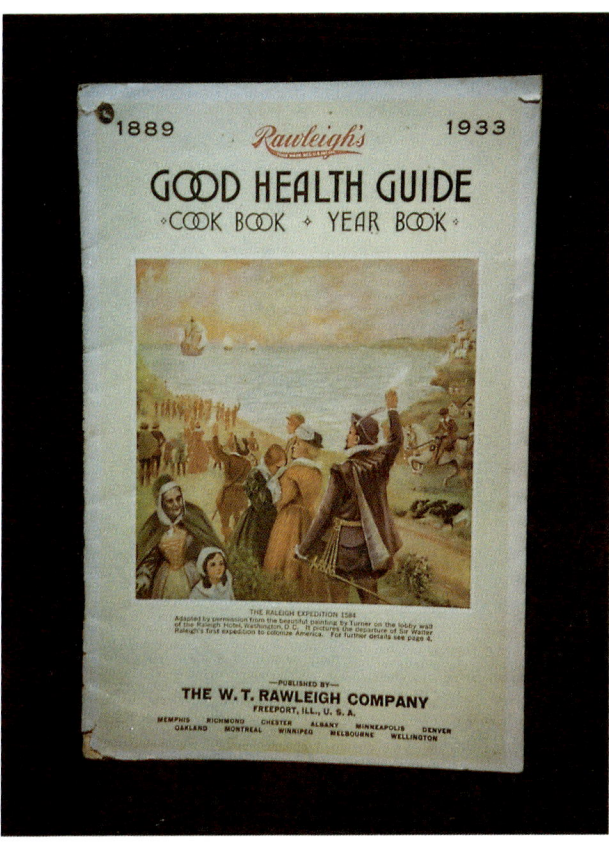

"For 45 years Rawleigh's Medicines and other Products have stood the test of actual use and proven their superior value and usefulness. They now have a world-wide sale. They have given good satisfaction in millions of families, who for two generations have recommended them to their relatives, neighbors and friends."

"Raw materials are bought in the world's best markets, then tested in our own laboratories for purity and strength by pharmaceutical and analytical chemists who are kept busy the year around supervising manufacture and making important researches to make Rawleigh Products still more valuable, reliable and useful."

"To give consumers the utmost in values and service it is the general policy (insofar as practical) to make everything — bottles, boxes, soaps. Fluid Extracts, Tinctures, Tablets, etc., are made directly from the roots, herbs, barks, and other raw materials. All under the careful control of one management with a fixed purpose and determination to give consumers the utmost protection and benefits."

"Millions of dollars are invested in Rawleigh factories, branches, equipment, raw materials, stocks and other property in the United States, Canada, Australia and New Zealand."
Rawleigh's Good Health Guide Almanac - Catalog 1935, ©1934.

The Year 1936

"**This new book contains** valuable information to safeguard the health and welfare of every member of the family. It includes many favorite cooking recipes, how to make foods more tasty with spices, salad dressings, fine extracts and food flavors."

"It explains the usefulness of Rawleigh Products and the benefits from keeping them in your home and using them when needed. Please keep it handy to refer to often for the added benefits you get from Rawleigh Service."

"**An old Rawleigh policy** is to make everything from the best raw materials money can buy and to give the utmost in values. The Management is independent and competitive. There is no bonded or other indebtedness which would increase costs without adding anything to values. Despite world-wide business depression steady work has been given to some 10,000 employees and dealers who buy, make and sell some 40 million farm and home Products annually in a factory-to-home service which merits public confidence and generous patronage."

To protect Dealers and Consumers against higher costs, higher wholesale and retail prices, which are expected from inflation and a multitude of higher taxes, we have been heavy buyers of the most important raw materials, therefore you can depend upon getting the best qualities and values again this year."
Rawleigh's Good Health Guide Almanac Catalog.

The Year 1937

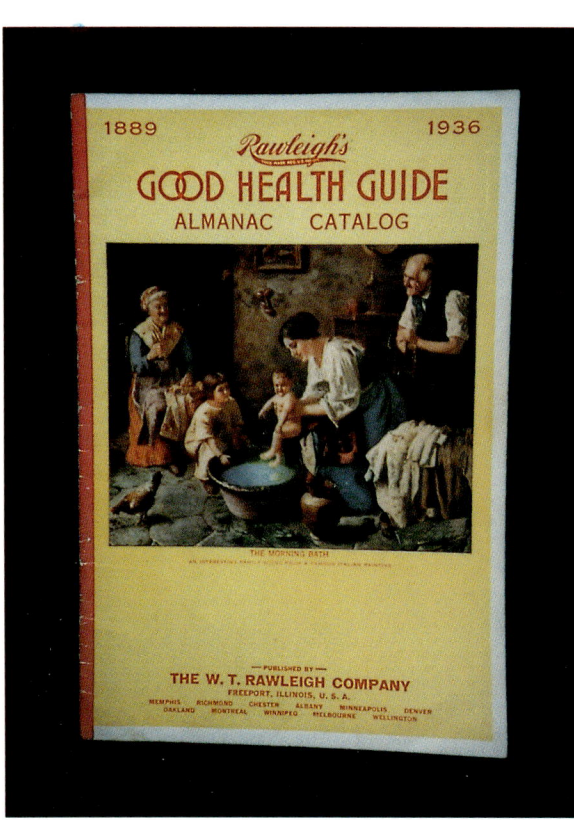

Rawleigh's Good Health Guide Almanac Catalog 1936. Published by THE W.T. RAWLEIGH COMPANY FREEPORT, ILLINOIS, U.S.A. $20-$25.

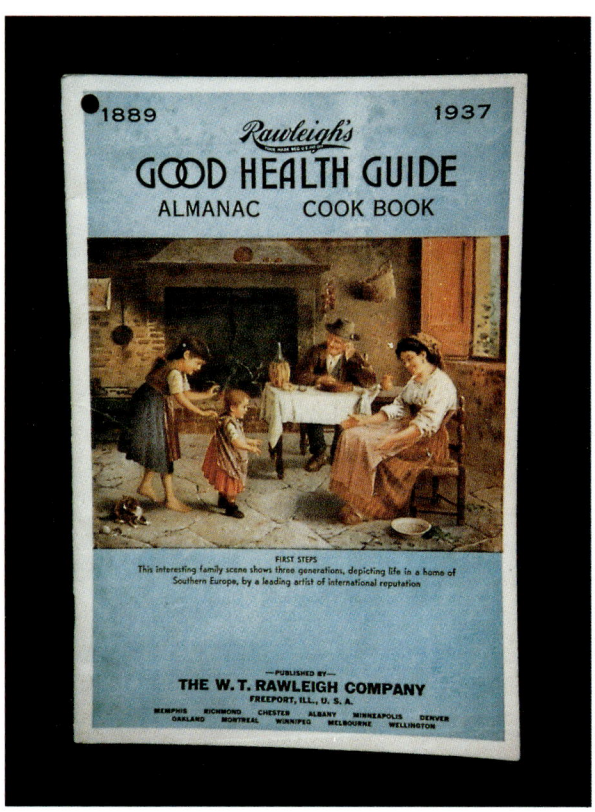

Rawleigh's Good Health Guide Almanac Cook Book 1937. Published by THE W.T. RAWLEIGH COMPANY FREEPORT, ILL., U.S.A. ©1936, The W.T. Rawleigh Company. $20-$25.

The Year 1938

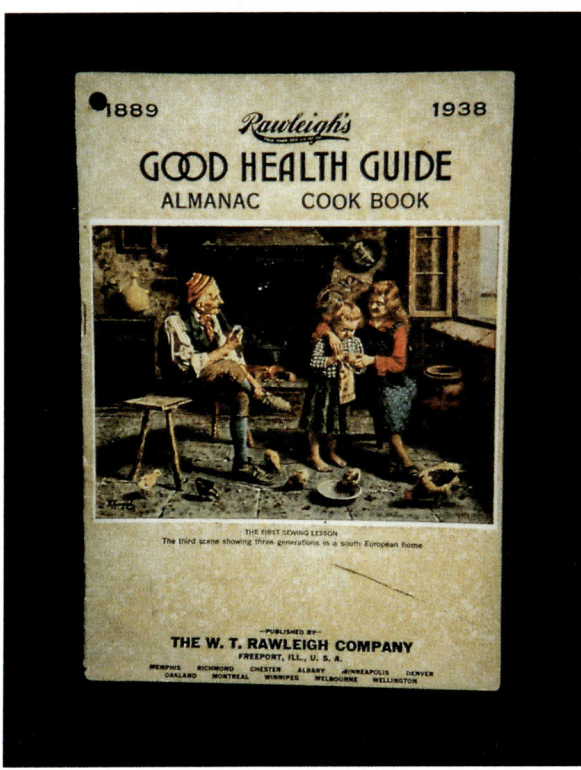

Rawleigh's 32 page 1938 Good Health Guide Almanac Cook Book. Published by THE W.T. RAWLEIGH COMPANY FREEPORT, ILL., U.S.A. ©1937, The W.T. Rawleigh Company. $20-$25.

"During nearly half a century we have invested millions in modern factories, equipment and stocks to make scientific and reliable products which give consumers maximum values, protection and benefits at minimum costs. For generations millions of families have learned to rely upon and keep these reliable medicines and other products on hand ready for emergencies to relieve sickness, pains, injuries and for their daily needs."

"Every year thousands visit our Freeport, Memphis, Montreal, Winnipeg, Melbourne and Wellington factories and farms. Old folks, who have been patrons for generations — mothers, fathers bring their children to see how thousands of carloads raw materials and products move in and out of our Factories and Branches annually."

"Here they see our laboratories test raw materials for purity, quality and strength — how trained chemists standardize, test, check and control every Product. How modern equipment corks, caps, labels without being touched, conveyed, loaded, shipped from coast to coast, with directions for consumers' use in English, French and other languages."

"The best materials money can buy come from nearly all countries. Most interesting to visitors are spices from Sumatra, Java, China, India, Africa, the West Indies; oils lemon and orange from California and Sicily and Vanilla from Madagascar and Java. Women visitors are especially fascinated with the exquisite natural oils made from the flowers of jasmine, orange blossoms, rose and lavender from sunny France, used in our fine creams, lotions and powders."

"Most of the herbs, roots, barks, buds used in making Cough Medicines, Tonics and Alternatives come from Europe, India, Ceylon, China, North America, the West Indies, Jamaica, Honduras and Asia. From Japan comes immense quantities of camphor and methyl for making medicines; hundreds of tons of pyrethrum flowers for insecticides to kill flies and insects."

"Visitors at the Rawleigh Industries see how we generate heat, light and power at Freeport, how we buy, make and sell some 42 million packages annually. Your and others' patronage provide work for some 10,000 employees and dealers who make and sell some 20 useful products, fresh from the factories, by the most economical factory-to-home service from producers to consumers."

The Year 1939

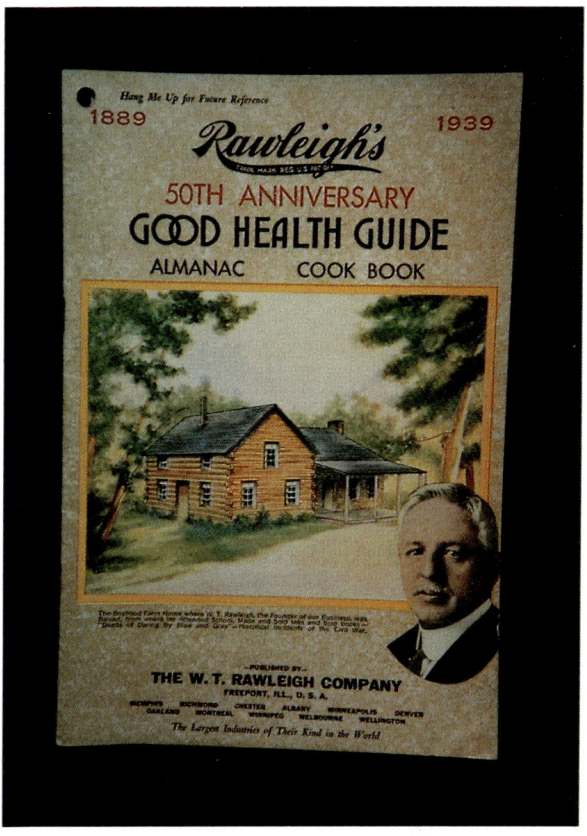

Rawleigh's 1939 50TH ANNIVERSARY Good Health Guide Almanac Cook Book. Published by THE W.T. RAWLEIGH COMPANY FREEPORT, ILL., U.S.A. $20-$25.

"Half a century is a long time in the life of a business under the same ownership yet on our 50th Anniversary we take pleasure in presenting this new book in sincere appreciation to millions of friends who have used the products of our laboratories for about a half century. Days of opportunity and service dawned for W.T. Rawleigh when he drove from his boyhood home in 1889. His service found welcome in the hearts of consumers, his free trial offers, guarantee of satisfaction or no sale and fair dealing with friends in ever widening circles."

"Great progress has been made since those early days when needs and desires were simpler. Men worked longer hours and thrift was a virtue. Living costs were low and there was great hospitality, more self-reliance, more economy and simple ways of caring for human welfare. Even in those early days no pains or reasonable expense was spared to make the most useful and reliable medicines. Consumers were given the utmost in values and superior service that has since made millions of steadfast customers, who have learned through long years of use that Rawleigh's are reliable, useful and superior quality Products."

"For 50 golden years we have faithfully practiced those old-fashioned ideals of honesty, of quality, values and satisfaction. Our methods have brought producers and consumers closer together, have helped save much sickness, suffering and expense, improved human relations, given some 10,000 dealers and employees steady work which has brought improved health and happiness in millions of homes."

"Today our greatest asset is the good will, loyalty, confidence and generous patronage which we treasure more highly than the miser treasures his gold. Now, after about a half century, from the bottom of our hearts we thank our millions of old friends for their confidence, loyalty and steadfast patronage which we have always tried to merit. This has made our business grow from a small beginning into one of the oldest and largest industries of its kind in the world. Rawleigh policies have always been independent, competitive and progressive."

"We now point with pride to our great factories and laboratories. They are monuments and evidence of the quality of Rawleigh Products and the value, convenience and practicability of our world-wide service from factory to home. In times of peace and war, in good years and lean years, we have endeavored to keep the faith and to give Dealers and Consumers the utmost in values, service and satisfaction. For all this we sincerely appreciate your loyalty and generous patronage which has made it possible to gradually extend our business into a great international organization." *Rawleigh's 50th Anniversary Good Health Guide Almanac Cook Book 1939.*

The Year 1940

Issue not available.

The Year 1941

"Fifty-two years ago our line of Products was small. Now there are some 200 reliable Medicines and Products. Increased material costs, greatly increased ocean freights and constantly increasing taxes have created many problems for us. But you can still get the most and best for your money and now is the time to stock up."

"In time of peace and war, to protect the health and pocketbooks of millions of families irrespective of costs we have regarded it our duty to consumers to maintain our high standards of quality, which millions have learned to rely upon for protection of their loved ones, livestock and poultry."

"In times of peace and war, to protect the health and pocketbook of millions of families irrespective of costs we have regarded it our duty to consumers to maintain our high standards of quality, which millions have learned to rely upon for protection of their loved ones, livestock and poultry."

"Expecting that wars would come again we have been heavy buyers of materials which come from nearly all countries. In times of war it is difficult to obtain raw materials from Europe, Asia, the East and West Indies, and from distant islands of the seas and oceans. Yet, within the year, we received and shipped over 3,000 carloads raw materials and Products from our U.S. and Canadian factories."

"Hundreds of tons of Insecticide materials, Camphor and Menthol came from far-away Japan and Brazil. Then there were large imports of Spices from Java, Sumatra, India, China and Africa. Many seeds, roots, herbs, barks came from France and Egypt. Oils Lemon, Orange and Eucalyptus from Italy, California and Australia. Vanilla came from Madagascar and Mexico; Cloves from Madagascar and Zanzibar."

"Rawleigh's Good Health Products have given good satisfaction everywhere they have been introduced. They save many drug and doctor bills. There is now world-wide sale and praise of their reliability, usefulness and good values."

The Year 1942

Rawleigh's 32 page 1942 Good Health Guide Almanac Cook Book. Published By THE W.T. RAWLEIGH COMPANY FREEPORT, IL., U.S.A. Cover photograph titled "Man's Most Faithful Friend Confidence Well Placed." $20-$25.

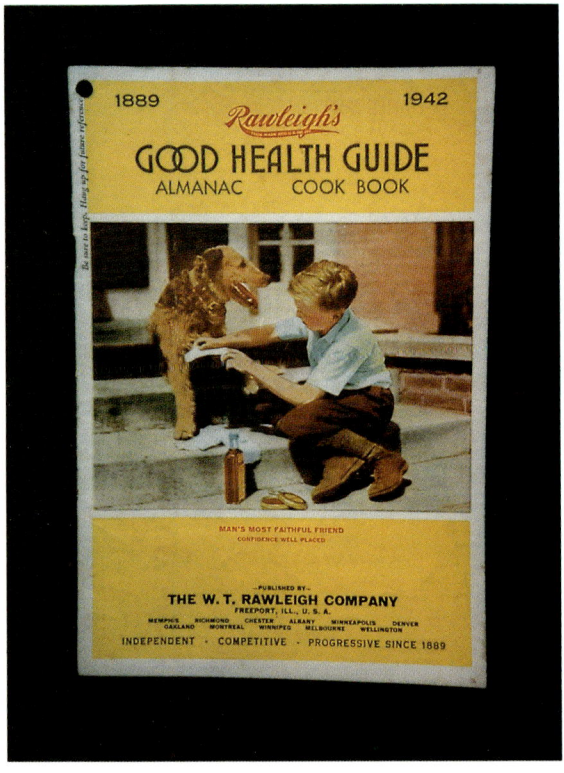

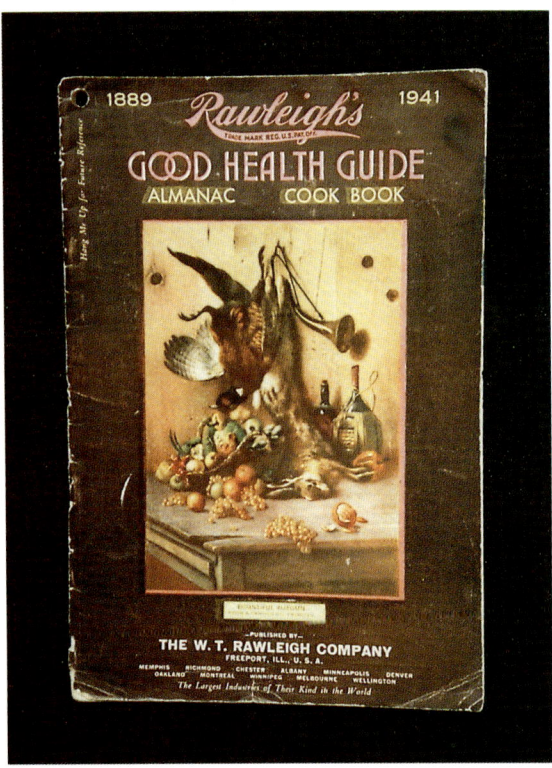

Rawleigh's 32 page 1941 Good Health Guide Almanac Cook Book. Published By THE W.T. RAWLEIGH COMPANY FREEPORT, IL., U.S.A. The Largest Industries of their kind in the World. Cover photograph from a famous oil painting titled "Bountiful Autumn." $20-$25.

"In beginning our 53rd year it is natural to look both backward and forward. Backward to our early struggles. Those were happy days, when most folks were poor, but honest. They worked full time for small pay. Then all industries were small, independent and competitive. There were no large corporations, except railroads and big city banks. There were no trusts, no radios, no telephones, no automobiles, airplanes or bombers to destroy life and property."

"The great Civil War, which freed the slaves, was followed by panics, but united the North and South in bonds of patriotism, brotherly love and toleration. Prosperity spread everywhere. The people were happy and the most contented in the history of the world."

"The Indians roamed the western prairie's with bows, arrows and scalping knives, chasing buffalo and frightening the pioneer settlers. That was right after the Civil War when I was born in 1870. Those were days of excitement, but the people were happy, prosperous, contented and rejoiced in their victory which re-united the entire United States and freed the slaves."

"Then came the great World War to end all wars and save the world for Democracy! It was a life and death struggle, in which many millions of men were killed fighting for their lives and liberties on the battlefields of France, Italy and the Balkans, which I have since seen. The people everywhere declared they would never go to war again."

"The most cruel war in all history is now raging again on the same battlefields of Europe, the Balkans, from Russia and the Black Sea ports to the Mediterranean and Egypt. Millions have lost their homes; thousands are prisoners or are enslaved and died of hunger."

"Many of raw materials come from Europe, Japan, China, the Dutch East Indies, and from the islands of the Mediterranean, the Indian Ocean and Pacific. All are now at war, ports are closed, travel dangerous, slow. Nearly all materials have become scarce and dear. But we shall continue to use all our capital and facilities to keep you supplied with everything in our line to protect your health and pocketbook, your loved ones, livestock and poultry."

"To faithfully serve our millions of friends you can depend that we will keep up the good fight, side by side, until peace, prosperity, freedom of the seas, justice, liberty and independence are restored to the people throughout the world."

The Year 1943

Issue not available.

The Year 1944

"You may be interested to know that our scientific staff includes chemical engineers, pharmaceutical and analytical chemists, bacteriologists and entomologists. Many thousands of dollars are spent each year to examine, test and analyze botanical drugs, roots, herbs, seeds, spices, chemicals, essential oils and other raw materials and to do research work to improve processes, materials and products, because we know that millions of people rely on the products of our laboratories to protect their loved ones, livestock and poultry. The result is uniform, high strength, purity, quality and reliability."

Rawleigh's 32 page 1944 Good Health Guide Almanac Cook Book. Published By THE W.T. RAWLEIGH COMPANY FREEPORT, IL., U.S.A. $20-$25.

The Year 1945

Issue not available.

The Year 1946

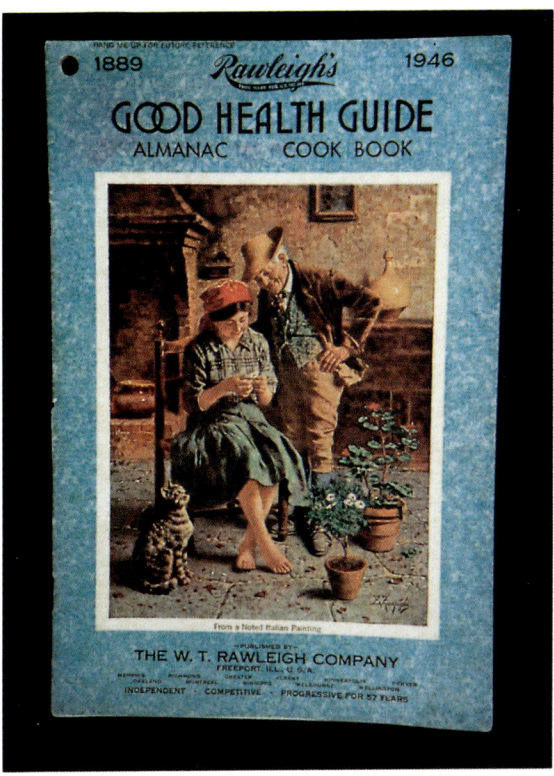

Rawleigh's 32 page 1946 Good Health Guide Almanac Cook Book. Published By THE W.T. RAWLEIGH COMPANY FREEPORT, IL., U.S.A. Cover photograph is from a noted Italian painting. $20-$25.

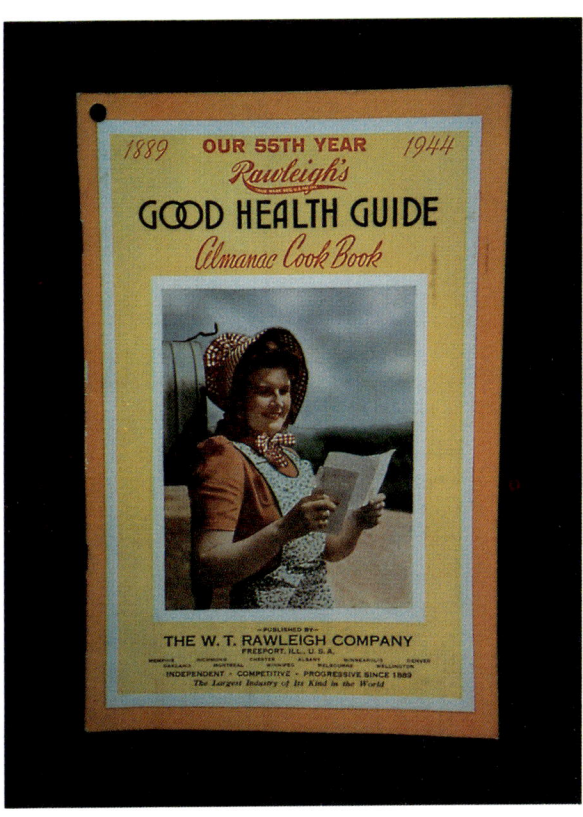

"For 57 years of peace and war, health and sickness, prosperity and depression, our world-wide industry has tried to serve you faithfully with supreme quality, reliable Medicines and other Products that devoted Dealers bring from our factories to your homes."

"Now there are many restrictions on trade and travel, heavy taxes and higher costs, but we still have fair stocks of nearly all materials to make nearly 200 Good Health Products. They are still sold at about the same prices they have been sold for many years. You can still get the utmost in supreme quality, big values, reliability and usefulness."

"While merchandise of nearly all kinds is scarce, rationed and restricted, your Dealer will continue to make free deliveries to your home to protect your loved ones, livestock and poultry and save your time, tires and gas."

"You should welcome your Rawleigh Dealer. When he calls ask him to explain the unusual value of his reliable Medicines for coughs and colds, Tonics and Alternatives, Extracts, Flavors, Spices, Food Products, Toilet Preparations (Creams, Powders, Lotions) — his big line of Vitamins and his Livestock and Poultry Tonics, Insecticides and Disinfectants."

The Year 1947

Issue not available.

The Year 1948

"From all over the world we gather the best materials, which come from Europe, Japan, China, Dutch East Indies, and from the islands of the Mediterranean, Indiana Ocean and the Pacific. All have recently been in the Second World War. Ports were closed, travel dangerous and slow, but even during the last war we were able to import many important materials from some of these countries."

"These materials come from old firms from whom we have bought or to whom we have sold for over a quarter of a century. Many materials are still scarce, dear and difficult to obtain, but we used all our capital and facilities to keep you supplied with nearly everything in our line during the last cruel, worldwide war, when there were many restrictions on trade and travel, heavy taxes and higher costs. But we will make nearly 200 Good Health Products, which are sold at about the same prices as they have been sold for many years. You can still get the utmost in supreme quality, big values, reliability and usefulness. Your Dealer will continue to make free deliveries to your home to protect your loved ones, livestock and poultry, and save you time, tires and gas."

The Year 1949

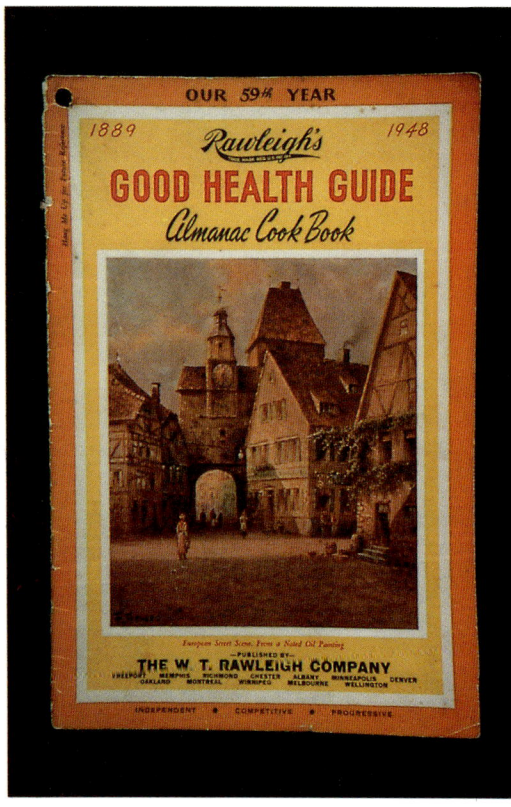

Rawleigh's 32 page 1948 Good Health Guide Almanac Cook Book. Published By THE W.T. RAWLEIGH COMPANY FREEPORT, IL., U.S.A. Cover photograph is from a noted oil painting "European Street Scene." The 1948 Introduction is repeated from the 1946 Introduction with additional paragraphs. $20-$25.

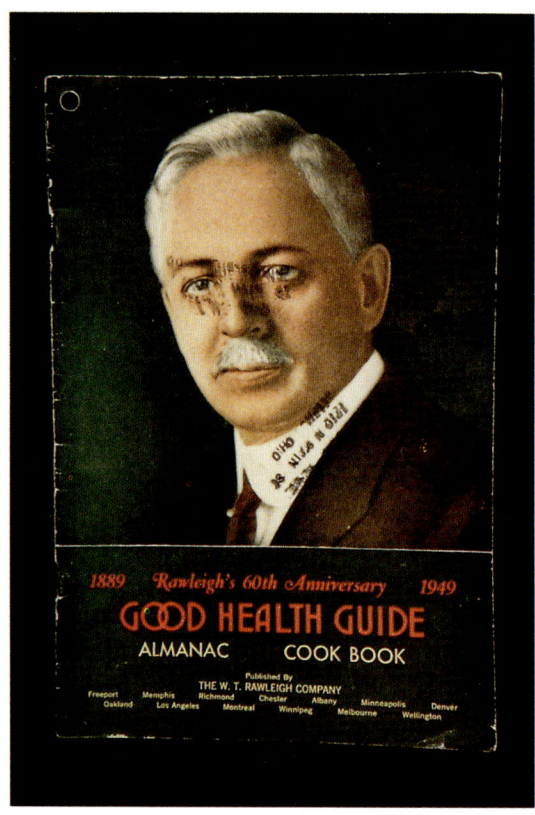

Rawleigh's 60th Anniversary 32 page 1949 Good Health Guide Almanac Cook Book. Published by THE W.T. RAWLEIGH COMPANY FREEPORT - MEMPHIS - RICHMOND - CHESTER - ALBANY - MINNEAPOLIS - DENVER - OAKLAND - LOS ANGELES - MONTREAL - WINNIPEG - MELBOURNE - WELLINGTON. $20-$25.

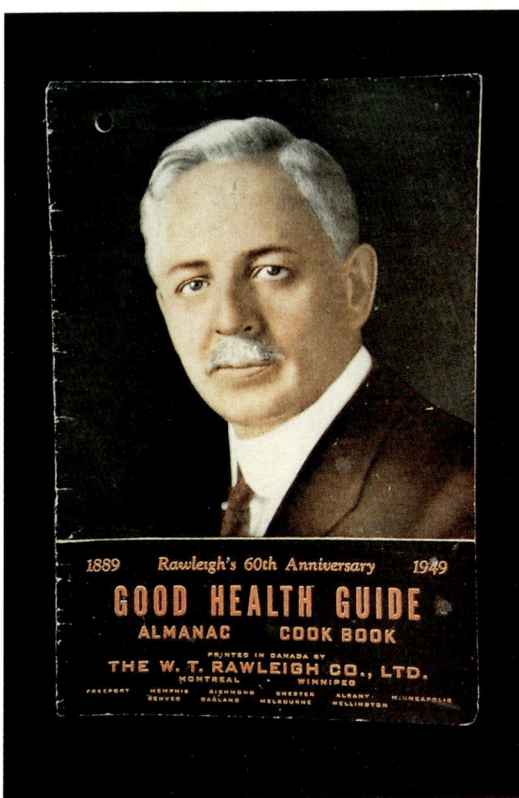

Rawleigh's 60th Anniversary 32 page 1949 Good Health Guide Almanac Cook Book. Published by THE W.T. RAWLEIGH COMPANY MONTREAL - WINNIPEG - FREEPORT - MEMPHIS - RICHMOND - CHESTER - ALBANY - MINNEAPOLIS - DENVER - OAKLAND - MELBOURNE - WELLINGTON. The same information appeared in both publications. $20-$25.

The Year 1950

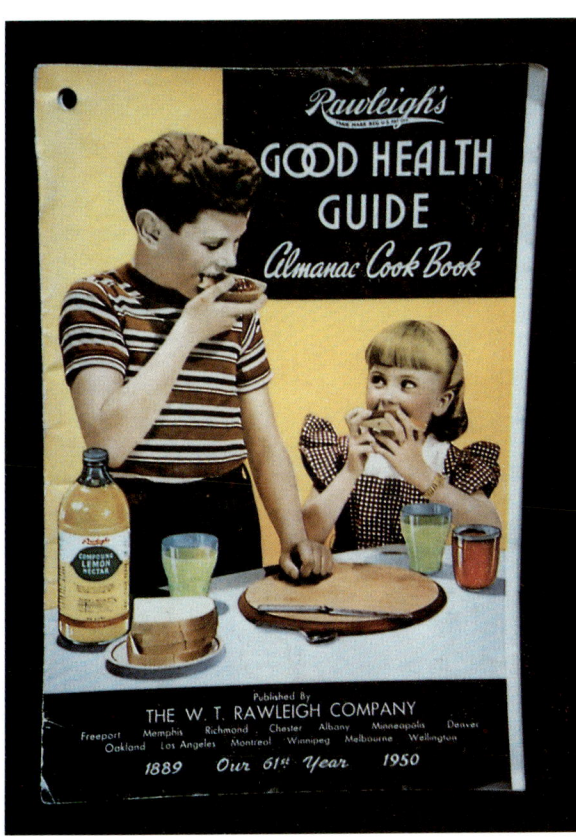

The Year 1951

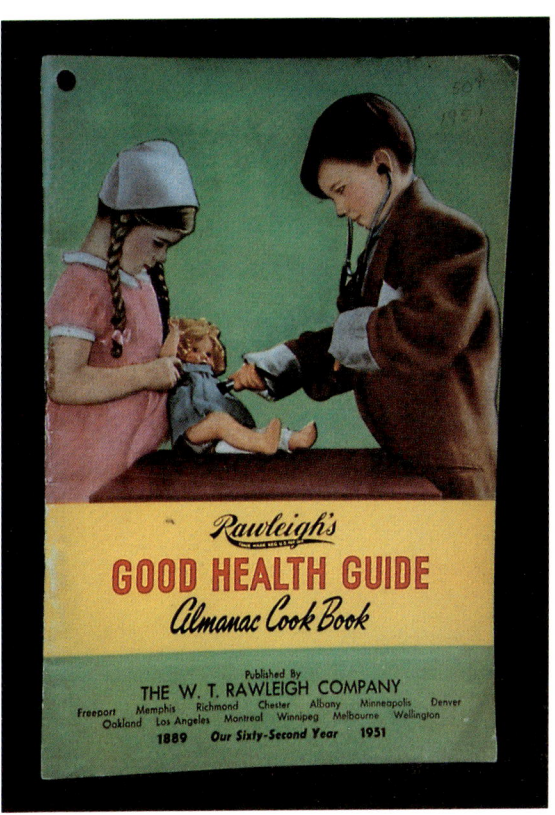

Rawleigh's sixty-second year 1951 Good Health Guide Almanac Cook Book. This would be W.T. Rawleigh's last address to his customers through the Almanacs. Mr. Rawleigh died on January 23, 1951. $15-$20.

"Another year of progress brings use to the sixty-second year of the business which I founded way back in 1889."

"Truly, your patronage has made this great business possible; and to you I promise that in the future, as in the past, you will always be uppermost in our minds."

"You have shown your approval of the new Products we introduced during the past year. Other new Products are on the way which I believe will please you as well."

"New factory processes will help us to continue the big values you have come to expect of Rawleigh's. All our studies and efforts are still devoted to bringing you the best values you can obtain anywhere in quantity, in quality and price."

"It is good to know that in all parts of the United States, Canada, Australia and New Zealand, millions of fine folks like you have come to know that Rawleigh's means the best. We sincerely appreciate your loyalty and patronage. You can depend on both your Rawleigh Dealer and the Company to continue to serve you faithfully."

"This book has been carefully prepared to bring you much information of permanent value. I am sure you will want to keep it handy and refer to it often. A new feature is the list of important pages you see at the right (shown below). This will help you to find any particular feature you are looking for."

Rawleigh's 30 page 1950 Good Health Guide Almanac Cook Book. Our 61st Year. $15-$20.

The Year 1952

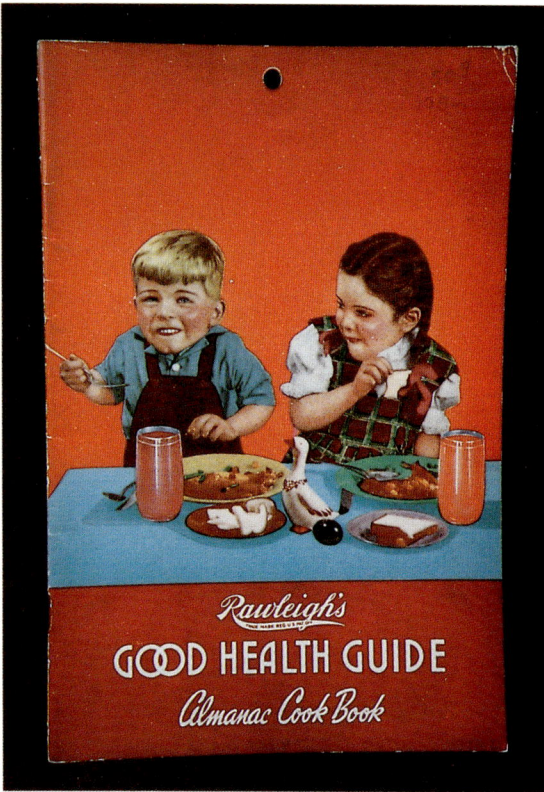

Rawleigh's 32 page 1952 Good Health Guide Almanac Cook Book. No Introduction appeared and no public notice of W.T. Rawleigh's death was printed in this issue. $15-$20.

The Year 1953

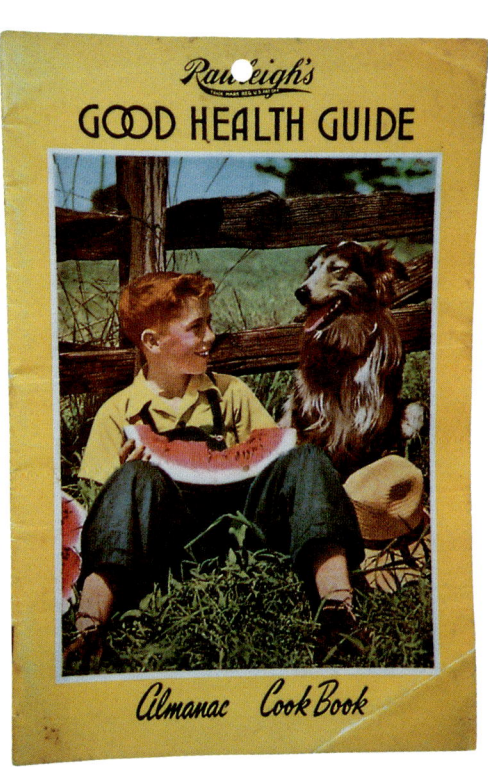

Rawleigh's 32 page 1953 Good Health Guide Almanac Cook Book. No Introduction appeared in this issue. $15-$20.

The Year 1954

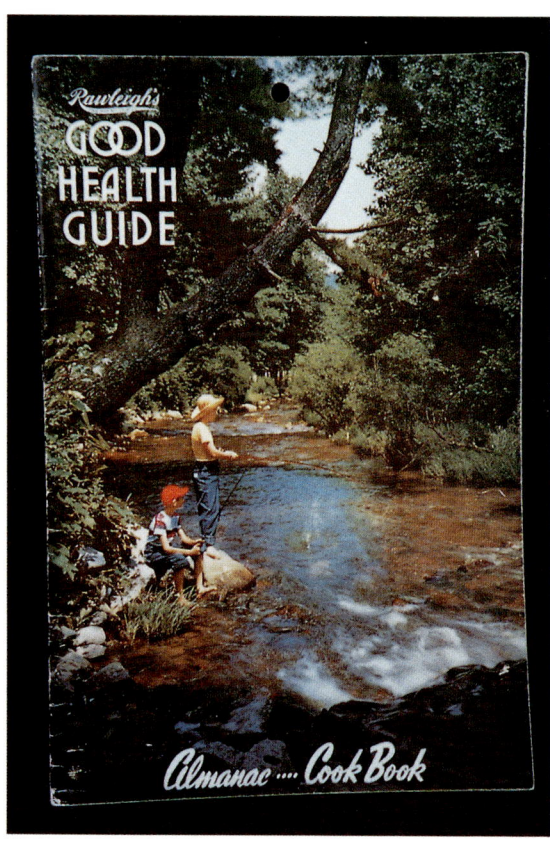

Rawleigh's 32 page 1954 Good Health Guide Almanac Cook Book. No Introduction appeared in this issue. $15-$20.

The Year 1955

Rawleigh's 32 page 1955 Good Health Guide Almanac & Cook Book. No Introduction appeared in this issue. $15-$20.

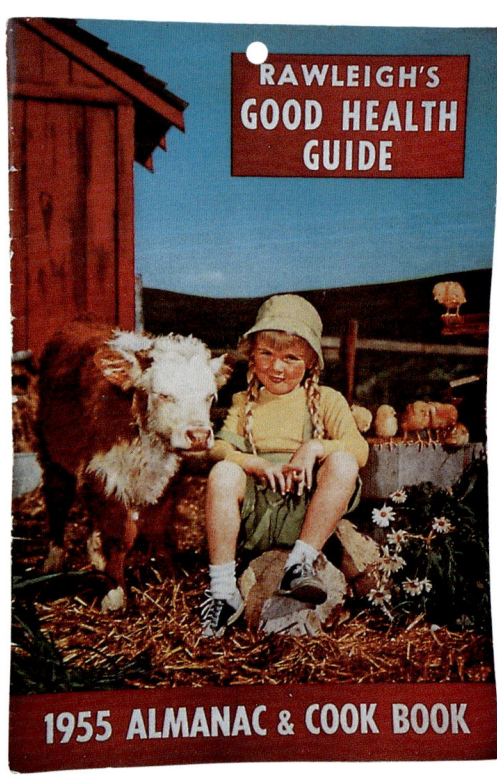

The Year 1956

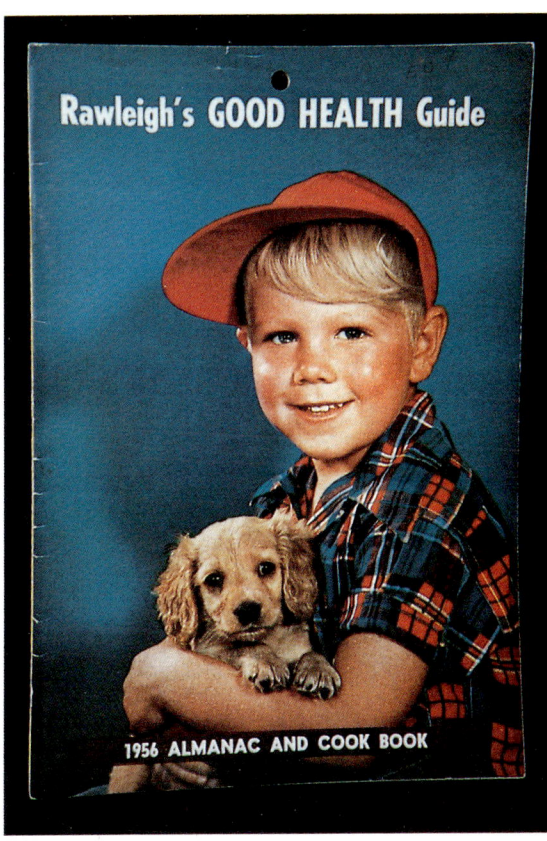

Rawleigh's 32 page 1956 Good Health Guide Almanac and Cook Book. No Introduction appeared in this issue. $15-$20.

The Year 1958

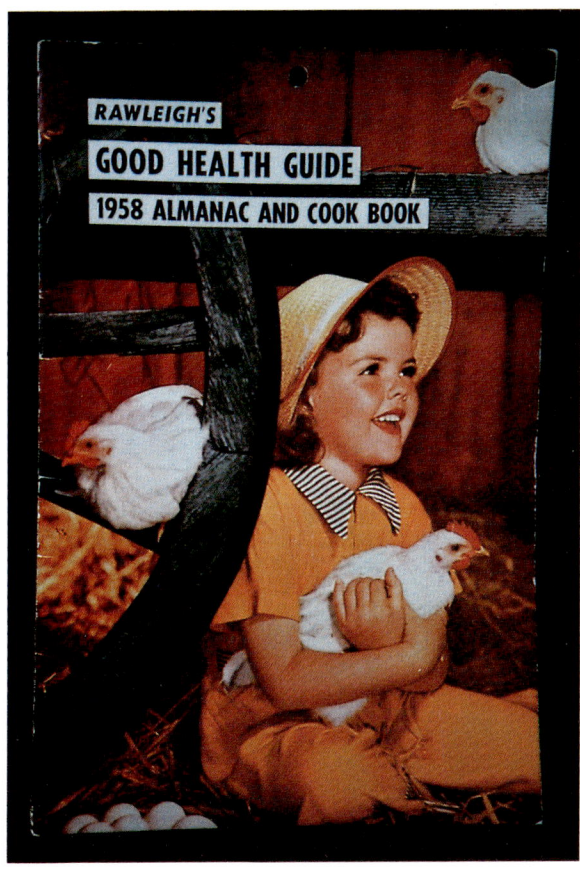

Rawleigh's 32 page 1958 Good Health Guide Almanac and Cook Book. No Introduction appeared in this issue. $15-$20.

The Year 1957

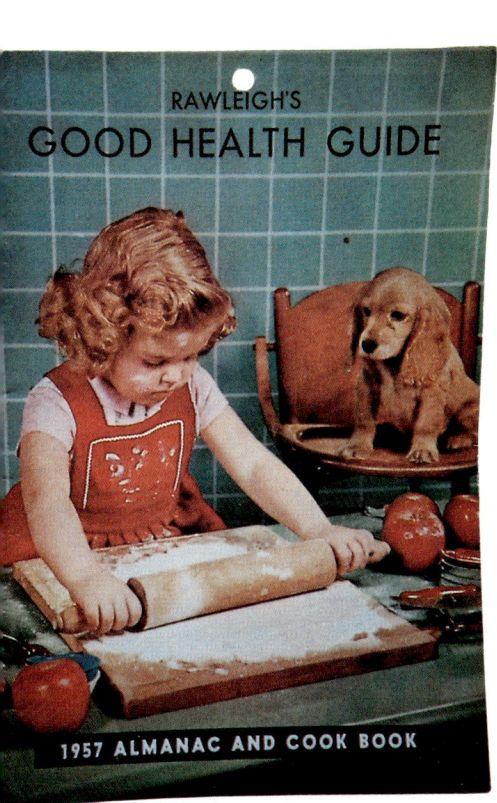

Rawleigh's 32 page 1957 Good Health Guide Almanac and Cook Book. No Introduction appeared in this issue. $15-$20.

The Year 1959

Rawleigh's 32 page 1959 Good Health Guide Almanac Cook Book. 70th Anniversary Issue. $15-$20.

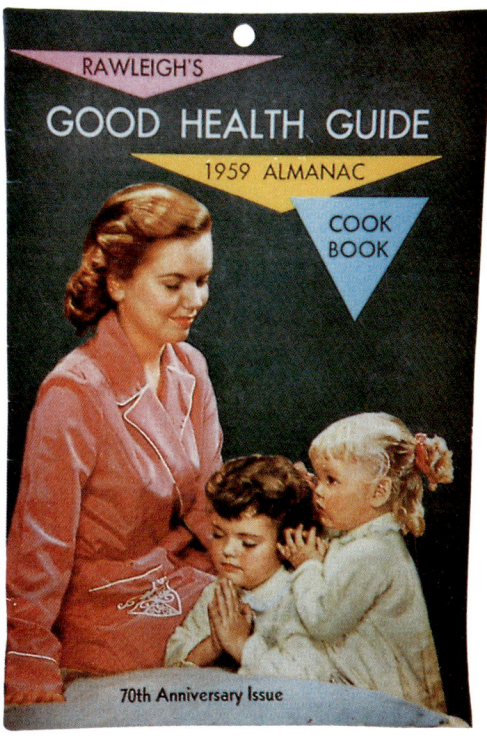

An Introduction appeared in this issue for the first time since Rawleigh's death in 1951. This introduction had the signature of J.D. Gilbert, the new company president.

The Year 1960

Issue not available.

The Year 1961

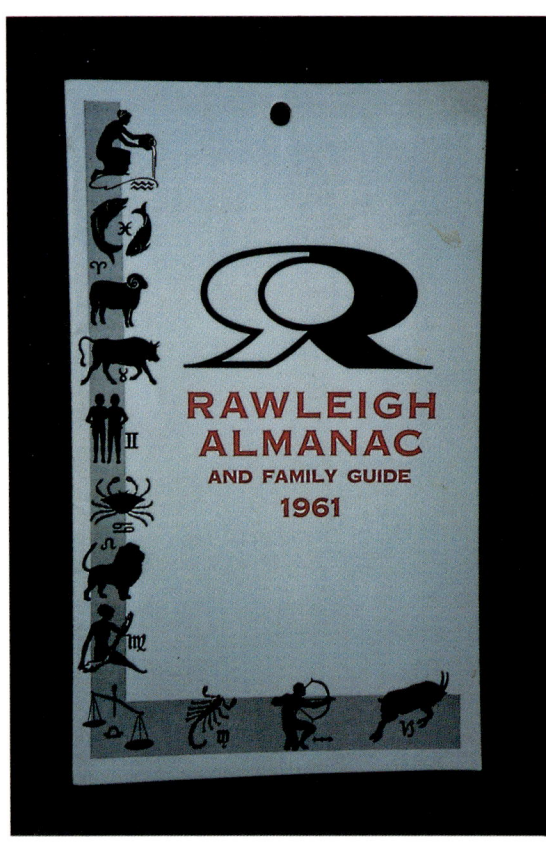

Rawleigh 24 page Almanac and Family Guide 1961. No Introduction appeared in this issue. $10-$15.

The Year 1962

"This is the 63rd consecutive annual edition of the Rawleigh Almanac...the oldest one continuously published by any home service company in America."

"The Dealers of our Company started serving housewives and farmers of Stephenson County, Illinois, with medicines, household products and livestock remedies 'way back' in April of 1889. Not until the turn of the century was our first 'Almanac, Cook Book and Medical Guide' published."

"Since that time our business has expanded to the extent that Rawleigh Dealers are now calling on farm and city homes in four great English-speaking countries; United States, Canada (1912), Australia (1928), and New Zealand (1931)."

Rawleigh 24 page Almanac and Family Guide 1962. $10-$15.

"The Dealer who handed you this Almanac and Family Guide sincerely appreciates your patronage as do we also who make the products. We trust that the information contained in this book will be of much help and guidance to you and your family during 1962. If you want an Almanac for a relative or friend, please ask you Rawleigh Dealer or write direct to me at Freeport, Illinois. I'll see that one is mailed promptly to his or her address." Signed Yours sincerely J.D. Gilbert, President.

The Year 1963

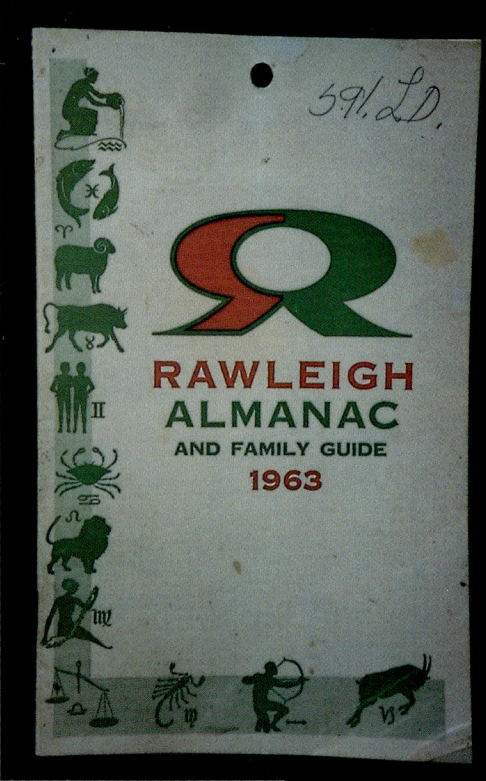

Rawleigh 24 page Almanac and Family Guide 1963. $10-$15.

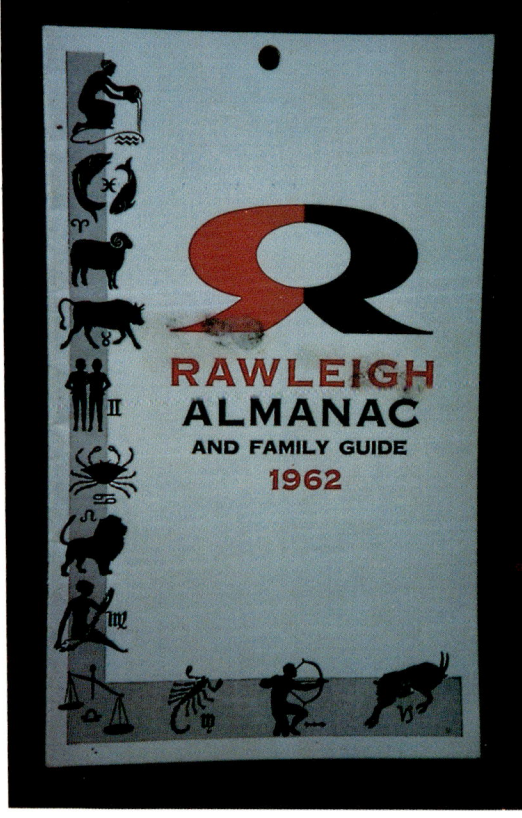

The Year 1964

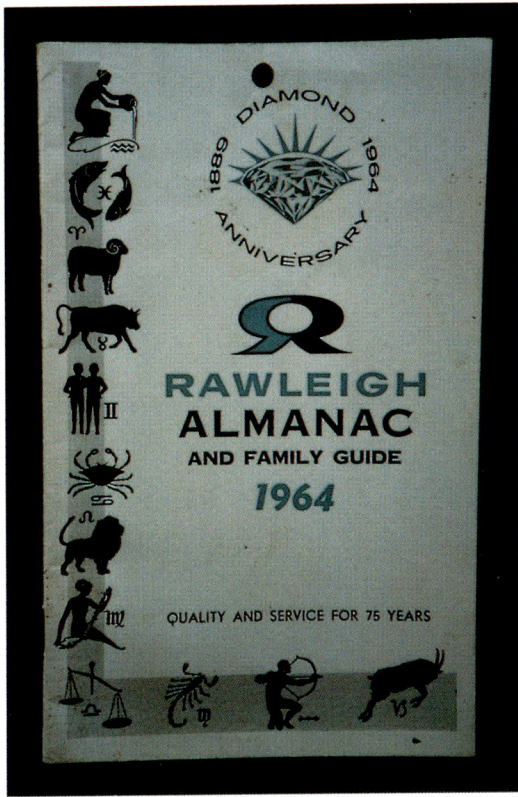

Rawleigh 24 page Almanac and Family Guide 1964. $10-$15.

"Since 1889 the United States has had 13 presidents. Rawleigh's now observing its 75th anniversary, has in the same span of time had only three presidents."

"But under the successive leadership of Founder W.T. Rawleigh, H.P. Ousley, and myself (J.D. Gilbert), Rawleigh's has grown to the point where it has 14 factories and branches in four English-speaking countries, serving a total population of over 216,000,000."

"During this 75-year period of growth there is a single publication that has marketed each step of the way - the annual Rawleigh Almanac and Family Guide. Generation after generation of Rawleigh customers have started the year with a Rawleigh Almanac hanging on the kitchen wall."

"The first American almanac, a one-leaf broadside, was compiled and printed in Cambridge, Massachusetts in 1639 on the first printing press used in this country. The production of almanacs increased as more printing presses were built and as the country grew. The almanac followed the pioneers west, leaving New England far behind. It also went beyond its original features - astronomical calculations, weather predictions, tide tables and snatches of philosophy - and began to provide its readers with poetry and stories, jokes, recipes, cures for minor ailments and advice for farmers and tradesmen."

"During the 19th century the almanac provided more about new roads, distances between larger towns, news of the courts, new agricultural machinery and domestic gadgets. Before 1825 the almanac carried no advertisements. It was supplied by subscription and purchase because its purpose was to educate and entertain."

"From 1832 on, the old-time American almanac began to change in character. It began to carry advertising for patent medicine manufactures, temperance organizations, anti-slavery groups and political parties."

"After the Civil War newspapers and magazines took over the once humble role of the annual almanac. Also booksellers, printers, insurance companies, seedsmen and many of our large manufacturers began compiling their own private almanacs."

"Though the original American almanac may have died about 130 years ago, its commercial cousins are carrying on in the grand 20th century manner. This year's Rawleigh Almanac and Family Guide is our 65th consecutive annual edition - the oldest one continuously published by an home service company in America. We trust that it helps to guide you and your family safely through another year and that the products your Rawleigh Dealer brings you will help you to easier housekeeping, better and tastier food, and a healthier and better-groomed family." Signed Yours sincerely, J.D. Gilbert, President.

The Year 1965

Issue not available.

The Year 1966

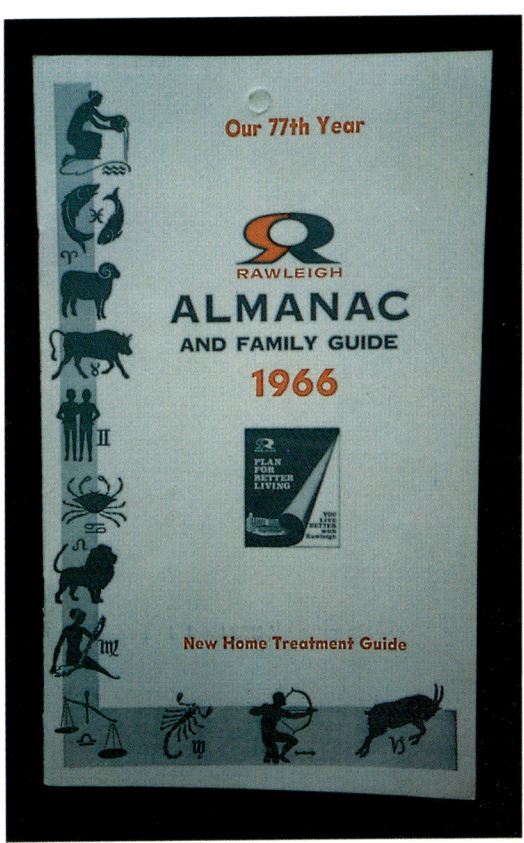

Rawleigh 24 page Almanac and Family Guide 1966. $10-$15.

"To our patrons and friends:"

"In our modern society, you, the American homemaker, are constantly exposed to the winds of change. Countless new products - and new forms of old products - vie for your attention."

"You cannot help but feel confused (and too often unheard) as you seek the best values for the hard-earned dollar you spend."

"In that never-ending search for values, Rawleigh Products have stood the test for more than 77 years:"

"(1) Quality is the factor that built our business into a worldwide industry. Should any single Rawleigh Product not measure up to your standard - not perform as it should - we want to know about it. Please tell your Dealer or write us at once so that we can make the changes necessary to assure you of continuing good performance from Rawleigh Products."

"(2) Quantity is important when you compare price per ounce. Many Rawleigh Products come in large packages to give you a better buy."

"(3) Price. Your Dealer brings you Rawleigh Products direct from our factories and branches. There are no jobbers, brokers or wholesale adding their profits to the price you pay."

"Again - we'll consider it a favor if you'll write us if any product should not give you full benefit. It is only by means of the cooperation of you, the user, that we can continue to supply best values to you and the other homemakers of America." Signed The W.T. Rawleigh Company.

The Years 1967 - 1969

Issues not available. $10-$15 ea.

The Years 1970 - 1976

Issues not available. $10-$15 ea.

The Year 1977

"One day a young man from California came into our offices and said the citrus growers in his state had developed an even finer grade of lemon oil. We investigated, found his claim to be true, and immediately began buying our lemon oil from California. If we should learn tomorrow that someone else has bettered the California quality, you can be sure we'll be the first in line to use it. That's how committed we are to using only the finest ingredients in Rawleigh products."

"Although selecting top-quality ingredients is tremendously important, so are the ways in which those ingredients are processed. The best ingredients in the world can be ruined by low-grade processing. Rawleigh's famous Black Pepper offers a dramatic example. After we have selected an aromatic, flavorful blend of the finest pepper berries available, the processing begins. The easiest thing to do would be to grind up each batch exactly as it comes from the fields - a mixture of berries, leaves stems, and anything else which may have fallen into the crop as it was harvested. But we could never retain Rawleigh's superior flavor and fragrance if we did that." *Rawleigh 1977 Almanac and Cook Book.*

The Year 1978

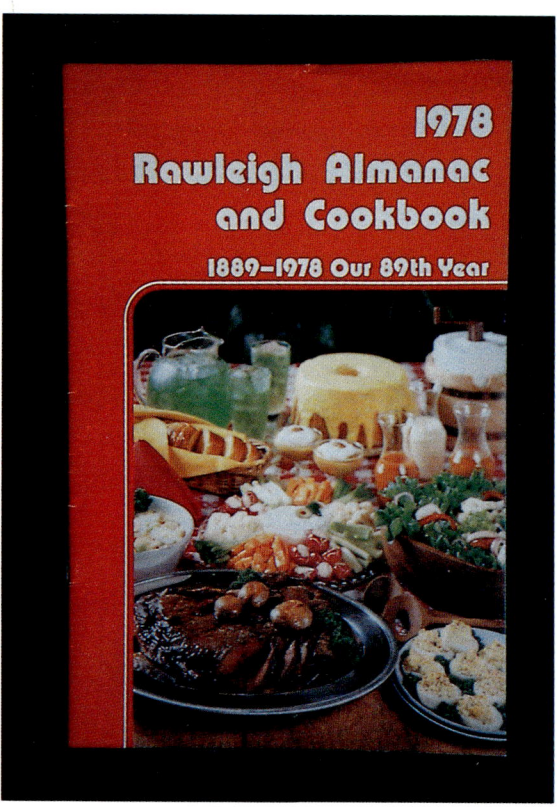

Rawleigh 89th Year 35 page 1978 Almanac and Cookbook, © 1977 by The W.T. Rawleigh Co., Freeport, IL 61032. *Bushue Collection.* $5-$10.

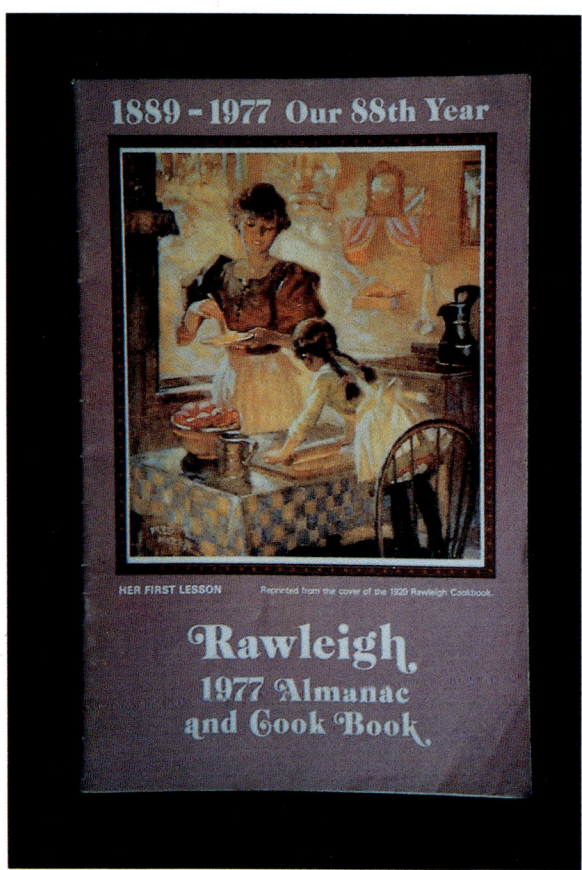

Rawleigh 88th Year, 34 page 1977 Almanac and Cook Book. Cover photograph is reprinted from the cover of the 1920 Rawleigh Cookbook. ©1976 by The W.T. Rawleigh Co., Freeport, IL 61032. *Bushue Collection.* $5-$10.

The Year 1979

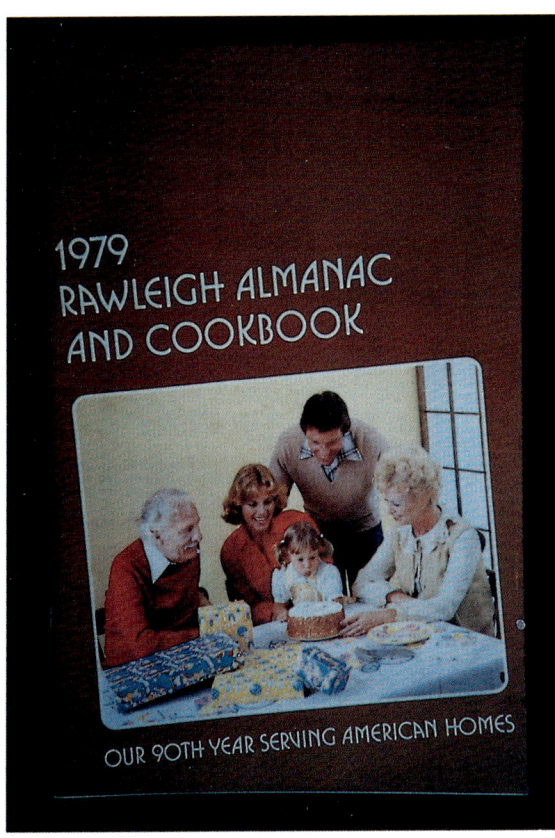

Rawleigh 90th Year 35 page 1979 Rawleigh Almanac and Cookbook. *Bushue Collection.* $5-$10.

The Year 1980

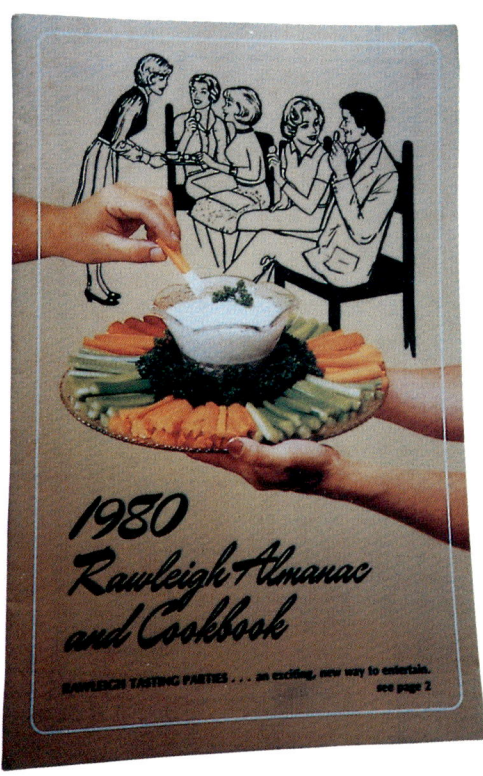

"Many Rawleigh distributors and customers are benefiting from an exciting new way to share the delicious taste of Rawleigh food products. We call it a Tasting Party. It's a unique opportunity to enjoy the company of friends and experience the many flavor sensations of Rawleigh food products. It's really very easy! As a Tasting Party hostess you invite a number of your friends and neighbors to your home to sample a variety of Rawleigh foods and discover the superior quality and many uses they offer. Your Rawleigh distributor does all the party preparation; even helps you make up your guest list."

"You can receive valuable gifts for being a Tasting Party hostess. And you'll be sharing a wonderful time with others. Sound like fun? It is! Your Rawleigh distributor will be glad to explain more about Tasting Parties. Why not ask today?" *Rawleigh 1980.*

See "Rawleigh Tasting Party" in Miscellaneous Documents in this Chapter.

The Year 1981

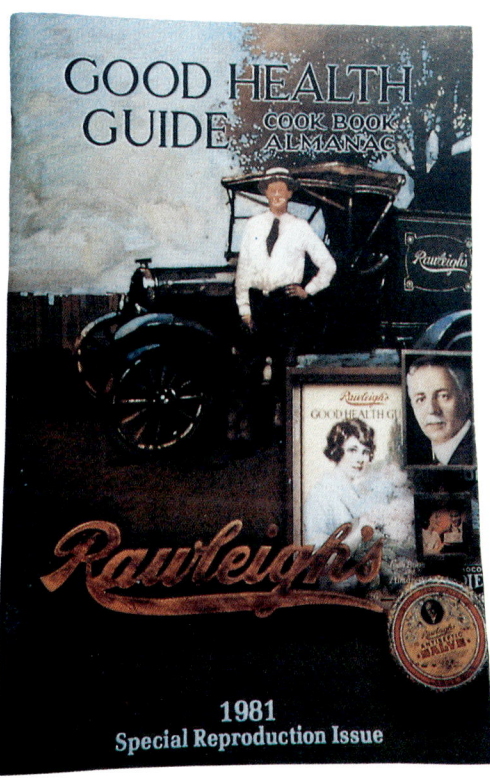

Rawleigh's 34 page Special Reproduction Issue Good Health Guide Cookbook Almanac. ©1924/1980. This 1981 guide contains pages from the 1925 edition and is sought by Rawleigh collectors. The 1925 and 1981 calendar have identical dates. The cover is an original by Tom Bookwalter, an Iowa artist. The original hung in the lobby of the Freeport headquarters; present whereabouts is unknown. *Bushue Collection.* $10-$15.

The Years 1982 - 1989

Issues not available. $10-$15 ea.

Rawleigh 35 page 1980 Almanac and Cookbook. ©1979 by The W.T. Rawleigh Company, Freeport, IL. 61032. *Bushue Collection.* $5-$10.

Cookbooks

As early as 1900, The W.T. Rawleigh Company published several selected recipes for the benefit of the thousands of customers they had at that time. The majority of recipes were part of their yearly Rawleigh Almanac. I have provide only those cookbooks that have been made available to me.

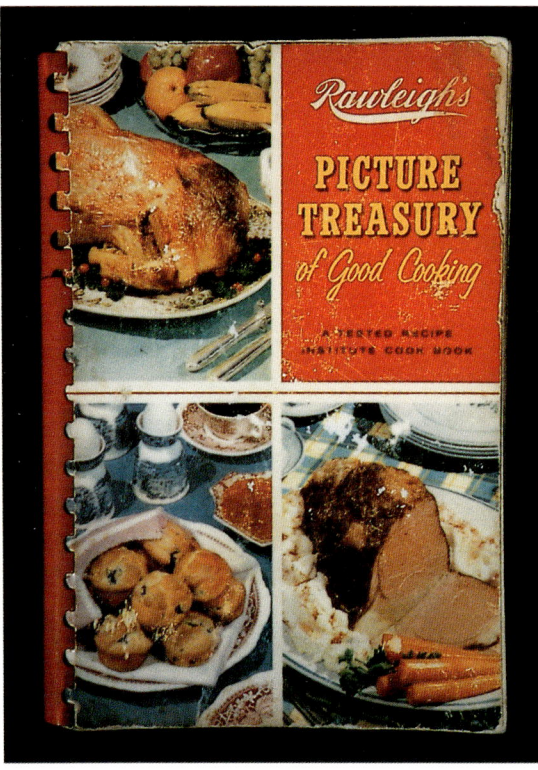

"Rawleigh's Picture Treasury of Good Cooking A Tested Recipe Institute Cook Book For The W.T. Rawleigh Company Freeport, Illinois. © 1959 by Tested Recipe Institute, Inc." Plastic spiral bound, 128 pages, 104 colored photographs, approximately 6-1/4" x 9". *Dupler Collection.* $40-$50.

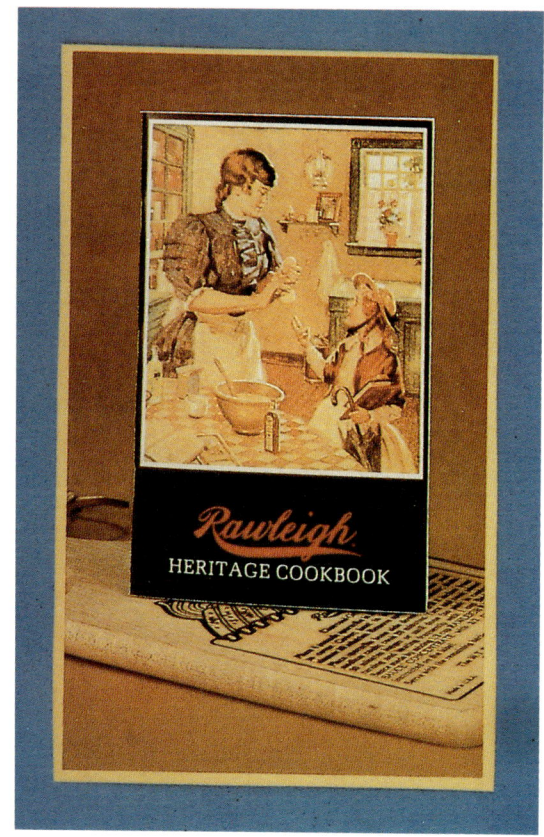

Rawleigh's Heritage Cookbook was an award winning cookbook containing recipes in every category from soups to pies and cookies. It was available during the mid-1980s and sold for $4.95. Rawleigh's Heritage Cookbook was also offered as part of a gift set during the mid-1980s, shown elsewhere in this publication. This Cookbook was still available in 1991 through Golden Pride International. $10-$15.

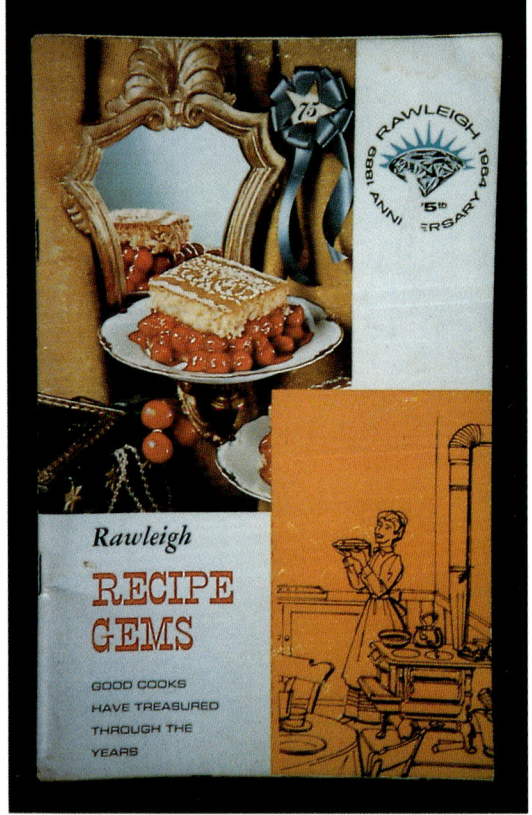

In honor of their 75th Anniversary, Rawleigh included several treasured recipes from the past which had been requested by generations of Rawleigh customers. This 55-page 5-1/4" x 8-1/2" "Rawleigh Recipes Gems" provide cooks with those treasured recipes. © The W.T. Rawleigh Company, Freeport, Illinois, 1964. $20-$30.

Highly sought by collectors is the Golden Pride International Heritage Plate. These limited edition collector's plates portray the Golden Pride International tradition of quality products brought to the home. Golden Pride International offered two plates; a gold edge with black back stamp and a gold edge with gold back stamp. The black back stamp sold for $59.95; the gold back stamp sold for $139.95 in 1991. These plates were only available through a Golden Pride/Rawleigh Independent Distributor. Photograph not available. $175-$200 ea.

Calendars

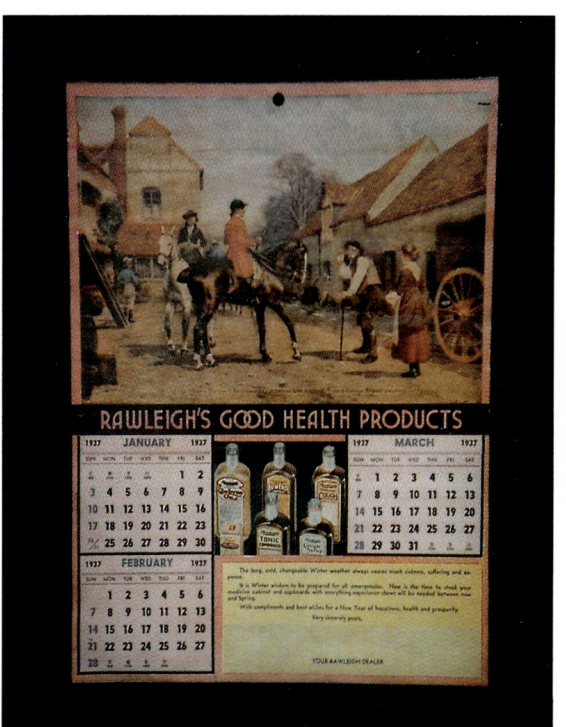

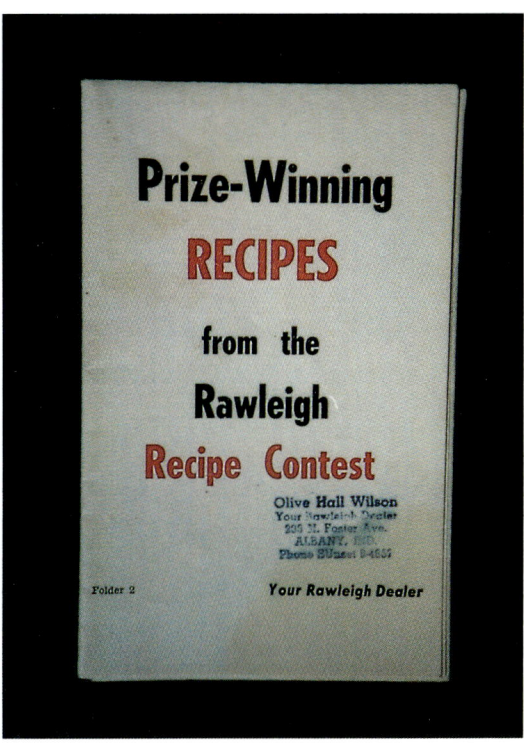

"Prize-Winning Recipes from the Rawleigh Recipe Contest." The is marked Folder 2. A selection of customer recipes were provided inside. *Dupler Collection.* $5-$10.

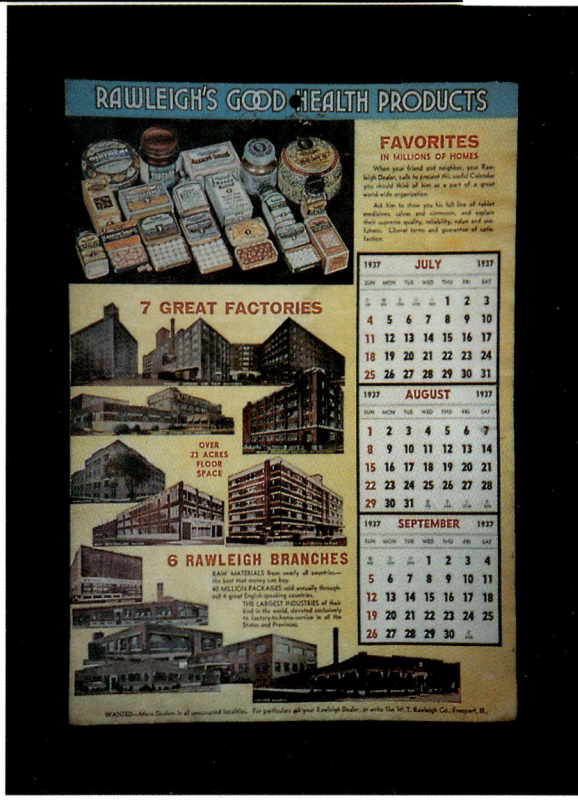

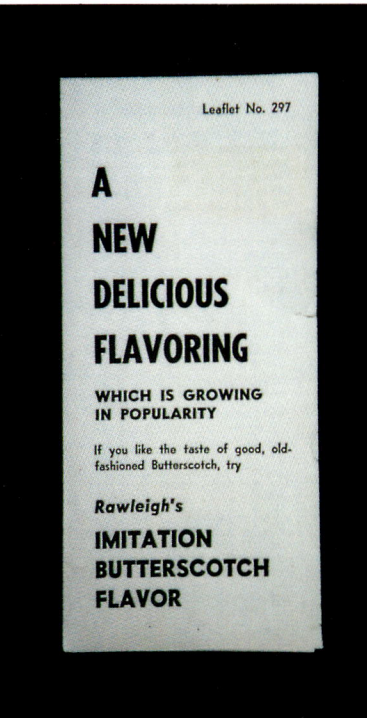

"A New Delicious Flavoring Which Is Growing In Popularity" This Leaflet No. 297 promoted Rawleigh's Imitation Butterscotch Flavor. *Dupler Collection.* $5-$10.

Rawleigh's Good Health Products 1937 Calendar. January through March appears with "The Old Huntsman's Story," a familiar scene in England taken from a famous English painting. April through June appears with "A Venetian Wedding." July through September appears with seven great Rawleigh factories and six Rawleigh branches. October through December appears with a copy of a mosaic, representing an Italian shoemaker whose wife is reading to him. W.T. Rawleigh also appears in this section. *Dupler Collection.* $75-$100.

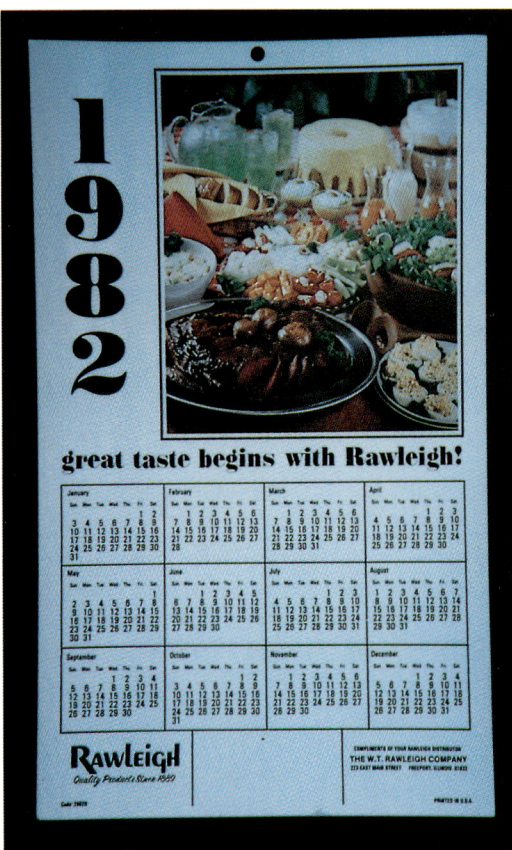

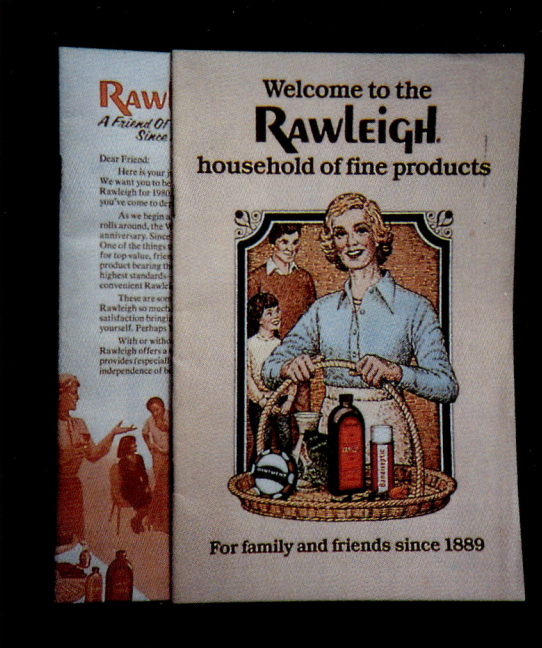

Two Rawleigh 19 page 1980 Shopping Guides. Both guides are identical, with the exception that the right one is missing the additional cover. ©1980 The W.T. Rawleigh Company Freeport, Illinois 61032. *Bushue and Dupler Collection.* $10-$15 ea.

Rawleigh's 8-1/2" x 14" single sided 1982 Calendar, "Compliments of your Rawleigh Distributor The W.T. Rawleigh Company, 223 East Main Street Freeport, Illinois 61032." *Dupler Collection.* $5-$10.

In September 1987, the new '88 Rawleigh calendar was available. It was the perfect "thank-you" gift for retail customers. The 11" x 17" calendar featured the same illustration used on the cover of the new Rawleigh Shopper's Guide. Photograph not available. $5-$10.

Miscellanoues Documents

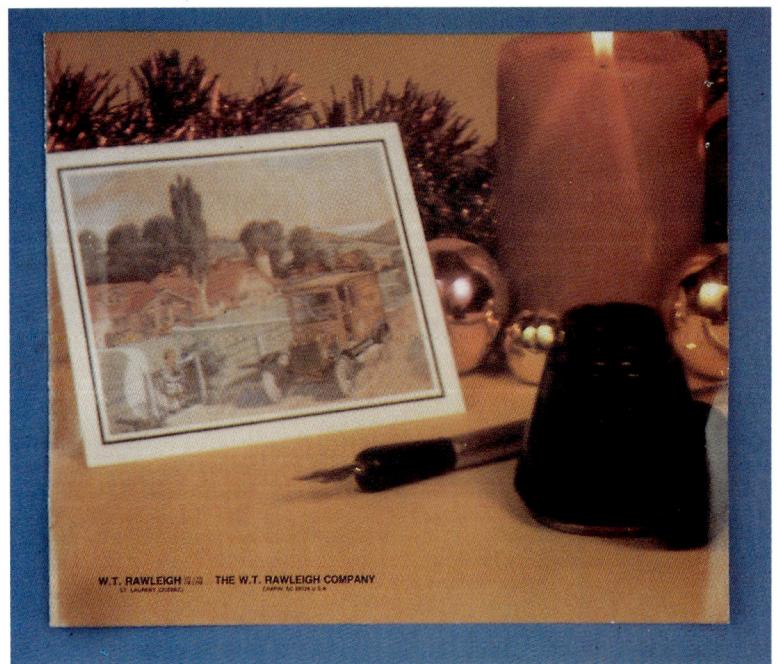

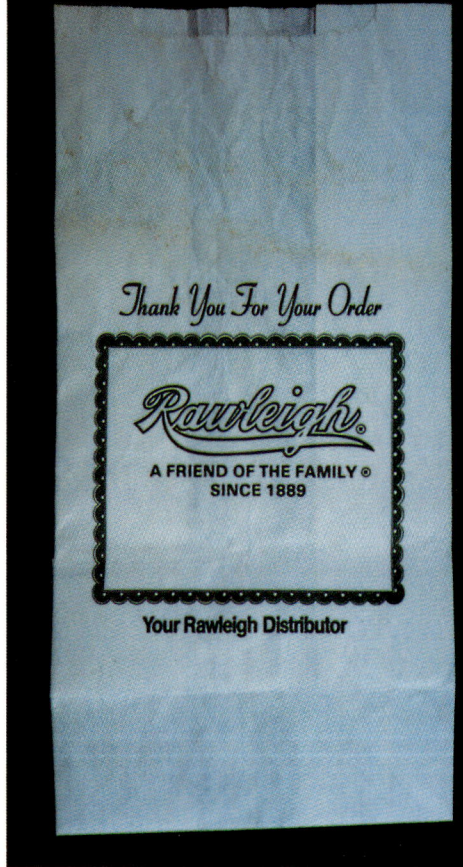

This delivery bag was used to deliver Rawleigh merchandise to customers. Approximately 7" x 13-3/4", delivery bags are available in various sizes. *Dupler Collection.* $2-$4.

An original advertisement for Rawleigh "Limited Edition" note cards that featured illustrations from the 1925 Rawleigh Almanac & Good Health Guide on the front and recipes from the 1935 edition on the back. These nostalgic cards came with their own envelopes and were packaged in boxes of 25. Circa 1987. $10-$15 complete.

Below is the original text that appears on the cover, shown on the left in this photograph.

"Here is your just-off-the-press 1980 Rawleigh Shopping Guide. We want you to be among the first to see all that's new and exciting in Rawleigh for 1980, along with all the fine Rawleigh products which you've come to depend on through the years."

"As we begin a new decade, it occurs to us that, before another one rolls around, the W.T. Rawleigh Company will have celebrated its 100th anniversary. Since 1889, our Rawleigh family has grown world-wide. One of the things that brings us all together is our common appreciation for top value, friendly service and trust. That will never change. Every product bearing the Rawleigh name will always conform to only the highest standards — you can be sure of it. Just as you can be sure of convenient Rawleigh service."

"These are some of the reasons we enjoy our association with Rawleigh so much. In addition to the income it provides, we get real satisfaction bringing Rawleigh's many benefits to nice people like yourself. Perhaps YOU would enjoy such an opportunity yourself."

"With or without previous business experience, you'd find that Rawleigh offers a wonderful opportunity. Not only for the income it provides (especially welcome in these inflationary times), but also for the independence of being your own boss — owning your business. And . . . there's no better time than right now to join Rawleigh because we've just introduced an appealing new concept that's really catching on. It's the Rawleigh Tasting Party, and it's making the Rawleigh opportunity more profitable and downright fun than ever before. The idea is that you arrange with hostesses to have Tasting Parties. They invite their friends and neighbors, and you bring the Rawleigh goodies. Once the guests get a taste of Rawleigh's flavor magic, they usually want to buy, and you're busy taking orders. See what we mean about the fun of being Rawleigh Distributors these days? When we go to "work," we go to a party. And get paid for it!"

"There's a lot more we can tell you about the benefits of being a Rawleigh Distributor . . . how you can start earning extra money for yourself right now and build toward a solid, long-term future of greater independence and security. And enjoy yourself while doing it."

"How about you? Would you like more of the good things of life? We'll show you an exciting way you can get them for yourself and in a pleasant, dignified and respected business based on a worthwhile service to others. Believe us, it's worth your consideration!"

"We'll look forward to serving you in 1980, and if you wish, we'll discuss Rawleigh Tasting Parties and distributor opportunities with you."

"Meanwhile, thank you very much for shopping with us, and now, enjoy your 1980 Rawleigh Shopping Guide; then give me a call." *Rawleigh Shopping Guide 1980.*

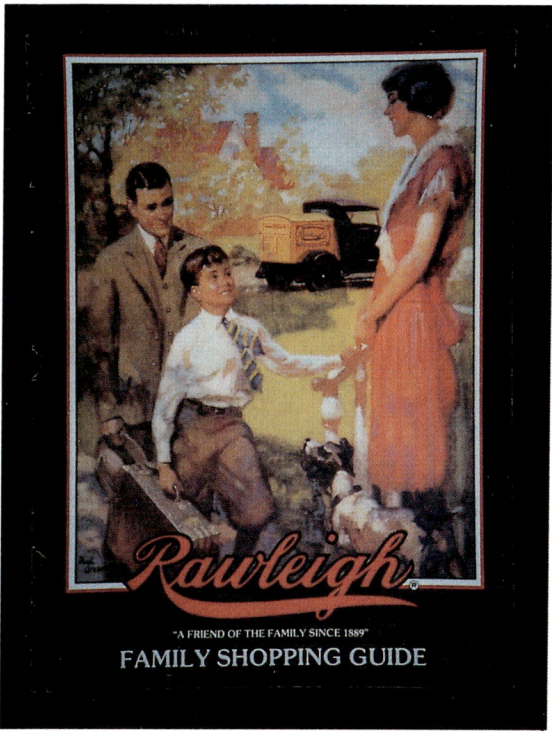

"Rawleigh 1985 Family Shopping Guide." Twenty-three pages approximately 8-1/2" x 11"; this guide featured famous health aids, spices and extracts, household, personal care, food and pet care products. ©1985 The W.T. Rawleigh Company Freeport, Illinois 61032 U.S.A. *Bushue Collection.* $5-$10.

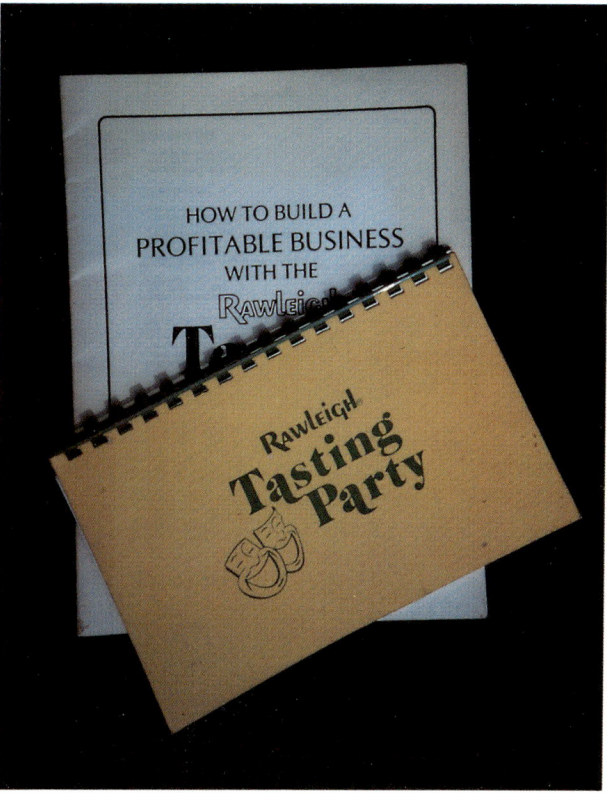

"Rawleigh Tasting Party" and "How To Build A Profitable Business with Rawleigh Tasting Party". This lecture was provided to independent dealers to use as a guide in developing a Rawleigh Tasting Party business in their own community. It was a unique method of appeal and beneficial to all participants. The guide and accompanying materials included a step-by-step format that could be put into immediate use. ©1979 The W.T. Rawleigh Co. *Bushue Collection.* $10-$15 ea.

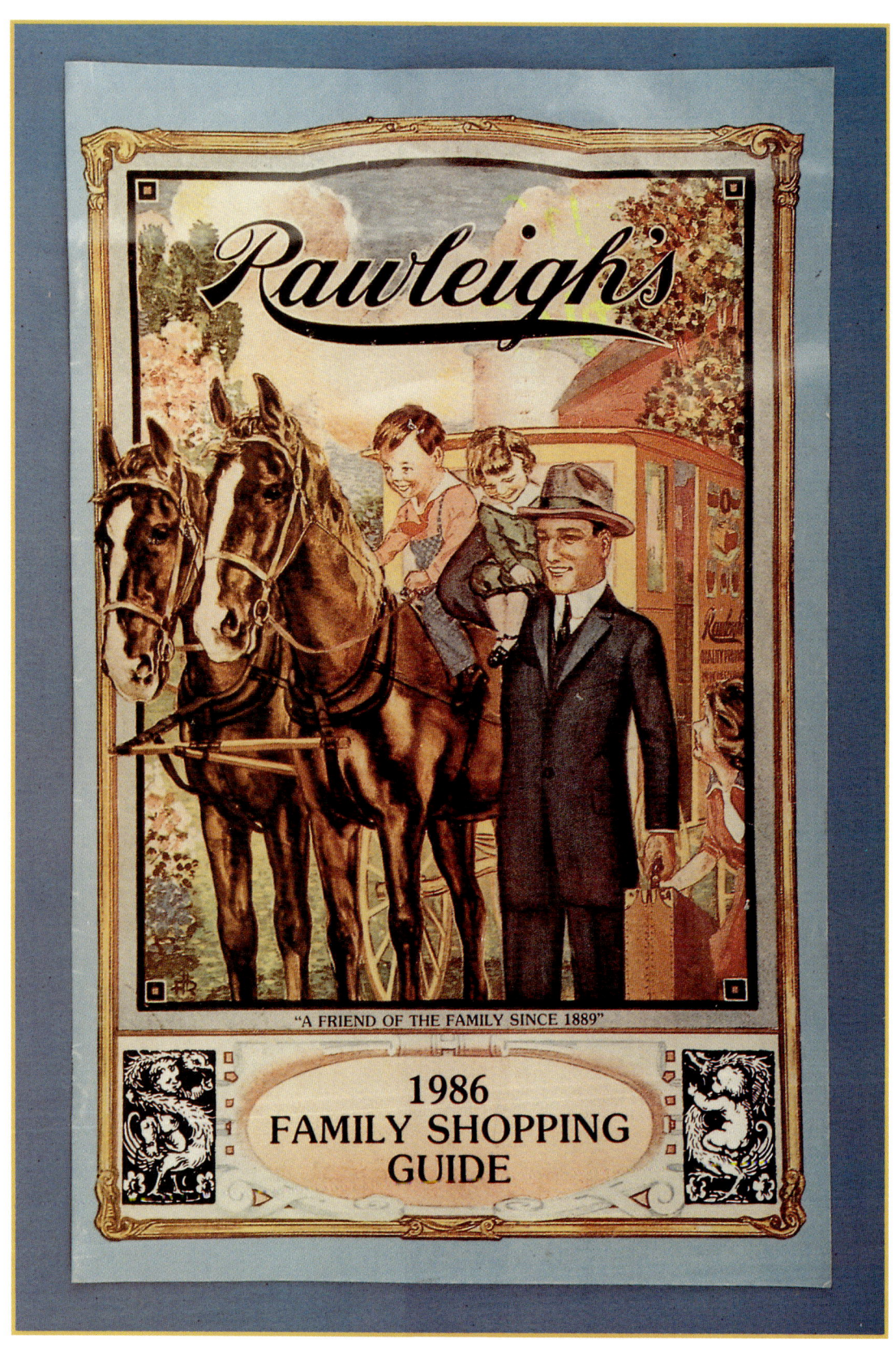

Rawleigh's 31 page 1986 Family Shopping Guide. *Bushue Collection.* $5-$10.

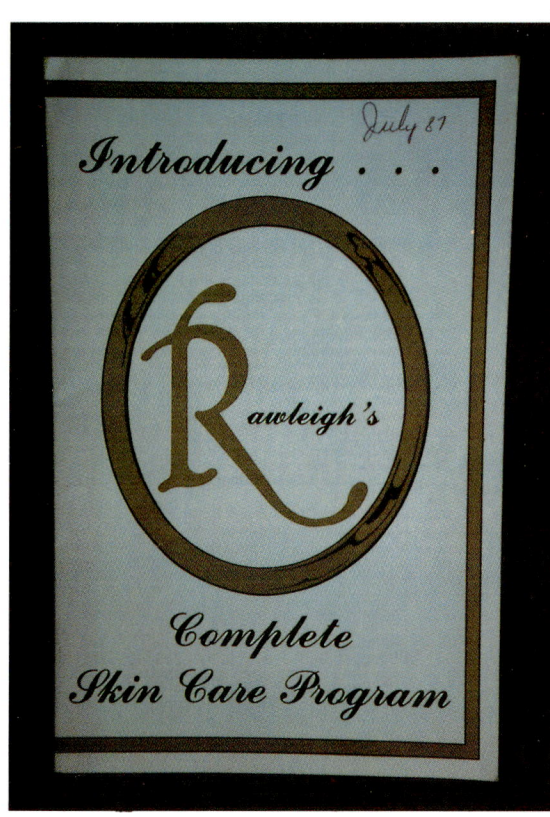

"Introducing Rawleigh's Complete Skin Care Program" booklet. A variety of Rawleigh cleansing products were promoted in this booklet. Someone has written in pen the date of July '87. *Bushue Collection.* $5-$10.

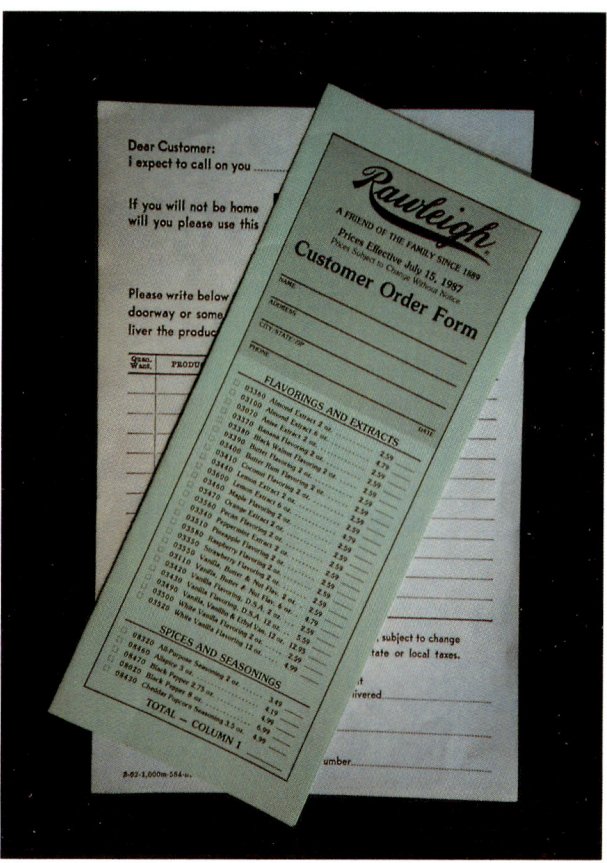

Two different Rawleigh customer order forms. Circa 1962 and 1987. *Dupler Collection.* $5-$10 ea.

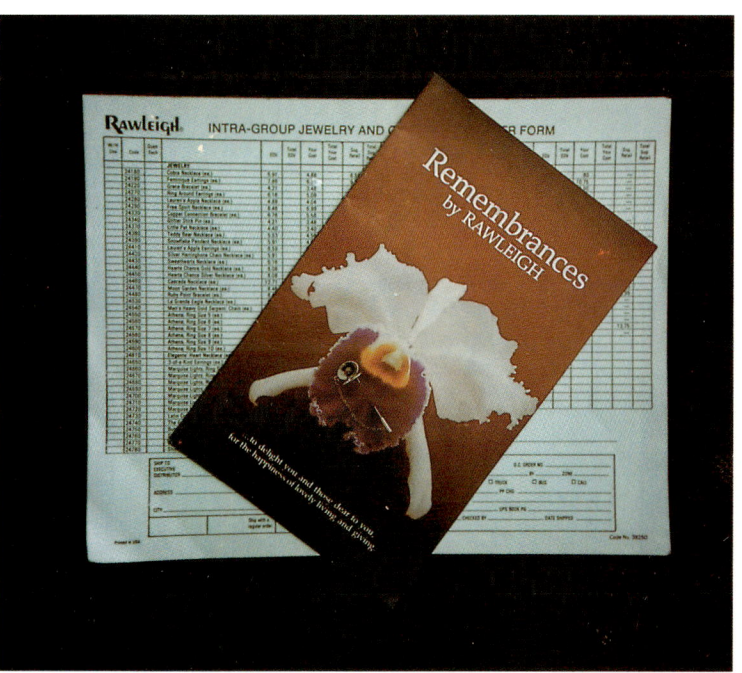

"Remembrances by Rawleigh" booklet and a pad of original Rawleigh "Intra-Group Jewelry and Other Gifts Order Form." ©1979 The W.T. Rawleigh Co. *Dupler Collection.* $15-$20 ea.

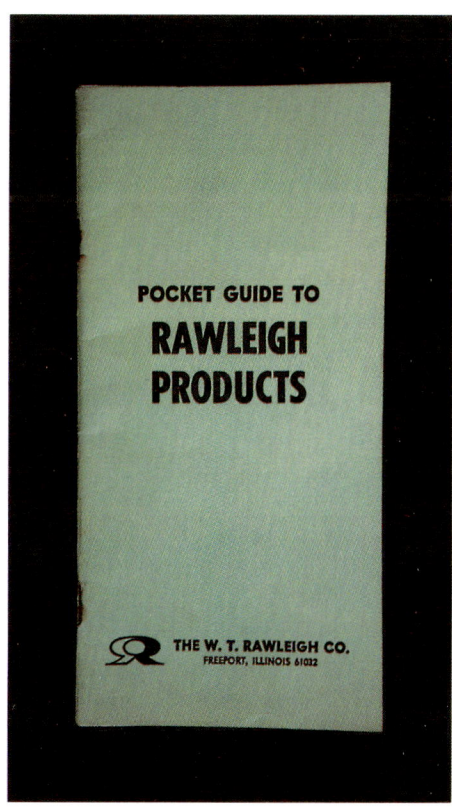

"Pocket Guide to Rawleigh Products." This guide provided condensed descriptions of Rawleigh products that helped dealers to learn important points about each item. Circa 1970s. *Dupler Collection.* $15-$20.

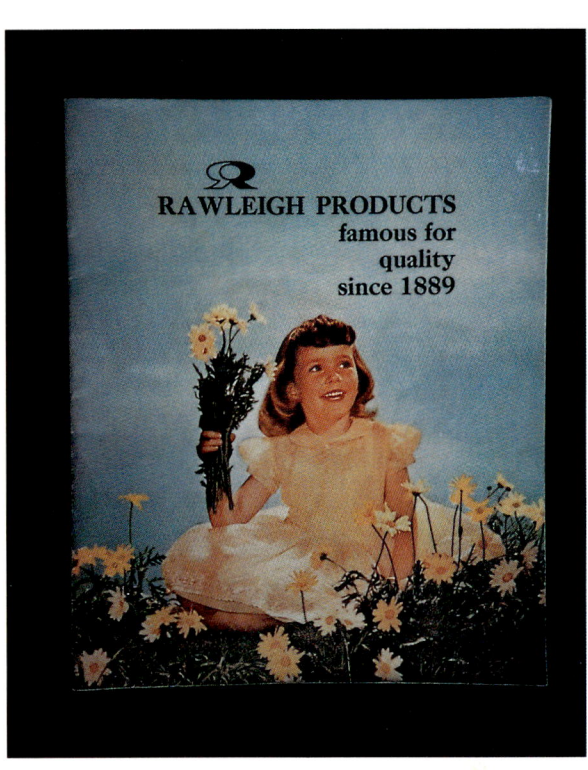

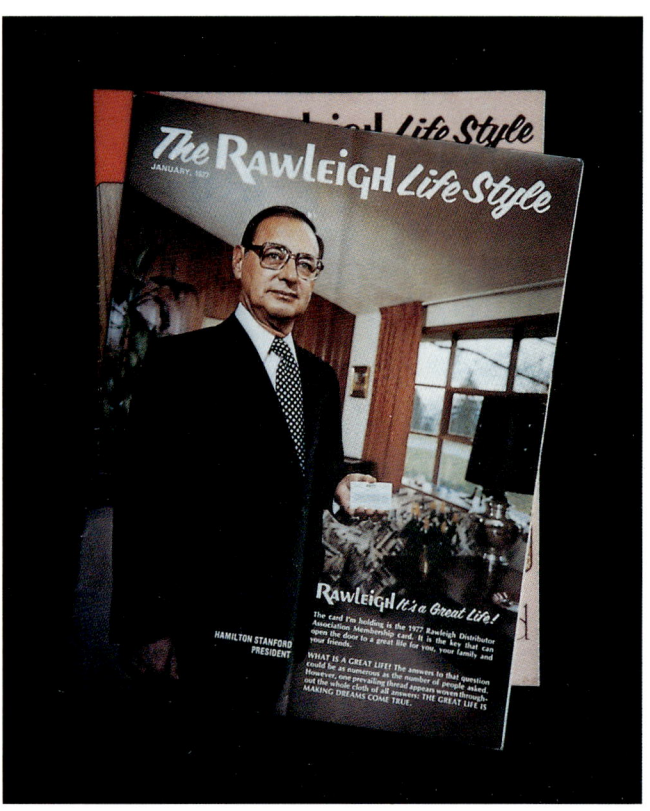

"Rawleigh Products famous for quality since 1889." Approximately 8-1/2" x 10-1/4" with 24 pages of Rawleigh products. Circa 1960s. *Dupler Collection.* $15-$20.

Issues of "The Rawleigh Life Style" January 1977 and April 1979. © The W.T. Rawleigh Co. Life Style was a publication available to Rawleigh dealers showing in photographs and stories how other dealers were making their dreams come true through their Rawleigh business. *Bushue Collection.* $8-$10 ea.

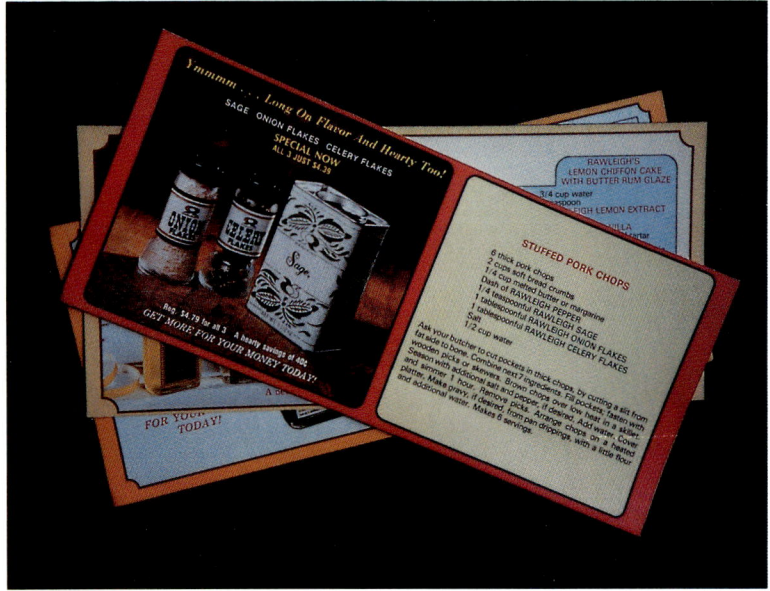

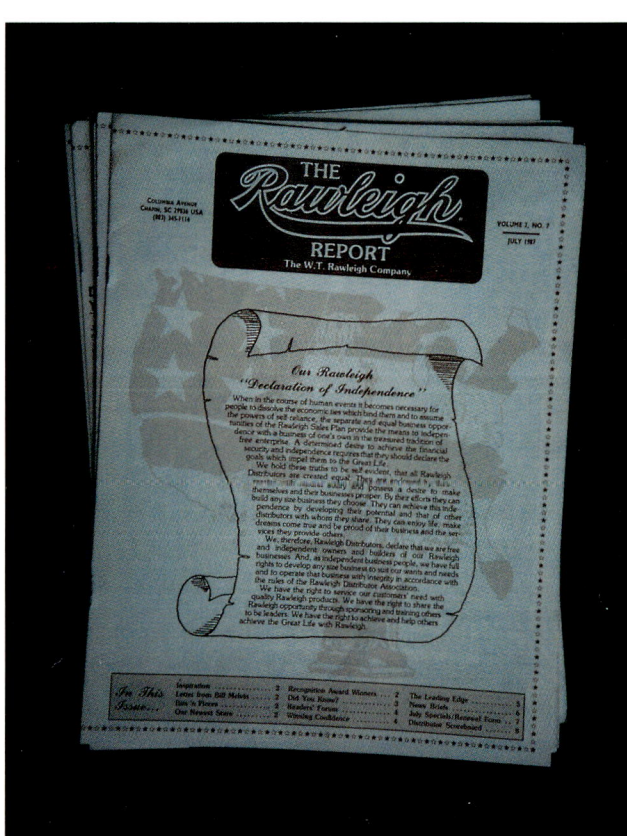

This series of flyers could be mailed directly to a customer's residence or hand delivered. Folded three times various Rawleigh products were promoted inside and out on each flyer. Circa 1970s. *Bushue Collection.* $3-$5 ea.

"The Rawleigh Report" a monthly publication to independent dealers. *Bushue Collection.* $8-$10.

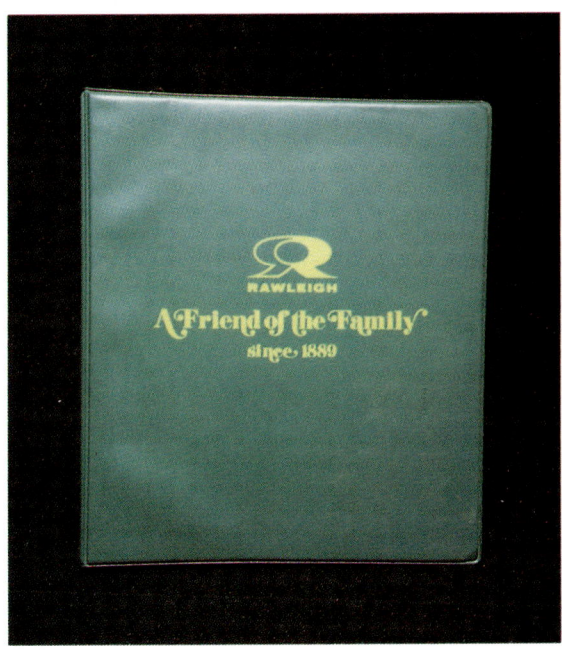

Rawleigh provided an array of modern sales aids and literature. These sales tools were designed to help show the benefits of Rawleigh products and to help explain the Rawleigh opportunity to others. The green plastic ledger was one of the tools available to dealers. *Bushue Collection.* $15-$20.

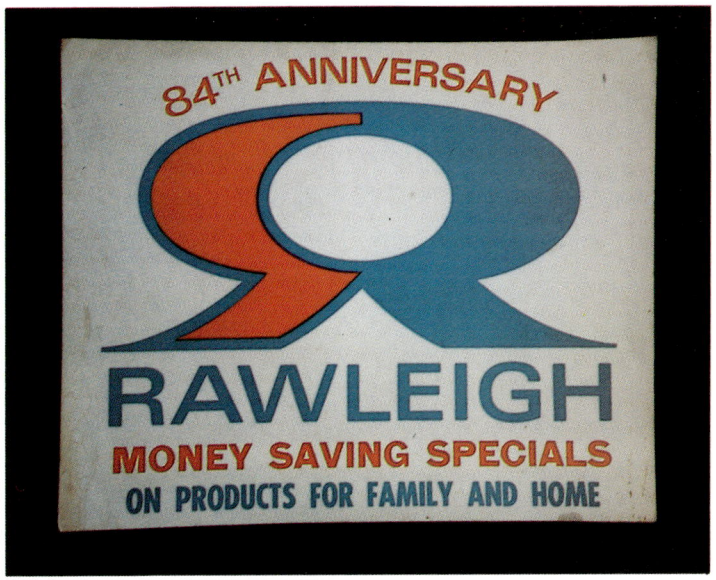

The 8-3/4" x 11" "84th ANNIVERSARY RAWLEIGH" sign could be fasten on the inside of the dealer's car window. 1973. $15-$20.

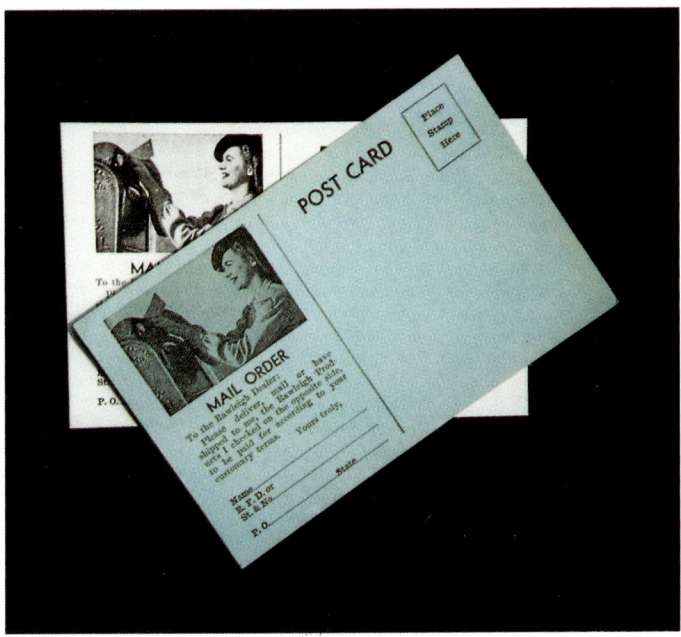

These postcards could be mailed directly to a Rawleigh Dealer. Instructions were provided on one side to "Deliver, mail or have shipped to me, the Rawleigh Products I checked on the opposite side, to be paid for according to your customary terms." Circa 1951. $20-$25 ea.

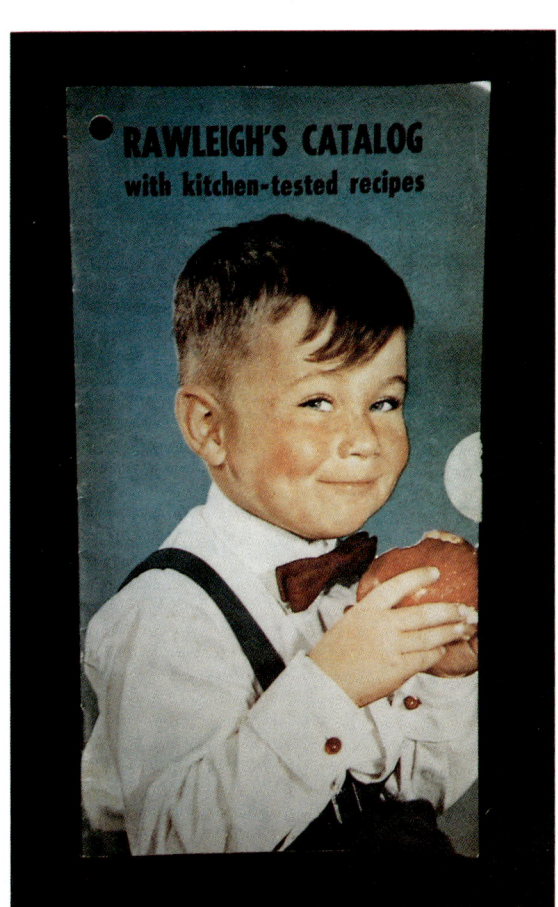

"Rawleigh's Catalog with kitchen-tested recipes." *Dupler Collection.* $15-$20.

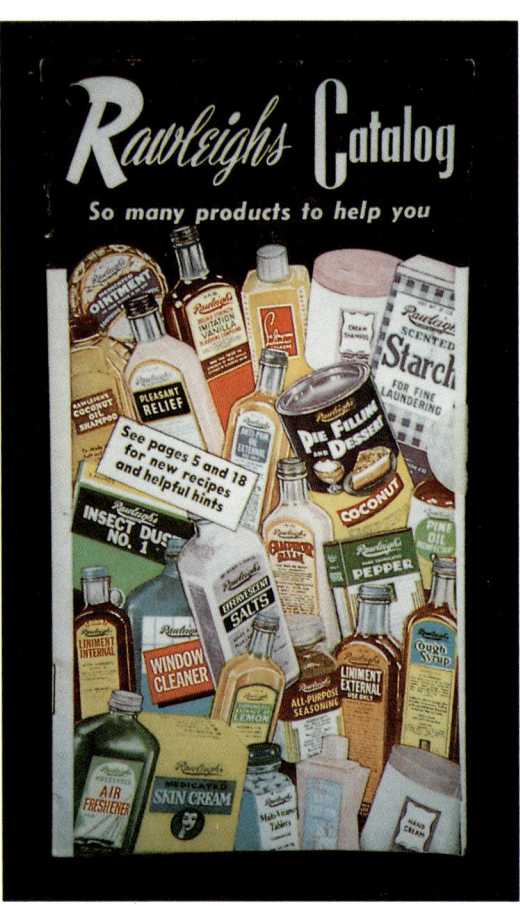

"Rawleigh's Catalog So many products to help you." *Dupler Collection.* $15-$20.

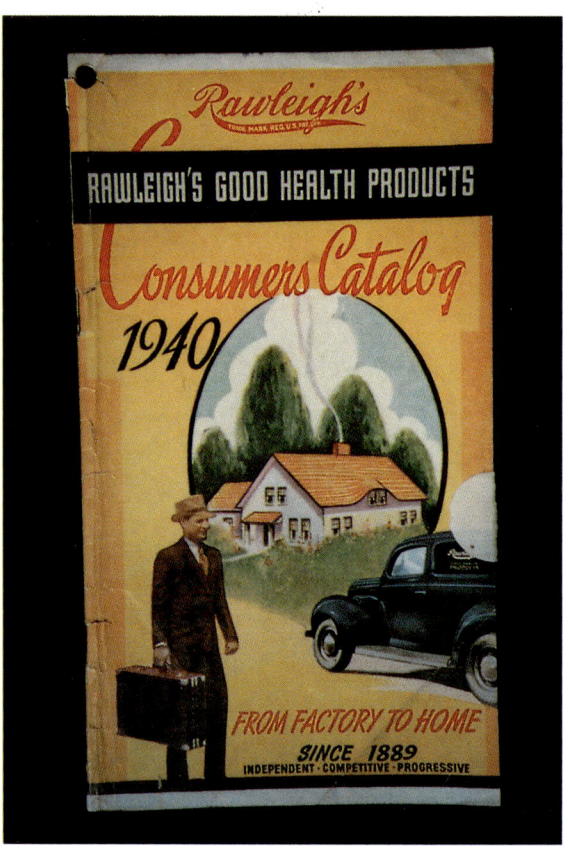

"Rawleigh Good Health Products 1940 Consumers Catalog." *Dupler Collection.* $15-$20.

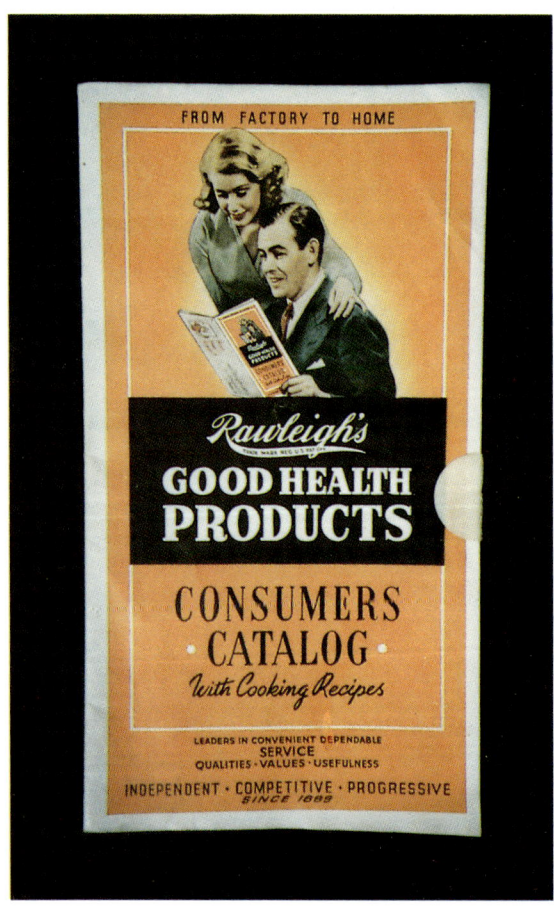

"Rawleigh's Good Health Products Consumers Catalog with Cooking Recipes." *Dupler Collection.* $15-$20.

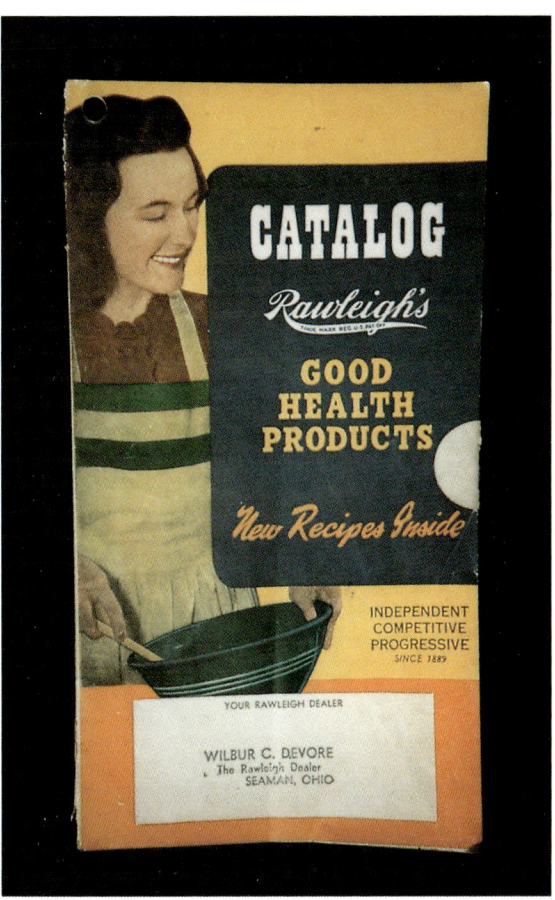

"Rawleigh's Good Health Products Catalog New Recipes Inside." *Dupler Collection.* $15-$20.

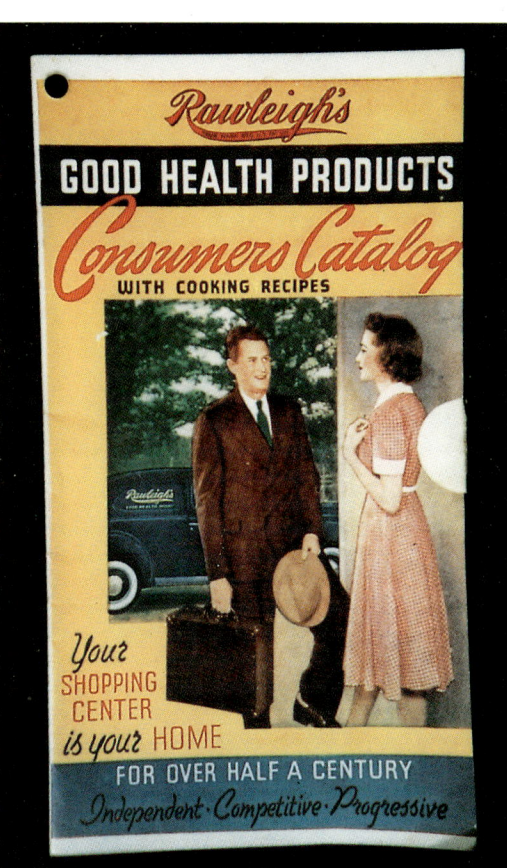

"Rawleigh's Good Health Products Consumers Catalog with Cooking Recipes." *Dupler Collection.* $15-$20.

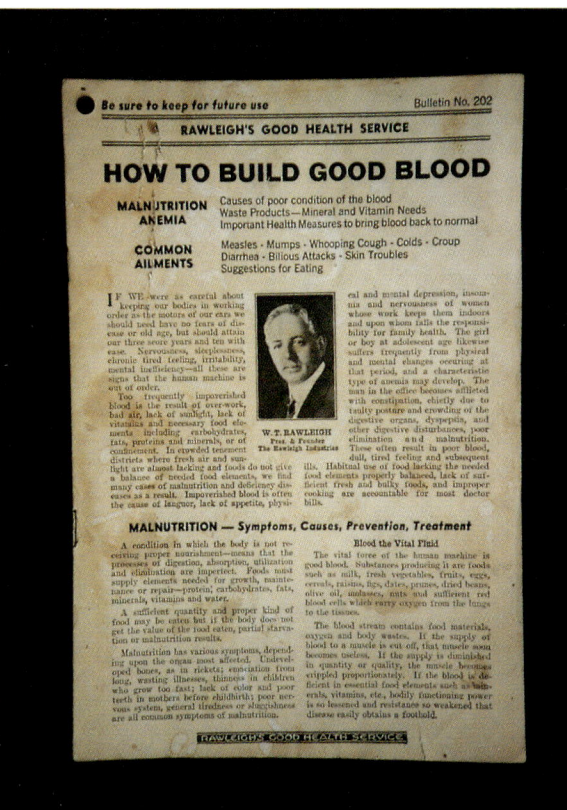

Bulletin No. 202 "How To Build Good Blood." *Dupler Collection.* $15-$20.

Chapter 4. Trading in Foreign Countries

In the beginning, when Rawleigh was small, no foreign buyers were needed. All of the materials required by the company were purchased in the near-by markets.

As the business grew, the demands increased and larger quantities were required. W.T. Rawleigh sought out the domestic importers and producers. As the business expanded nation wide, the company began buying American grown materials direct from producers. They imported camphor and menthol from Japan, essential oils from Sicily, perfume materials and vanilla beans from France and Mexico. Other minor commodities were acquired from other countries.

Rawleigh sent buyers to many foreign countries. In 1921 the largest importation of vanilla beans ever made by an American manufacturer was acquired by Rawleigh.

Rawleigh had business connections and bank accounts in some of the most important foreign trade centers. Rawleigh's substantial financial standing and responsibility were well known.

In 1922, the company imported over 1,500 tons of essential oils, spices, waxes, and materials for making their insecticides and disinfectants, a total value at nearly $700,000 and freights and duties over $50,000.

During 1922, Rawleigh imported from foreign countries over 500 tons of mustard, cloves, ginger, pepper, and other spices. Six-hundred tons of pepper, cinnamon, allspice, nutmegs, and other spices were purchased from importers in domestic markets.

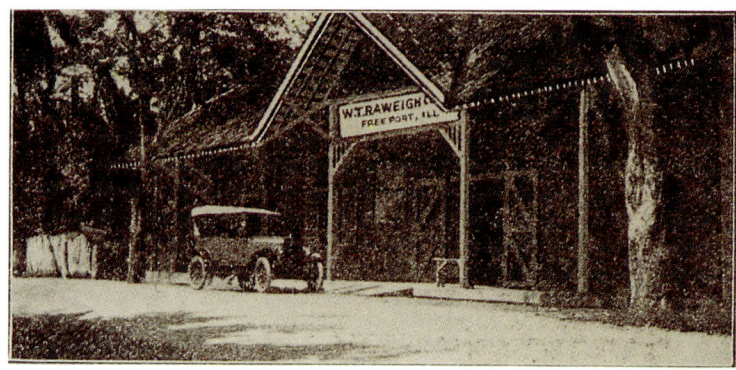

Offices and warehouses in Telok Betong, Sumatra, where the Rawleigh industries bought, inspected, cleaned, and shipped approximately 1000 tons of the best quality Lampong black pepper annually to their factories in the United States, Canada, and Australia.

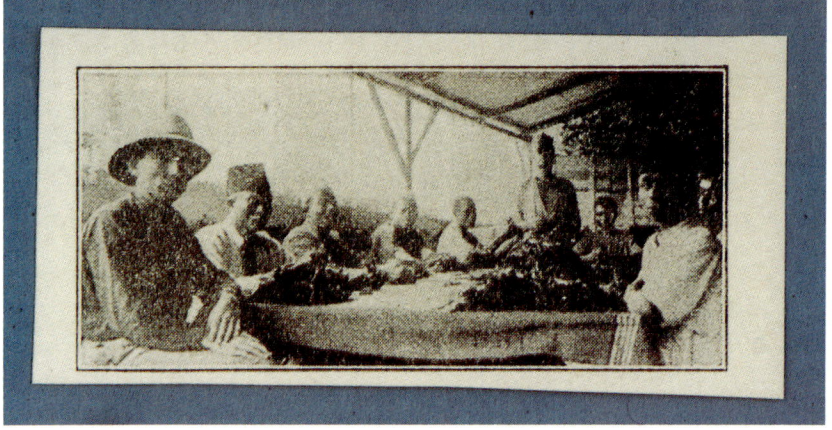

Vanilla beans are being sorted on Rawleigh's Moroi vanilla plantation on the Comore Islands.

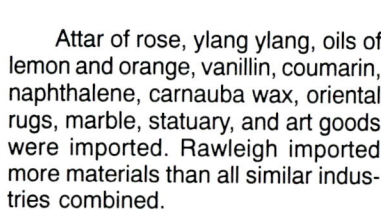

Attar of rose, ylang ylang, oils of lemon and orange, vanillin, coumarin, naphthalene, carnauba wax, oriental rugs, marble, statuary, and art goods were imported. Rawleigh imported more materials than all similar industries combined.

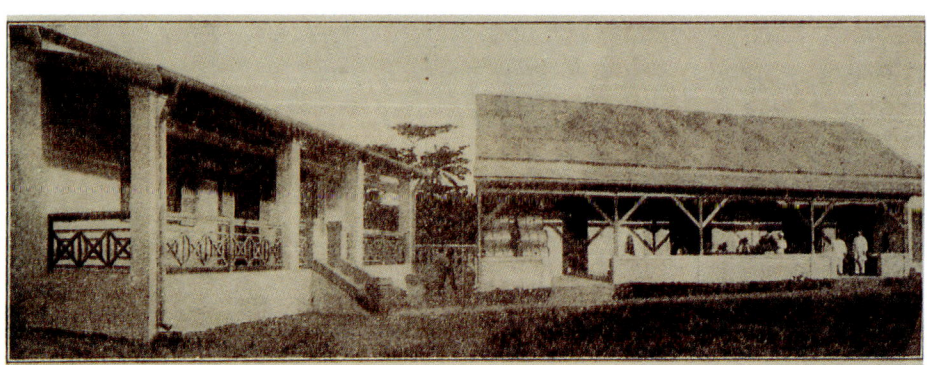

The new Tamative, Madagascar, offices and warehouses were the headquarters of the Rawleigh Industries for buying vanilla, cloves, oil of geranium, ylang ylang, and other raw materials and products in Madagascar, as well as the Comore and Reunion Islands — which are all French colonies located in the Indiana Ocean off the east coast of Africa. In 1931, these islands produced 85% of the world's supply of vanilla.

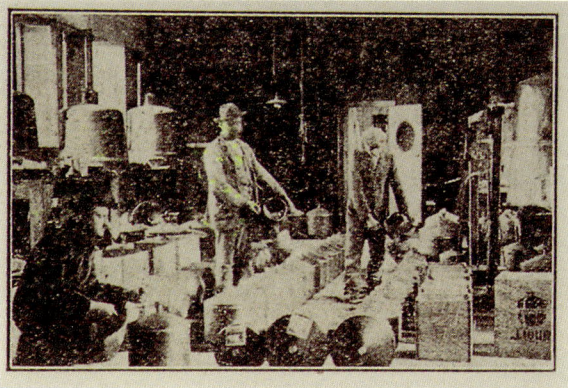

This historical photograph shows how lemon and orange oils are packed into hermetically sealed copper cans and made ready for shipment from Sicily to the Rawleigh industries.

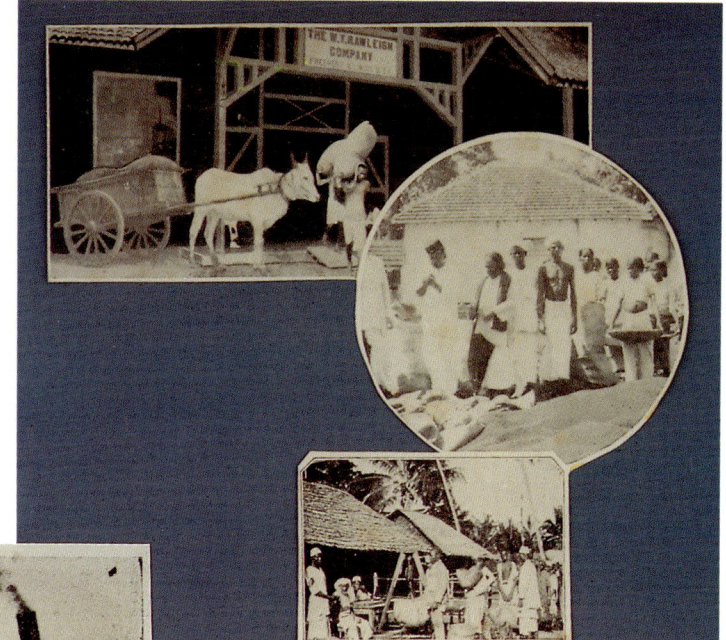

Photographs taken by Rawleigh employees while buying pepper on the Malabar coast of India and the Dutch East Indies, cloves from the Arbas in Zanzibar, vanilla in Madagascar and the Indian Ocean Islands, and caccia in Java and the Far East. Top to bottom: ox-cart in front of Rawleigh's office and warehouse in Sumatra; Rawleigh employees in "garbling" pepper in the Mallbar pepper districts of India; and weighing cloves in Zanzibar.

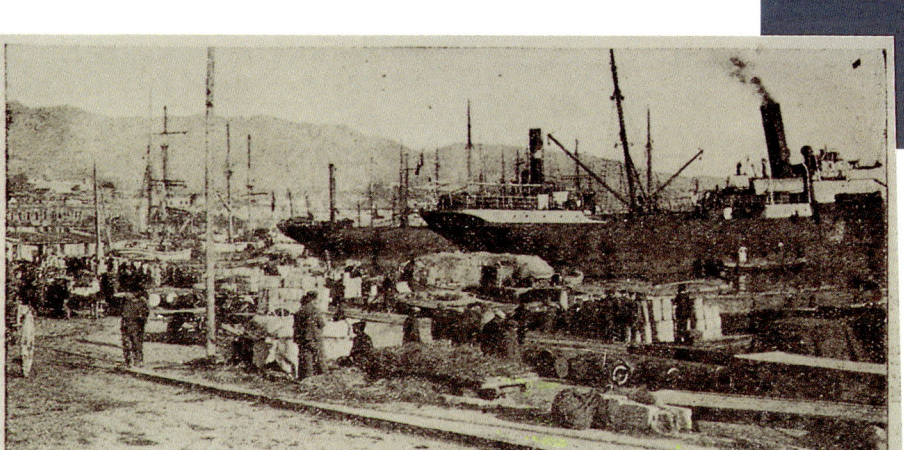

The harbor of Messina, Sicily, where immense quantities of lemon and orange oil used by the Rawleigh industries in making extracts and flavors were shipped to the Rawleigh factories in the United States, Canada, and Australia.

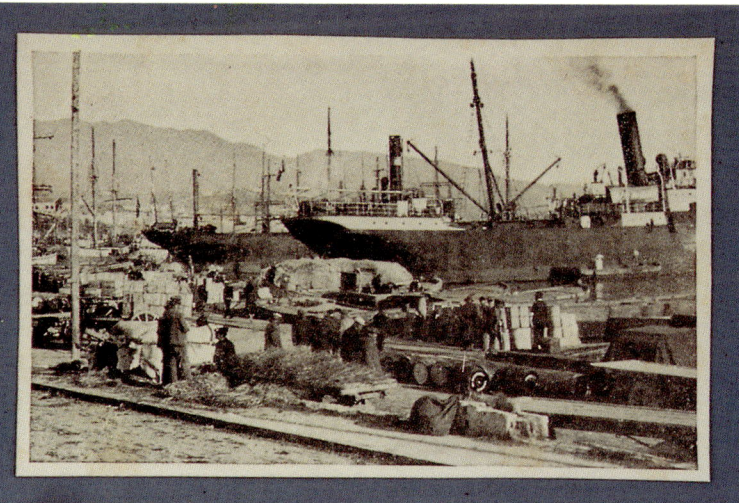

A closer look at the busy scene on the wharf of Messina. Circa 1942.

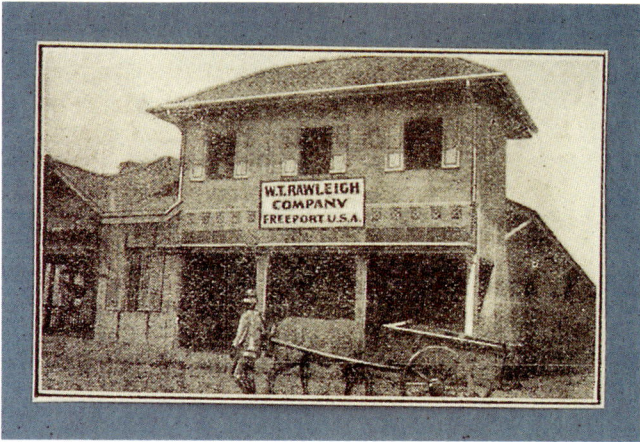

The Rawleigh pepper warehouse at Telok Betong, Sumatra, Java. Circa 1932.

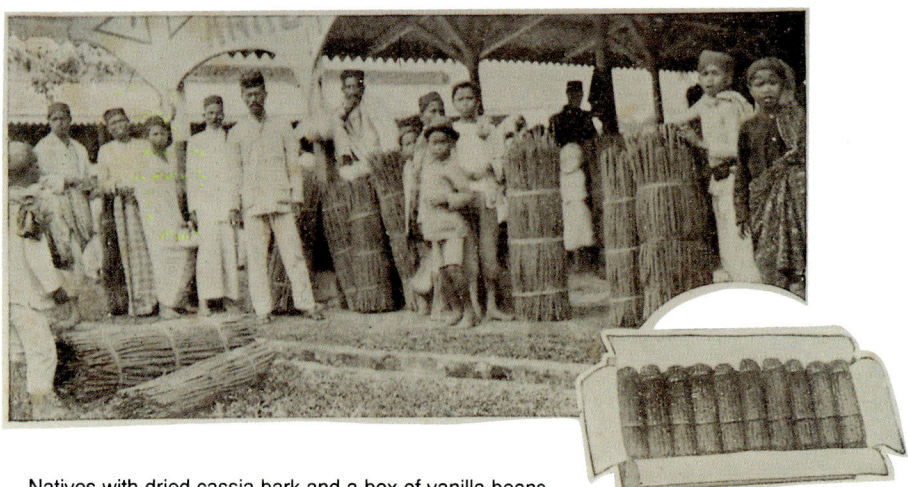

Natives with dried cassia bark and a box of vanilla beans.

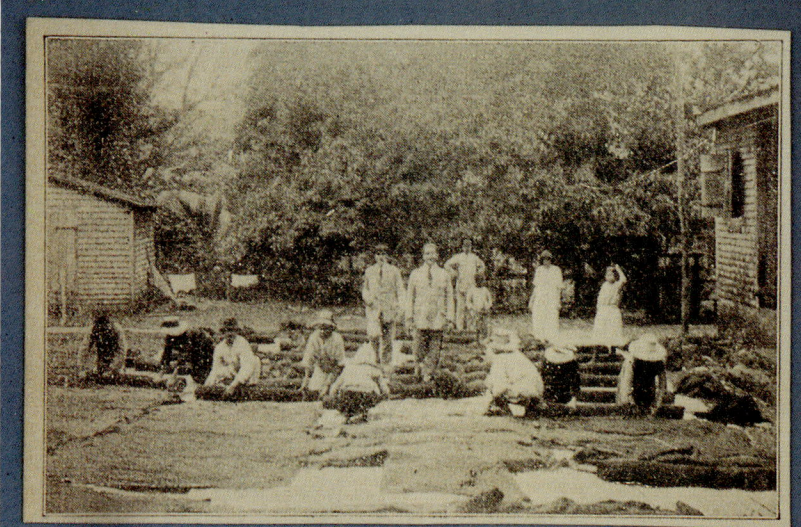

Curing vanilla beans in Madagascar. Circa 1939.

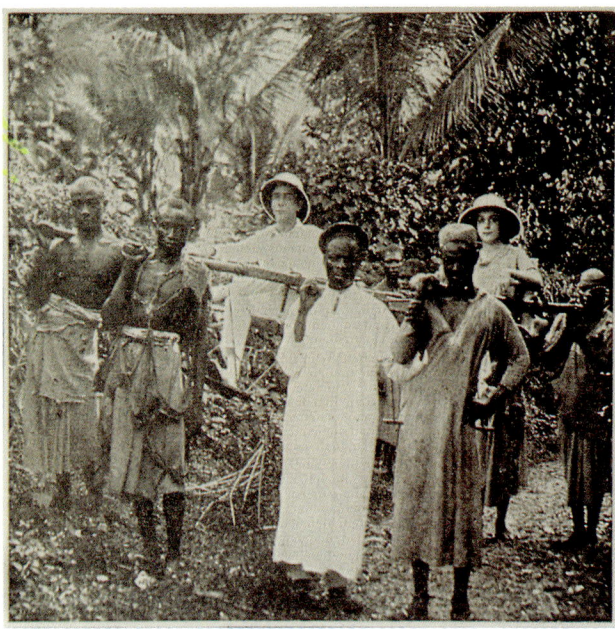

Rawleigh's vanilla plantation and curing house manager and his wife are each carried on a "filanza," a seat suspended on two poles and carried by four natives.

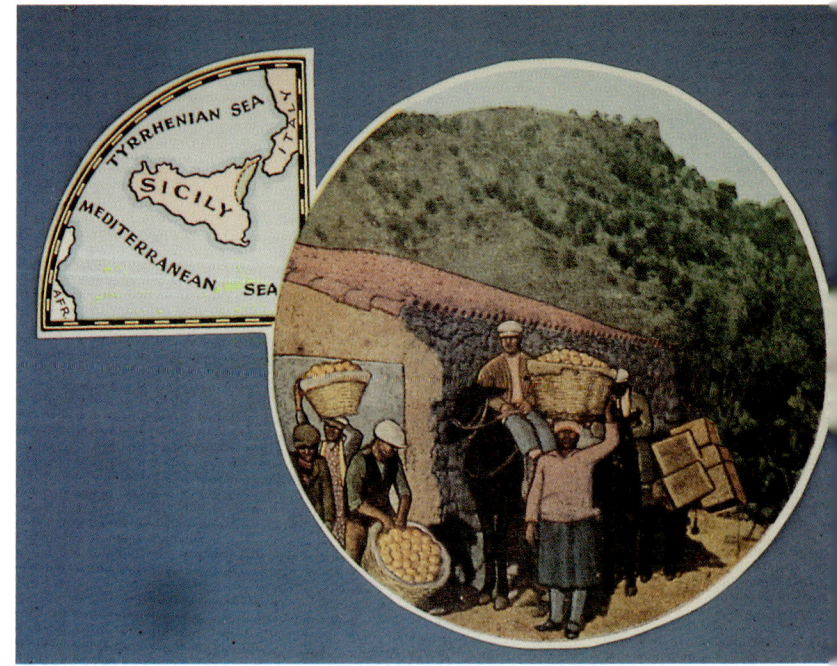

In this illustration, Rawleigh bought oils of lemon and orange in southern Italy.

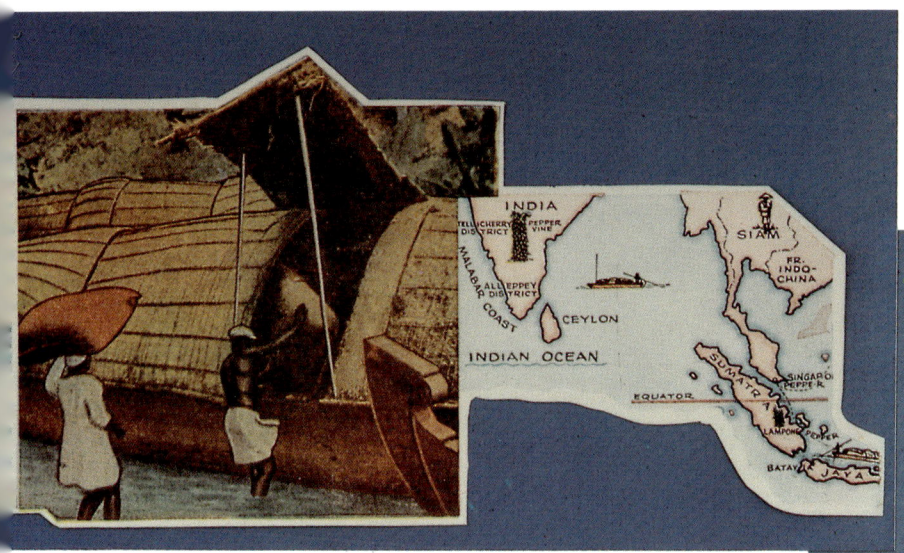

Pepper is loaded on native boats in southeast Sumatra. Rawleigh had a branch warehouse and cleaning mill for years at Telok Bentong.

Tropics to Table

During their journeys to foreign lands in quest of essential oils, vanilla beans, and other materials, Rawleigh buyers encountered "many adventures, hazards, and experiences."

Rawleigh acquired the oils for lemon and orange on the Island of Sicily in the Mediterranean Sea where these fruits are grown in abundance. The oils were taken from the rinds of the fruit by hand and machine, placed into large copper cans, and strapped across the backs of donkeys. Donkeys carried the oils from the interior to the nearest buyers, preparing it for market. It was then sold and exported all over the world.

In 1922, one of Rawleigh's foreign buyers returned from among the islands of the Indian Ocean to Freeport, Illinois, with over 500 cases of vanilla beans. The Rawleigh Company claims that this was the largest importation ever made by an American manufacturer to that time.

This 1922 world record consignment of 37 tons was shipped direct from Madagascar to the Freeport factories in two full carloads. The export and import duties, the ocean and rail freight, and the express charges amounted to over $23,000 dollars.

Securing materials for Rawleigh's extracts and flavors, buyers traveled from America to France through the Mediterranean and Red Sea, down the east coast of Africa to Madagascar and the Reunion Islands, and remained there for over a year. Rawleigh's buyer's watched the culture, growth, and curing of the product. They encountered a mixture of races and color, suffered from the deadly heat, and lived and worked in conditions different from any they had ever known. The most difficult encounter were with those they met who spoke no English; often an interpreter was called in.

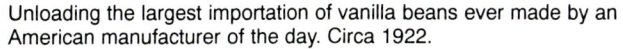

Unloading the largest importation of vanilla beans ever made by an American manufacturer of the day. Circa 1922.

The selection of historical photographs throughout this publication required patience. Old photographs have begun to attract the attention of document collectors and are beginning to escalate in value. Most photographs and/or documents will range from $1 to $100 each. Values are based on the condition of each item, whether the item is an original or a photograph from a magazine, and also on the rarity of the image. Purchase historical photographs whenever possible. Pass the image by once and it may be lost to you forever.

Carefully look the photographs over before buying. With today's high-tech reproduction equipment, it can, at times, be difficult to distinguish real photographs from clever reproductions. Always ask! However, that said, most honest copies are made through a local camera store or studio and are easily recognized by the Kodak™ trademark printed on the reverse side. Always look! There is nothing wrong with purchasing a reproduced photograph ... provided you are aware that you are purchasing a copy of the original image and not the original itself.

Old photographs provide an abundance of historical information. Look carefully, there are still great bargains to be found out there.

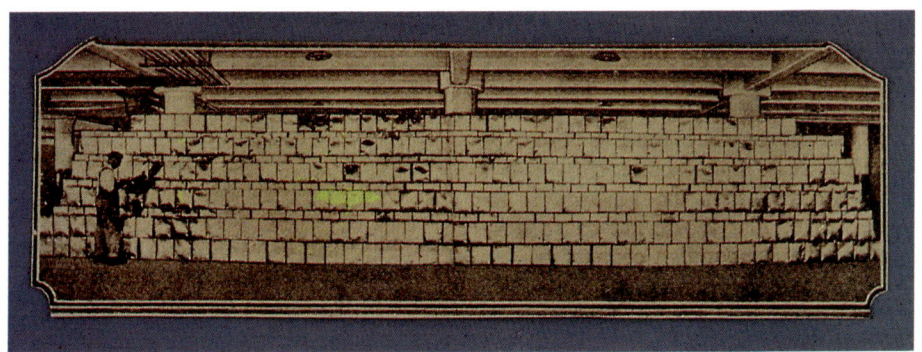

A 6-ton supply of oils of lemon and orange from Sicily. Circa 1922.

Food Products

Chapter 5. Collecting Rawleigh Products

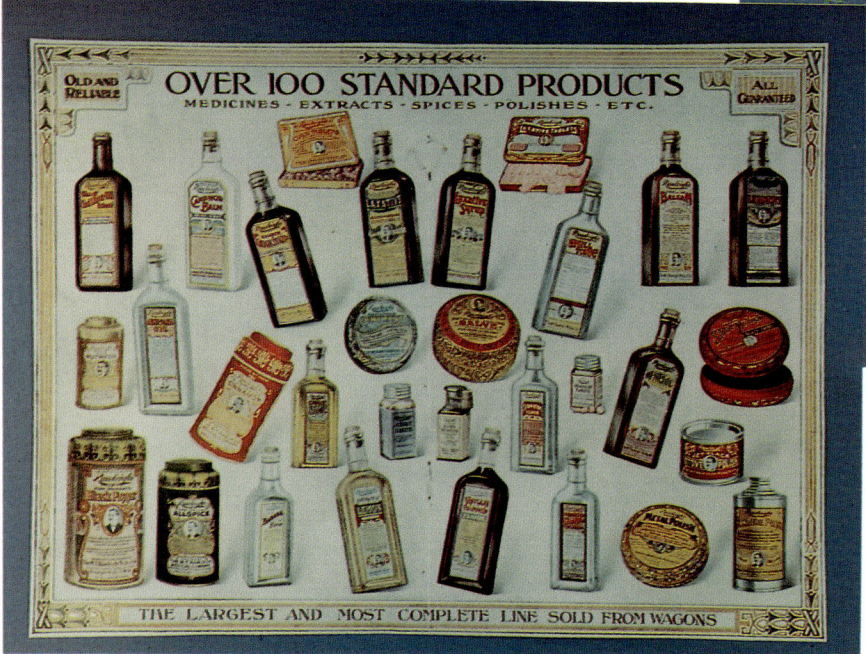

"Over 100 Standard Products" were promoted during 1915 - 1916. According to company literature, this was the largest and most complete line of products sold from wagons.

In 1942, Rawleigh promoted its products as "They're MIGHTY Good for me and my family."

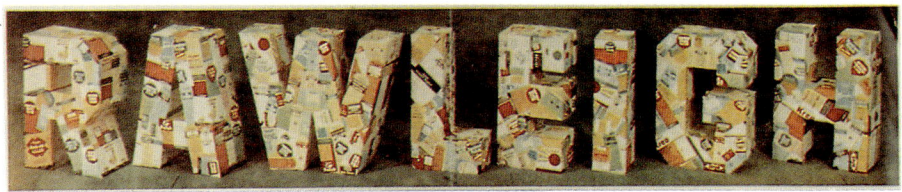

To spell their famous name, Rawleigh's artist used original labels to create the 3-dimension lettering. Circa 1957.

Food products that "gave variety and added attractiveness to the family table" were an interesting part of the necessities brought by the Rawleigh Dealer. Customers were invited to make trials and comparisons with similar preparations for, the Dealer would assert with confidence, this was the easiest way of learning superiority.

It is impossible to provide a complete list or photographs of all Rawleigh Food and Health Products. I have provided those in my own collection or those made available through other sources.

In 1986, the top ten Rawleigh Products were based on their records in both the United States and Canada. These reflected sales during the months of May - December 1986.

In the United States:
- #1.................Home Remedies
- #2.................Extracts/Flavorings
- #3.................Mr. Groom Products (Pet Care Products)
- #4.................Spices/Seasonings
- #5.................Household Products
- #6.................Pie Filling/Dessert Mixes
- #7.................Vitamins
- #8.................Laundry Aids
- #9.................Insecticides
- #10................Personal Care Products

In Canada:
- #1.................Home Remedies
- #2.................Household Products
- #3.................Spices/Seasonings
- #4.................Pie Filling/Dessert Mixes
- #5.................Extracts/Flavorings
- #6.................Mr. Groom Products (Pet Care Products)
- #7.................Laundry Aids
- #8.................Salad Dressing Mixes
- #9.................Insecticides
- #10................Soup Bases

Home Remedies were No. 1 in both the United States and Canada, even after nearly a century.

Baking Powders

Rawleigh made two baking powders. One was a pure phosphate baking powder and the other contained both phosphate and aluminum sulfate. They were priced about the same.

Rawleigh's Phosphate Baking Powder was sold as "especially healthful." It restored to flour the natural phosphates of wheat lost in milling but essential to proper nutrition. It was a "perfectly balanced leavening agent that produced uniform cellular structure in the baking, making it easily digested."

Using Rawleigh's Phosphate Baking Powder, cakes rose steadily, making for uniform consistency and size. Biscuits and cakes made from it did not readily dry out, deteriorate, or have a disagreeable taste.

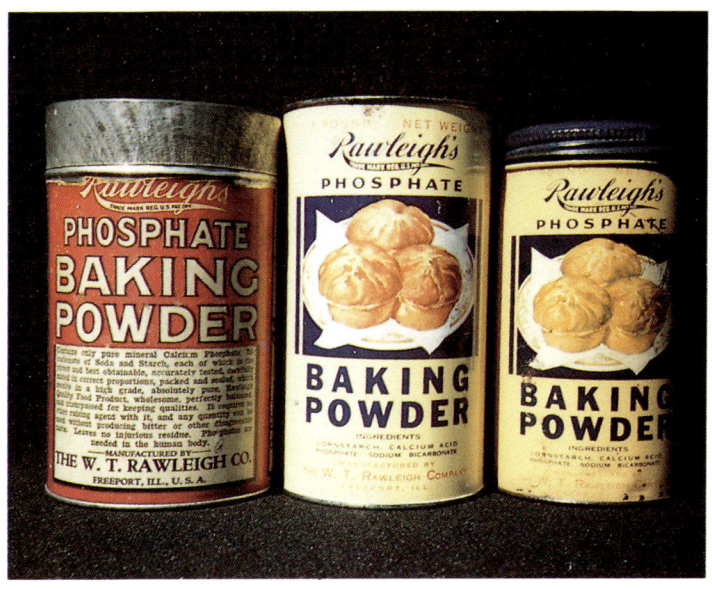

Three variations of "Rawleigh's Phosphate Baking Powder." These cylinder tin containers held 1 lb. On the reverse SIDE, directions and recipes were provided. MANUFACTURED BY THE W.T. RAWLEIGH COMPANY FREEPORT, ILL. $35-$40 ea.

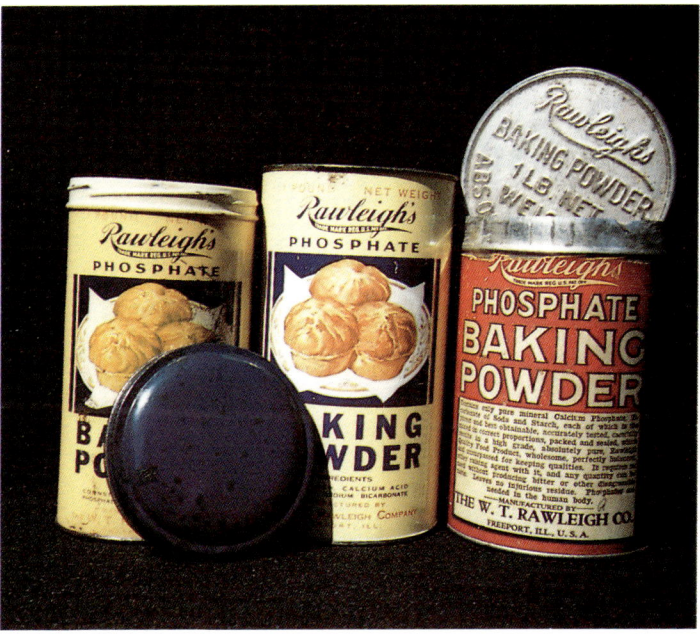

"Rawleigh's Phosphate Baking Powder." The container on the left has a screw on lid, the middle has a snap-on lid, and the right container features a highly embossed lid. $35-$40 ea.

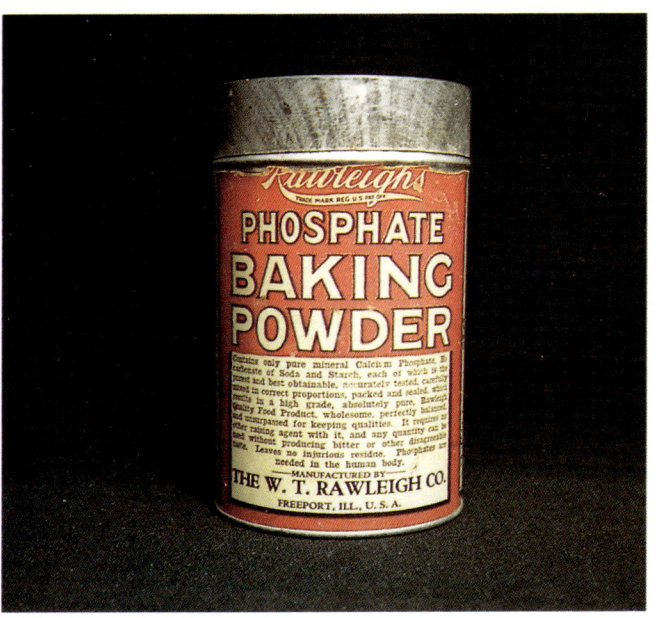

The metal cylinder "Phosphate Baking Powder" container is missing a portion of the original red paper label. Damaged or missing sections affect the selling price. This cylinder container has a metal embossed lid and was MANUFACTURED BY THE W.T. RAWLEIGH COMPANY FREEPORT, ILL., U.S.A. $60-$70 in mint condition.

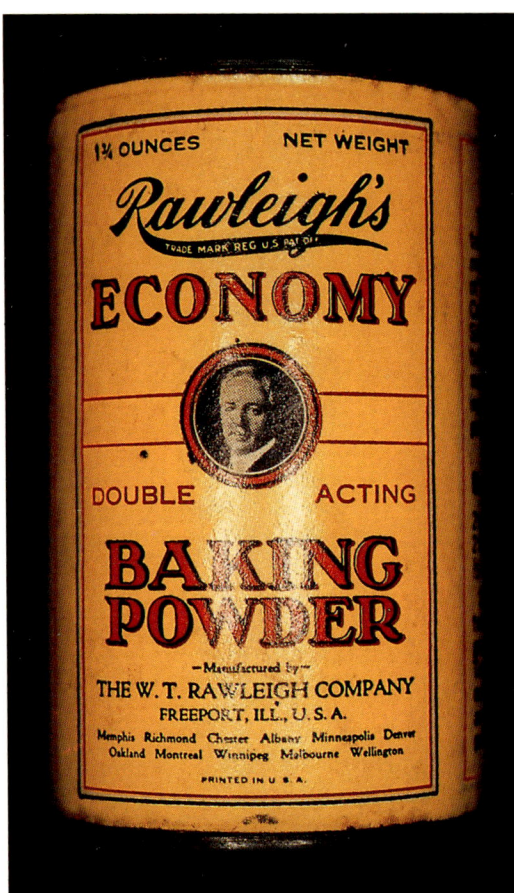

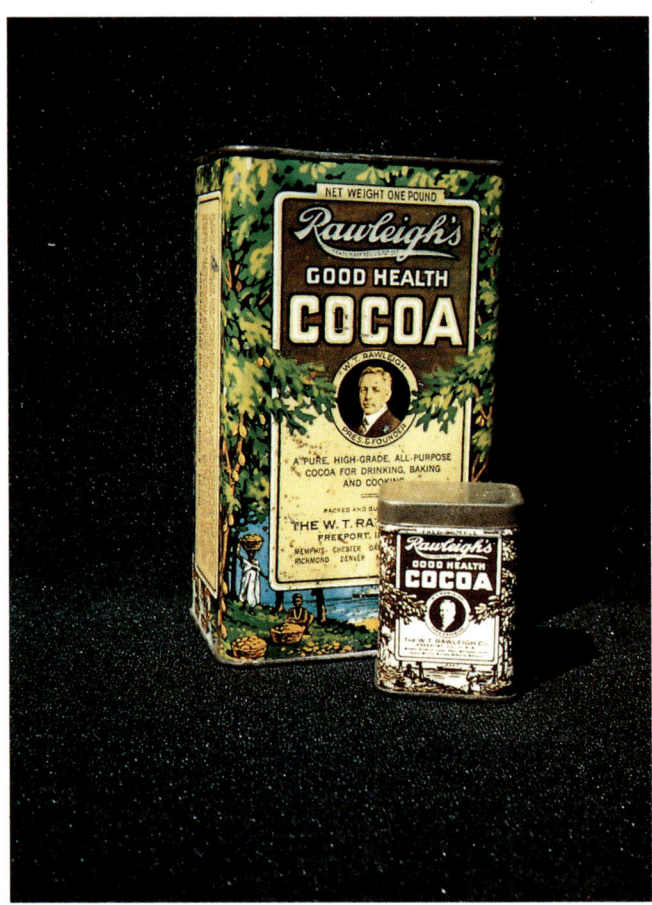

A 1-3/4 ounce metal and cardboard container of Double Action Rawleigh's ECONOMY BAKING POWDER. This could be a sample, given free to prospective customers. MANUFACTURED BY THE W.T. RAWLEIGH COMPANY FREEPORT, ILL., U.S.A. MEMPHIS RICHMOND CHESTER ALBANY MINNEAPOLIS DENVER OAKLAND MONTREAL WINNIPEG MELBOURNE WELLINGTON. Sample tins are highly sought by collectors and often demand more than the larger original tins. $50-$60.

A FREE SAMPLE of Rawleigh's Good Health Cocoa shown with a l lb. Cocoa container. Directions on the reverse side read, "Try this free sample your favorite way for using Cocoa or Chocolate. To make a delicious drink for each cup, mix one teaspoonful into a paste with hot water, add milk or water as desired and boil a minute." Sample tins are highly sought by collectors and often demand more than larger tins. $75-$100 sample tin.

Cocoa

Rawleigh's Cocoa was made from "selected cocoa beans, scientifically blended, roasted and ground, rich in a delicious flavor, and [was] a highly nutritious food." It had "the right amount of cocoa butter and the most desirable flavor, aroma and digestibility."

Rawleigh's Cocoa was standardized to meet the requirements for a breakfast cocoa, also for fineness, flavor, and quality. Rawleigh declared that its cocoa was more digestible than chocolate, stronger in flavoring and food value, and more convenient.

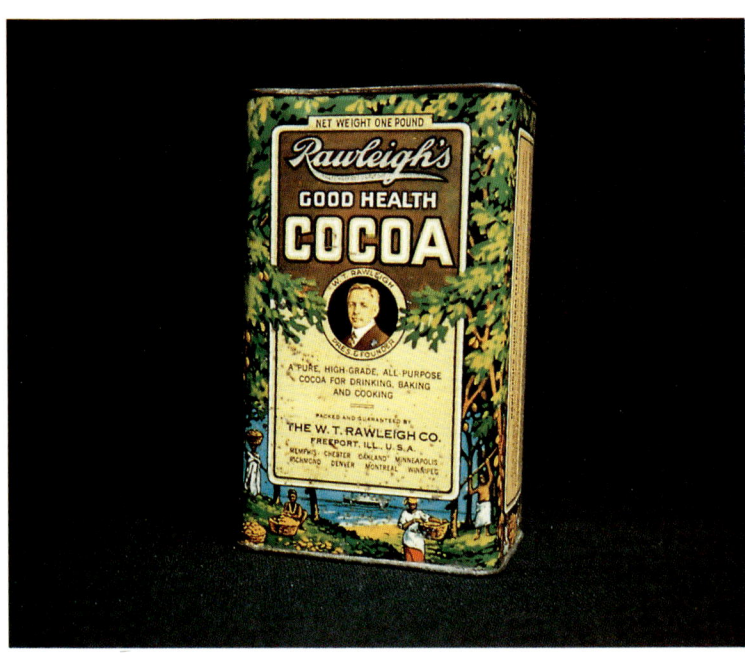

Packed and Guaranteed by The W.T. Rawleigh Co. Freeport, Ill., U.S.A. Memphis Chester Oakland Minneapolis Richmond Denver Montreal Winnipeg. This metal container held 1 lb., "Rawleigh's Good Health Cocoa," a pure, high-grade, all-purpose cocoa for drinking, baking, and cooking. A metal embossed snap-on lid kept the contents fresh. This cocoa appeared in the 1930s Rawleigh's Good Health Guide and could be even older. $35-$40.

Fruit Nectars

Rawleigh's Fruit Nectars made a delicious, refreshing, and healthful fruit drink. They were sold as costing only about half as much as drinks made from fresh fruit. These Fruit Nectars were available in Orange Nectar (which was prepared from the juice and pulp of tree-ripened Valencia oranges from California) and Lemon Nectar (containing the pure pulp juice of sun-ripened California lemons with natural oil of lemon and fruit acids added).

Rawleigh's Fruit Nectars could be used in frappe, sherbet, salads, puddings, pies, jellies, and frozen desserts.

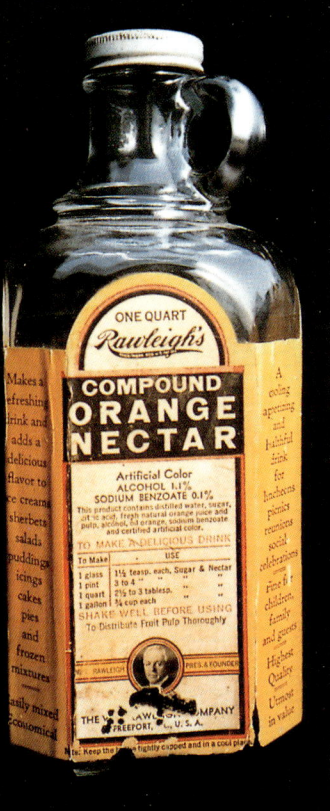

One quart bottle of "Rawleigh's Compound Orange Nectar." *Dupler Collection.* $40-$50.

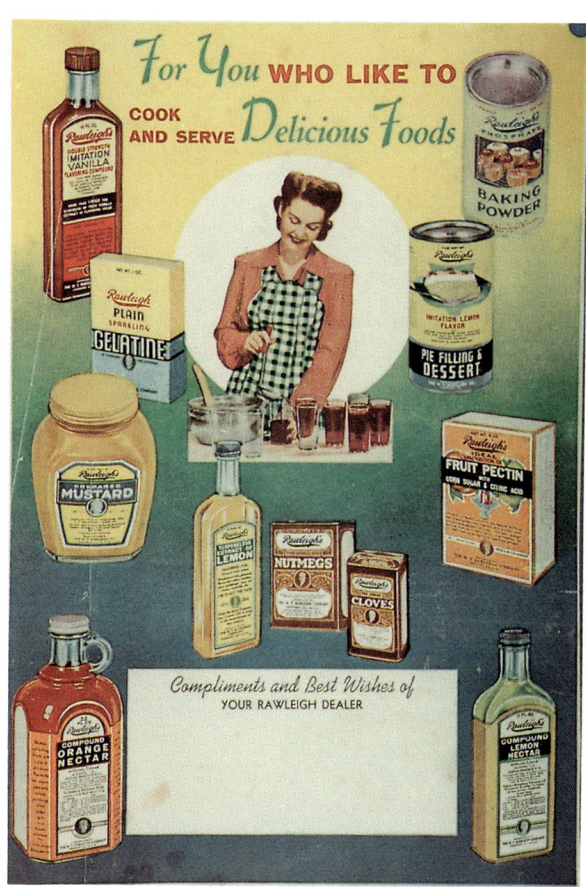

An original "For You Who Like To Cook and Serve Delicious Foods" advertisement for Rawleigh products. Note "Rawleigh's Compound Orange Nectar" in the lower left hand corner. Many of these products are shown throughout this publication. Circa 1946.

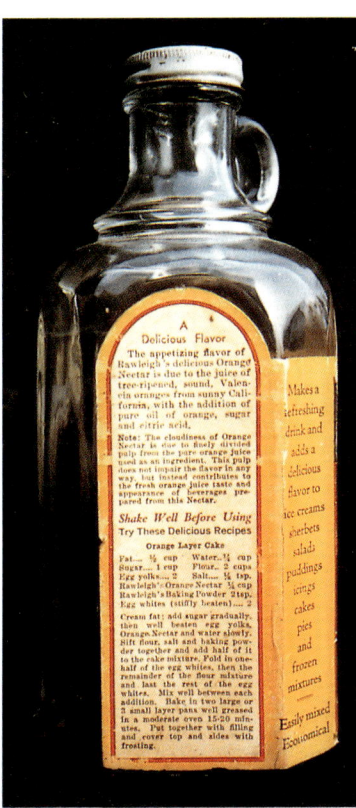

Directions, recipes, and instructions were provided on side panels for "Rawleigh's Compound Orange Nectar." *Dupler Collection.* $40-$50.

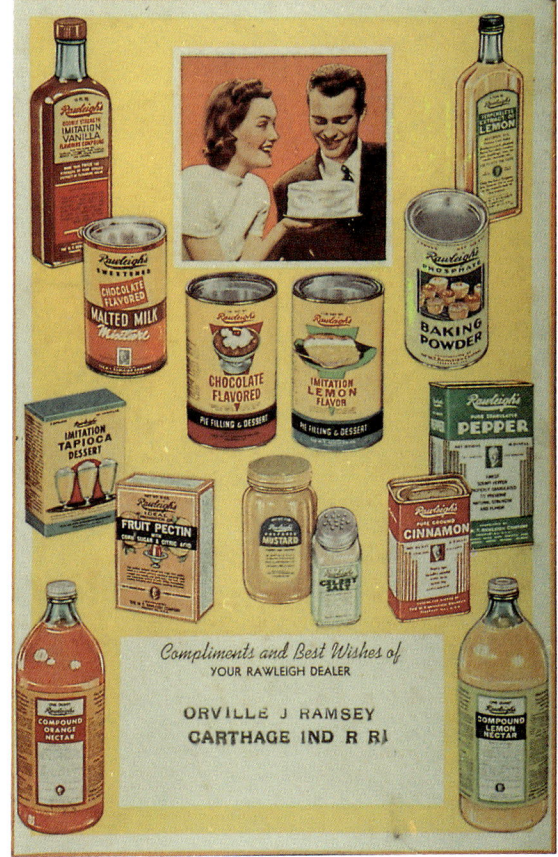

An original 1948 Rawleigh advertisement promoting various products. Note the Orange and Lemon Nectar bottles in the lower right and left hand corners. Also take note of the dealer's stamp at the bottom.

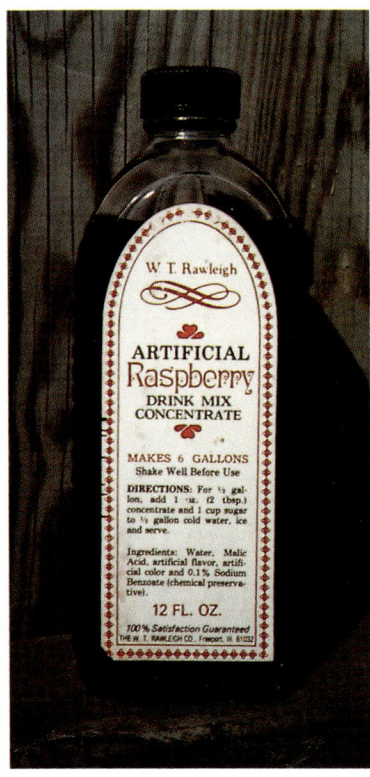

A 12 ounce bottle of W.T. Rawleigh Artificial Raspberry Drink Mix Concentrate. The W.T. Rawleigh Co., Freeport, Ill., 61032. *Dupler Collection.* $15-$20.

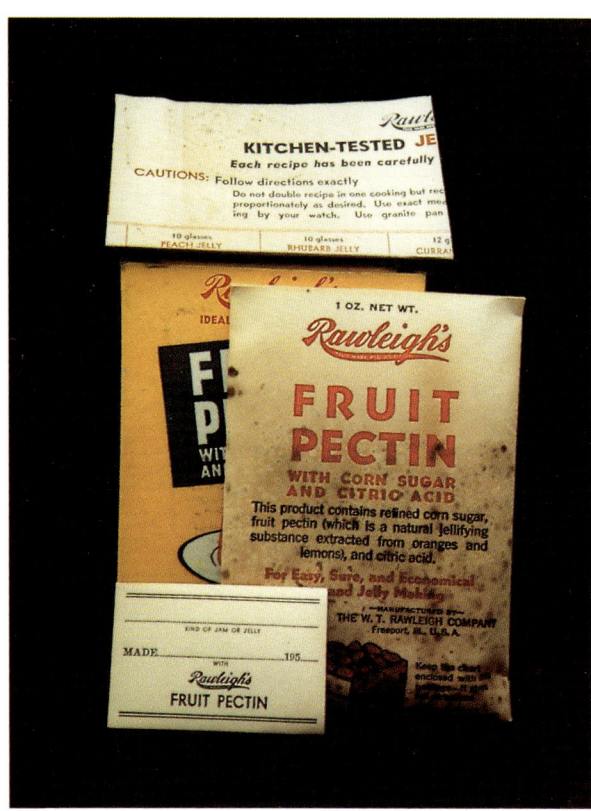

Fruit Pectin

Rawleigh's Fruit Pectin was introduced in 1932. It was a fruit powder made from the cell tissues of ripe fruit, and is the active principle that causes fruit juices to form into jelly. This made Fruit Pectin a valuable aid to housewives making jams and jellies.

Rawleigh's Fruit Pectin eliminated uncertainties of preserve making. Directions were provide on the package. With Rawleigh's Fruit Pectin "a housewife could make delicious jellies at any time of the year with fresh, canned, or dried fruit or Rawleigh's Extracts, Flavors, and Fruit Nectars."

This carton contained five original envelopes that made four or five 8 ounce glasses of jelly or eight to ten glasses of jam. This carton also has the original Rawleigh's "KITCHEN-TESTED JELLY RECIPE CHART" and "KITCHEN-TESTED JAM AND MARMALADE RECIPE CHART" inside. Each recipe had been carefully tested by Rawleigh's dietitian. $30-$40.

Gelatine

Rawleigh 1 ounce carton of plain sparkling "Gelatine." Manufactured For The W.T. Rawleigh Company Freeport, Ill., U.S.A. Four envelopes were enclosed with a new recipe pamphlet. One envelope of gelatin made six servings. $20-$30.

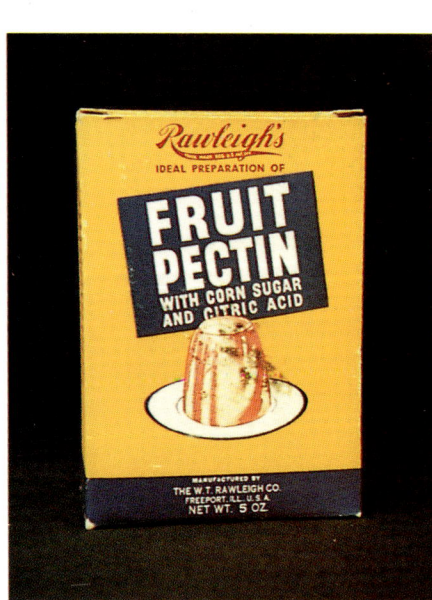

Rawleigh's Fruit Pectin with corn sugar and citric acid. Manufactured by The W.T. Rawleigh Co. Freeport, Ill., U.S.A. Net Wt. 5 ounces. A cardboard carton with directions on the reverse panels told "HOW THIS PECTIN HELPS YOU Make Better Jellies and Jams." $30-$40.

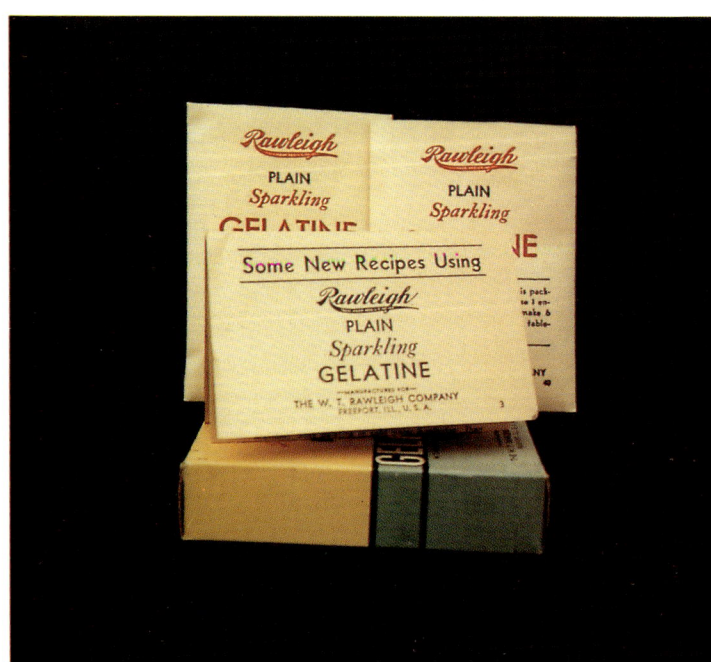

Shredded Coconut

Rawleigh's Shredded Coconut was preserved by drying and was prepared for keeping fresh and ready for use in making cakes, desserts, and confections. Photograph not available. $20-$30.

Pie Fillings

In 1927, Rawleigh Pie Fillings and Dessert Mixes were introduced. The company gave three reasons for their popularity: 1) Rawleigh Pie Fillings and Desserts Taste Great, 2) Rawleigh Pie Fillings and Desserts Make More Nutritious Servings, and 3) Rawleigh Pie Fillings and Desserts Are More Economical.

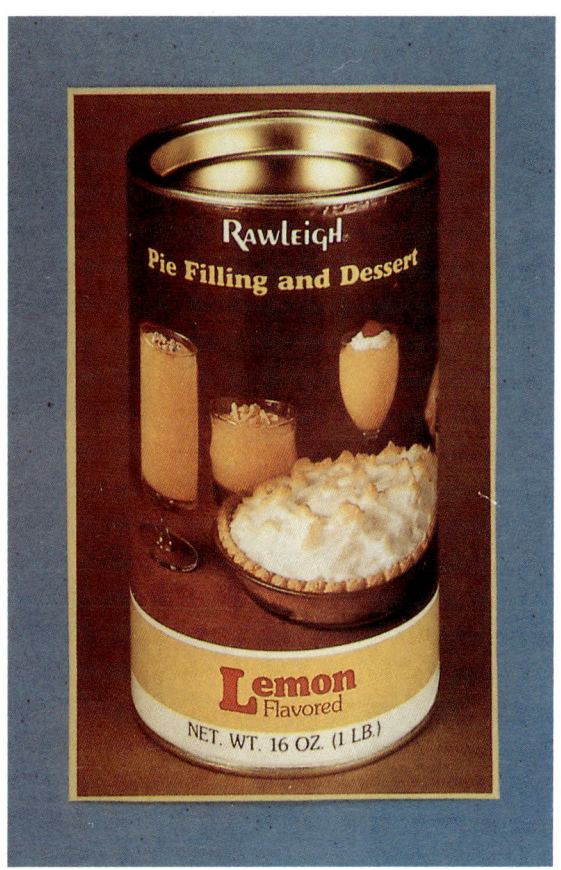

In 1986-1987, this original advertisement for Rawleigh Lemon Flavored Pie Filling and Dessert in a 1 lb. cylinder container was offered in the "Family Shopping Guide." One container made 6-9 pies or 36 to 54 servings of dessert. Available in Butterscotch, Chocolate, Coconut, Lemon, Tapioca, and Vanilla. Prices varied between $5.29 to $5.89.

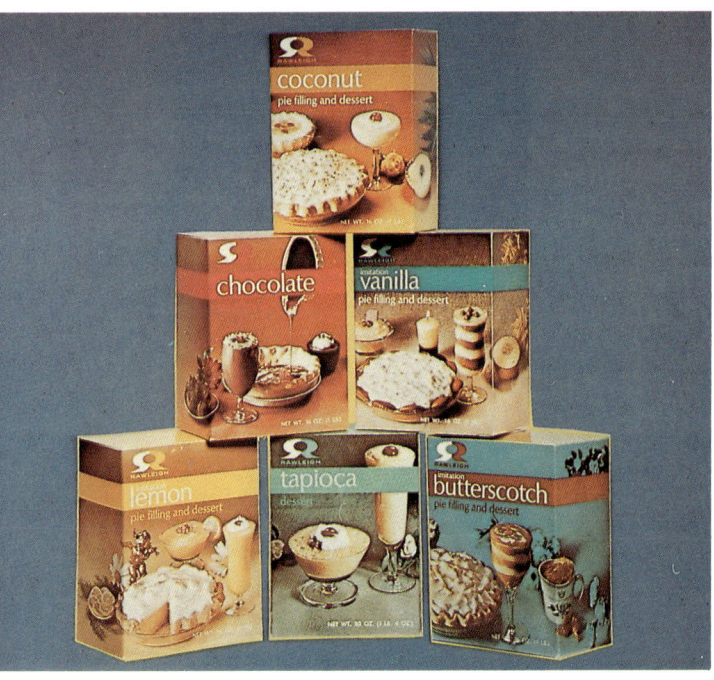

An original display of Rawleigh Pie Filling and Dessert mixes. "These mouthwatering desserts were great for puddings, cakes, sponge rolls, ice box cakes, cream puffs and many other homemade treats." These 16 ounce and 20 ounce cardboard containers in various flavors appeared in a ©1973 THE W.T. RAWLEIGH COMPANY brochure. Recipes were provided on each carton giving ideas for exciting desserts. $10-$15 ea.

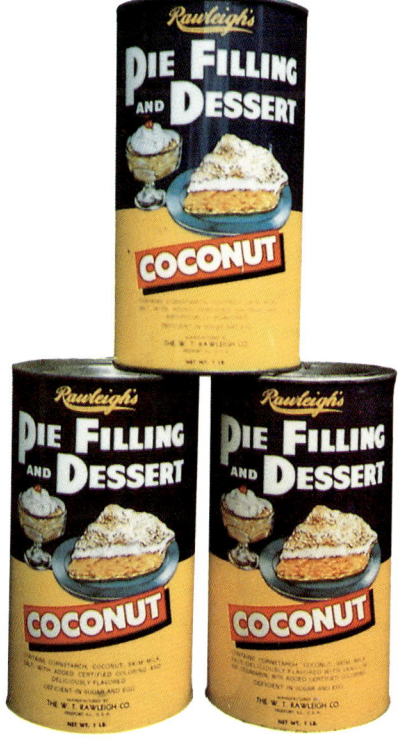

Three Rawleigh's "Coconut Pie Filling and Dessert." Each is a 1 lb., metal container with snap-on lid. Manufactured by The W.T. Rawleigh Co. Freeport, Ill., U.S.A. On the reverse, recipes were provided for coconut cream pie, pudding, fillings, fudge, and frozen dessert. $20-$30 ea.

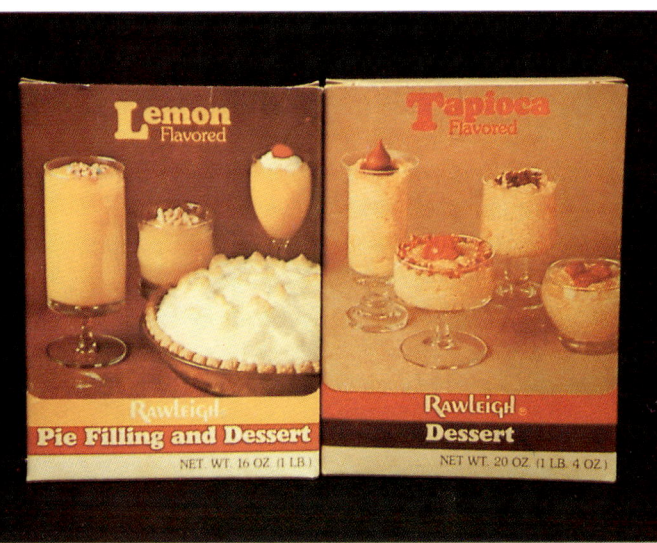

Rawleigh's "Lemon Flavored Pie Filling and Dessert" and "Tapioca Flavored Dessert." Both cartons "Manufactured by The W.T. Rawleigh Company Freeport, Illinois 61032." *Dupler Collection.* $20-$30 ea.

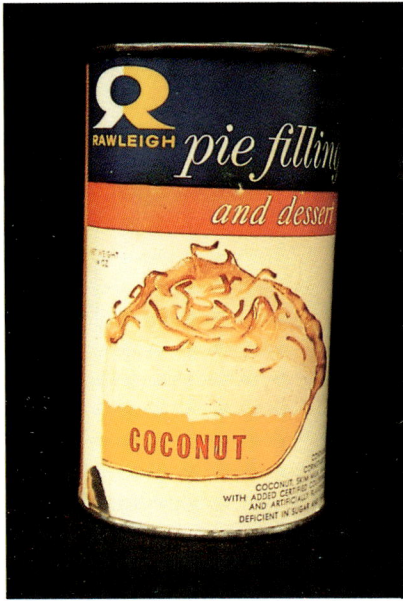

A 14 ounce metal with snap-on lid, paper label, Rawleigh "Coconut Pie Filling and Dessert." Manufactured by The W.T. Rawleigh Company Freeport, Ill., U.S.A. $20-$30.

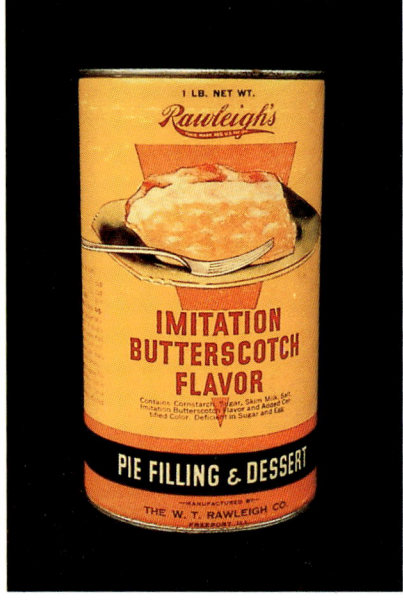

A 1 lb., cardboard container with snap-on lid of Rawleigh's imitation "Butterscotch Flavor Pie Filling & Dessert." Manufactured by The W.T. Rawleigh Co. Freeport, Ill. Two recipes are provided on the sides for pie, pudding, and frozen dessert. $20-$30.

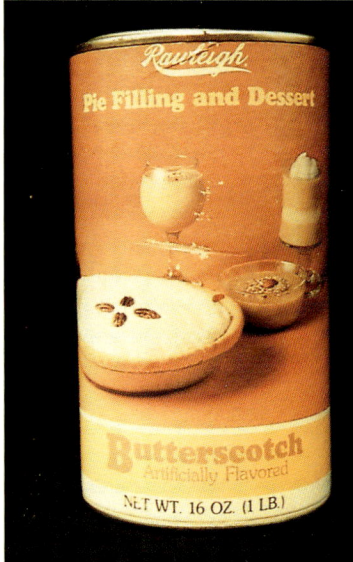

A 1 lb., cardboard container with snap-on lid of Rawleigh's artificially flavored "Butterscotch Pie Filling and Dessert." The W.T. Rawleigh Company Chapin, SC 29036 U.S.A. $20-$30.

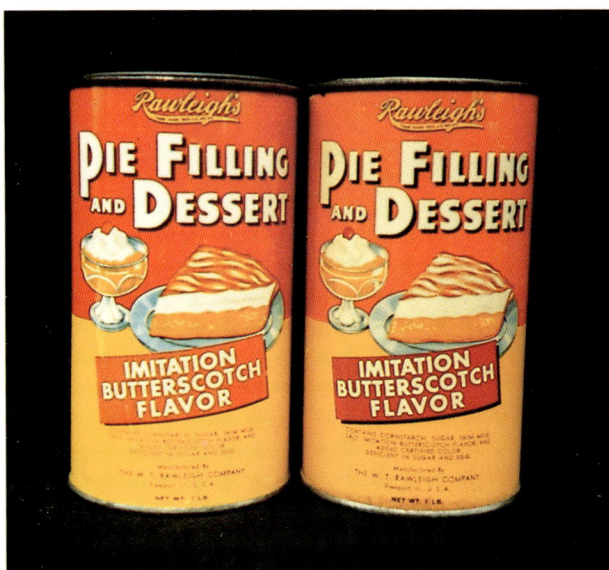

Two Rawleigh's imitation "Butterscotch Pie Filling and Dessert." Each is a 1 lb., metal container with snap-on lid. Manufactured by The W.T. Rawleigh Co. Freeport, Ill., U.S.A. $20-$30 ea.

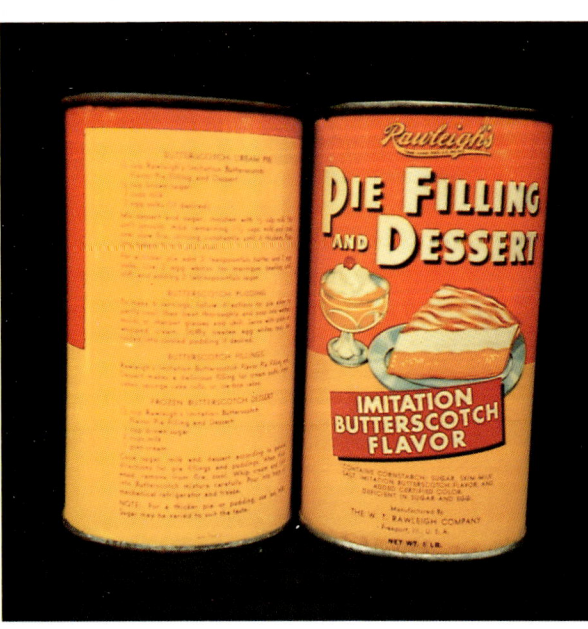

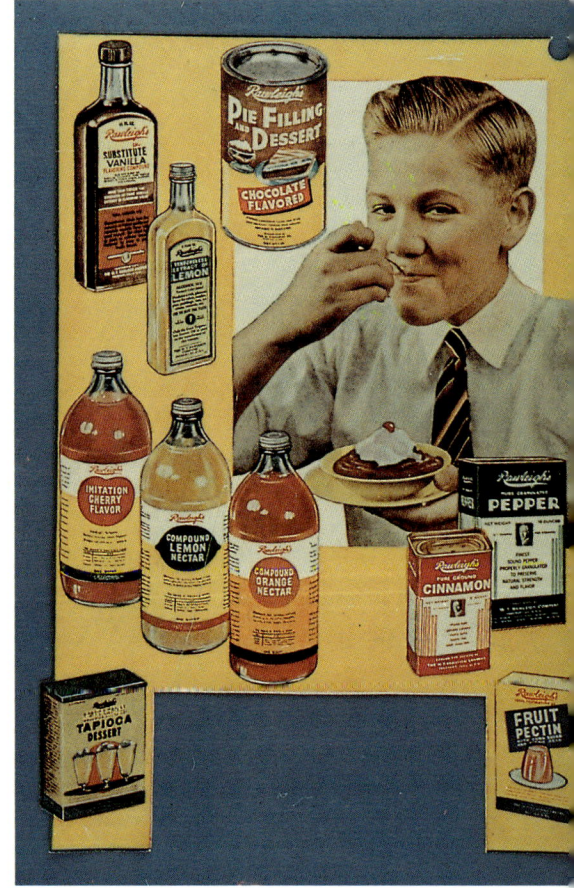

In 1949, Rawleigh promoted these products: "Extract, Pie Filling and Dessert, Imitation Cherry Flavor, Compound Lemon and Orange Nectar, Tapioca Dessert, Pepper, and Cinnamon and Fruit Pectin." $6-$8 advertisement.

Rawleigh's imitation "Butterscotch Pie Filling and Dessert." On the reverse, recipes were provided for butterscotch cream pie, pudding, fillings, and frozen dessert. $20-$30.

Tapioca Dessert

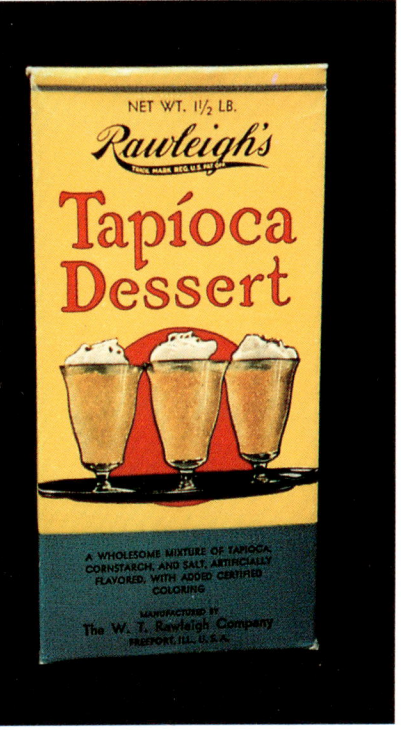

Rawleigh's Tapioca Dessert was a mixture of tapioca, cornstarch and salt. Artificially flavored with added certified coloring. This 1-1/2 lb. cardboard carton provided directions and additional recipes on the reverse panels. MANUFACTURED BY THE W.T. RAWLEIGH COMPANY FREEPORT, ILL., U.S.A. $30-$40.

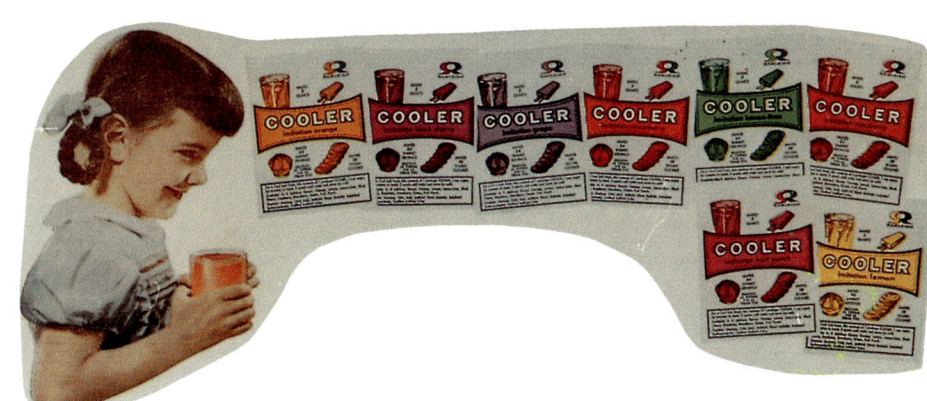

They were NEW cooler drinks a child could mix for about 2 cents a glass. Each envelope of Rawleigh COOLER made two quarts. "Imitation Fruit Punch, Orange, Lemon, Lemon-Lime, Black Cherry, Grape, Raspberry, and Strawberry." $10-$15 ea.

Spices

"The best spices the world grew were brought to the home as a part of the service of the Rawleigh Industries. The best varieties and grades were carefully selected by Rawleigh for their curing, cleaning, and condition upon arrival at the factories. Rawleigh always had many carloads of the world's best crops in stock."

"Rawleigh quality spices were manufactured on special mills and in prime conditions; they were properly prepared to retain their rich oils and full piquant flavors, then packed into airtight containers retaining their freshness." *Rawleigh's 1928.*

Concentrate Drink Mix

These Rawleigh's Drink Mix Concentrates appeared in a © July 1986 brochure. Rawleigh's Lemon-Lime, Raspberry, and Strawberry concentrate drink mixes in 12 fluid ounce containers made 6 gallons or 96 - 8 ounce glasses each. Rawleigh's 5.5 ounce Root Beer Drink Mix featured a full-bodied root beer flavor and made up to 5 gallons. $10-$15 ea.

Cream of Tartar

Rawleigh's Cream of Tartar was a food product useful for fine baking, cooking, pastries, and candies. Cream of Tartar came packed in 1/4 lb. cans with directions and recipes.

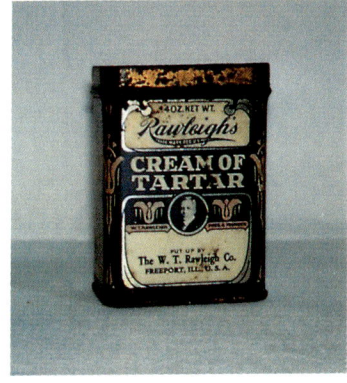

Rawleigh's 4 ounce Cream of Tartar. PUT UP BY The W.T. Rawleigh Co. Freeport, Ill., U.S.A. Metal snap-on lid tin. Circa 1930s. *Dupler Collection.* $30-$40.

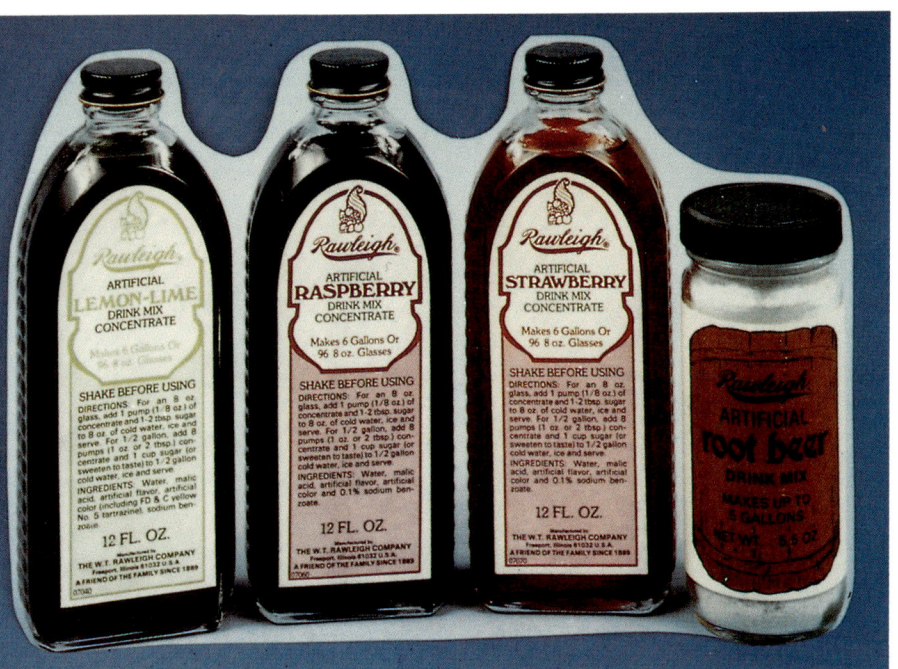

Celery Salt

Rawleigh's Celery Salt was made of finely ground celery seeds in pulverized salt. The flavor is most pronounced in the seeds. It was a popular seasoning, adding a savory taste to soups, stews, meats, dressings, salads, bouillon's, and croquettes.

Rawleigh's Celery Salt was the ninth new product introduced in 1932. A popular seasoning product that made insipid and bland foods appetizing. Rawleigh's Celery Salt gave a pleasing and appetizing taste to soups, dressings, stews, meats, sauces, gravies, vegetable salads, and pickles.

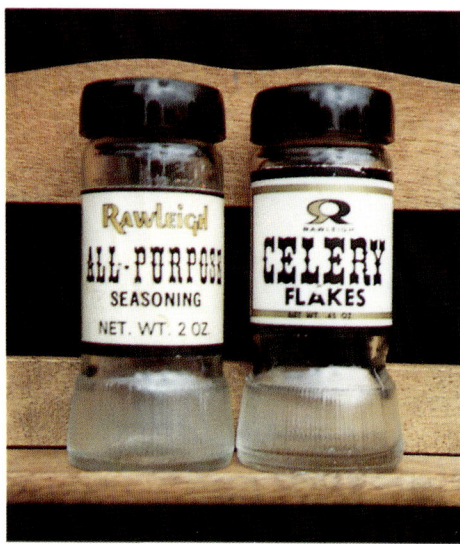

Rawleigh 2 ounce "All-Purpose Seasoning" and "Dehydrated Celery Flakes" in a 4.5 ounce glass jar with a black plastic screw on lid. W.T. RAWLEIGH CO. Freeport, Illinois 61032. Rawleigh's Dehydrated Celery Flakes were advertised in a 1970s brochure promoting Rawleigh's Sage, Onion Flakes, and Celery Flakes. All three could be purchased for $4.39. "A hearty savings of 40 cents." $15-$20 ea.

Onion Flavored Seasoning

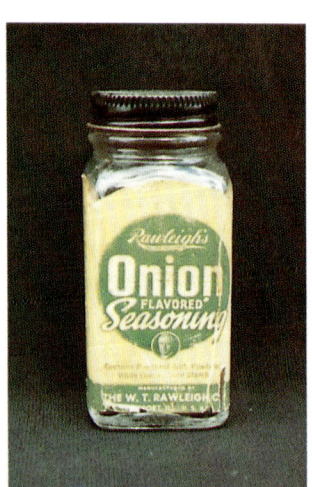

Rawleigh's "Onion Flavored Seasoning," a 4 ounce glass bottle with a paper label and black metal screw on lid. The insert liner under the lid that could be removed allowing the lid to be used as a shaker. Manufactured by The W.T. Rawleigh Co. Freeport, Ill., U.S.A. Rawleigh promoted this seasoning as "Enjoy one of our most popular flavors without a lingering onion odor on hands and utensils!" $15-$20.

Poultry, Garlic and Fish Seasoning

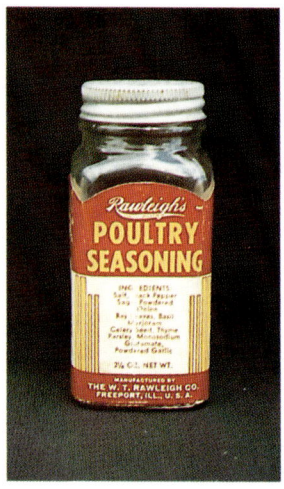

A 2-1/4 ounce glass bottle with paper label and metal screw on lid. A liner under the lid that could be removed allowing the bottle to be used as a shaker. Manufactured by The W.T. Rawleigh Co. Freeport, Ill., U.S.A. Rawleigh's Poultry seasoning was made exclusively of clean, fresh, sweet herbs, spices, and condiments. $15-$20.

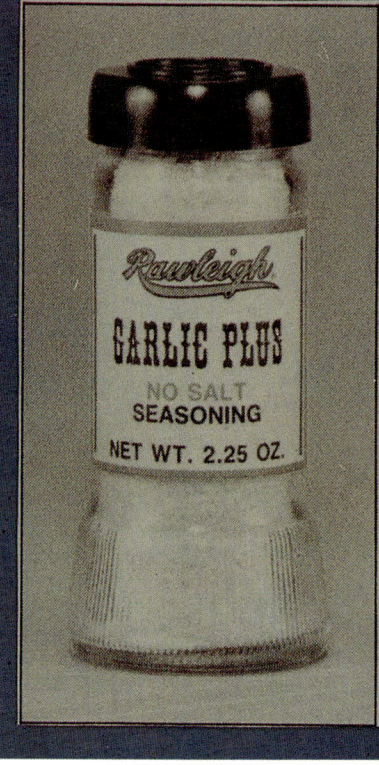

Rawleigh Garlic Plus Seasoning. Glass 2.25 ounce container with black plastic screw on lid. $15-$20.

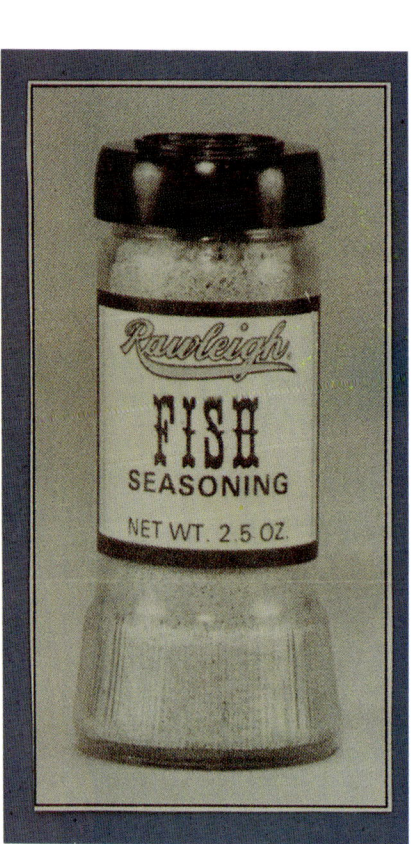

Rawleigh Fish seasoning. Glass container, 2.25 ounce, with black plastic screw on lid. $15-$20.

Cinnamon

Rawleigh's Cinnamon had a delightful, full, rich aroma, velvety smoothness, sweet, delicious flavor, and great strength. It came from the properly blending and preparing of three choice varieties including the expensive Saigon Cinnamon and the sweet Padang Cassia.

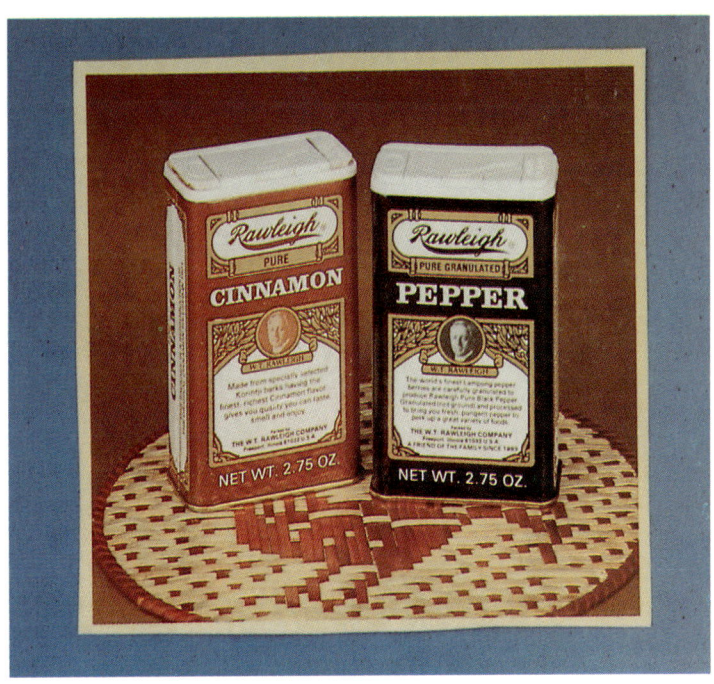

In 1986, this original advertisement promoted Rawleigh "Cinnamon" and "Pepper." The pure granulated pepper tin featured a 1921 recipe for pork sausage. The cinnamon tin featured a recipe for old fashioned cinnamon rolls, offered in either 8 or 2.75 ounce metal containers.

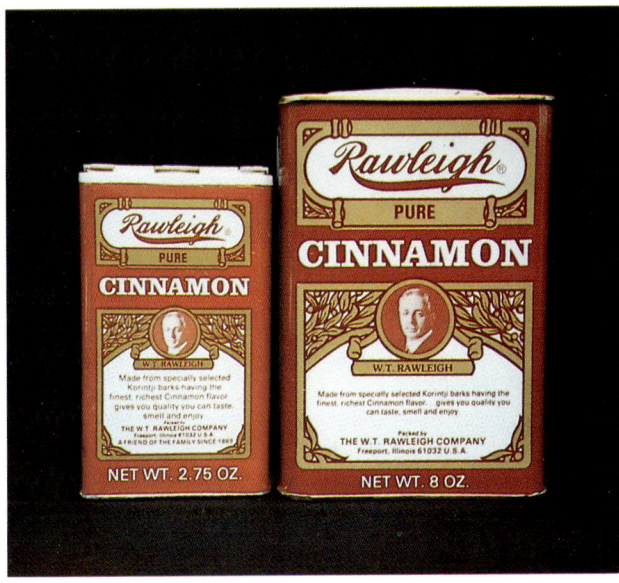

Two Rawleigh pure "Cinnamon" containers, 2.75 ounce and 8 ounce. Packed by The W.T. Rawleigh Company Freeport, Illinois 61032 U.S.A. Circa mid-1980s. $10-$15 ea.

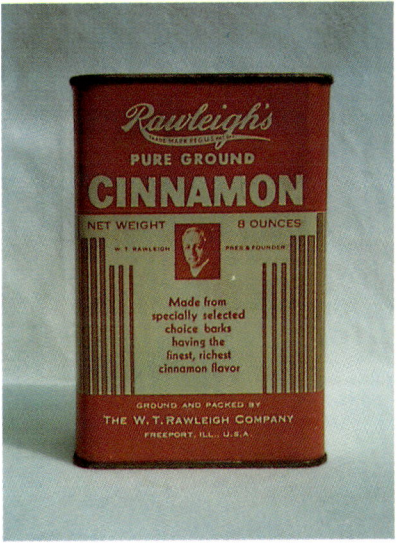

Rawleigh's 8 ounce pure ground "Cinnamon." Ground and Packed by The W.T. Rawleigh Company Freeport, Ill., U.S.A. This is a metal container. $15-$20.

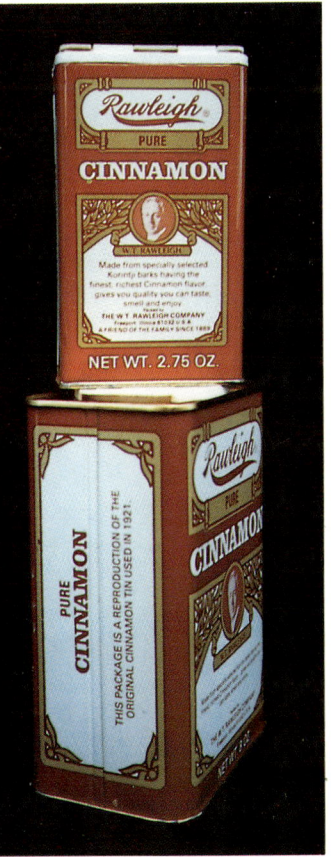

Rawleigh pure "Cinnamon" containers. The packaging is a reproduction of the original cinnamon tin used in 1921. This is noted on the side of the bottom container. $15-$20.

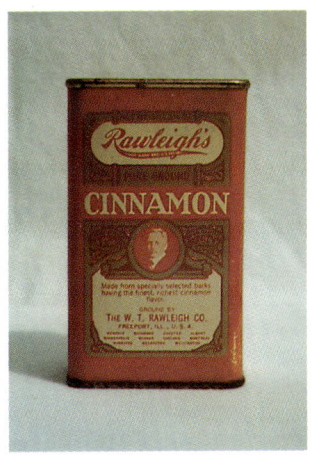

Rawleigh's 3-1/4 ounce pure ground "Cinnamon." Ground by The W.T. Rawleigh Co. Freeport, Ill., U.S.A. Memphis - Richmond - Chester - Albany - Minneapolis Denver - Oakland - Montreal - Winnipeg - Melbourne - Wellington. This is a metal container. $15-$20.

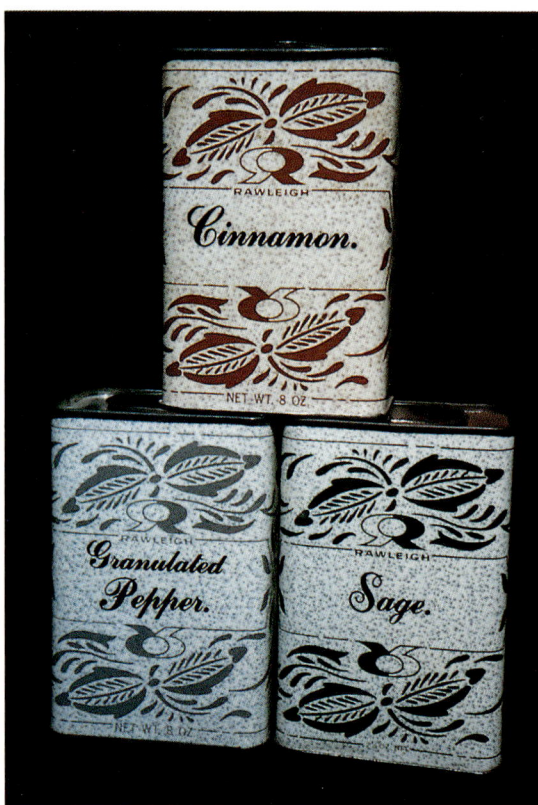

Rawleigh "Cinnamon, Granulated Pepper, and Sage." The unusual design on these containers is popular with collectors and appeared in numerous Rawleigh publications. The W.T. Rawleigh Co. Freeport, Ill. 61032. This design is shown again elsewhere in this chapter. $15-$20.

Cloves, Ginger and Allspice

Rawleigh's Cloves had a fragrant aroma, strength, and richness of flavor. It was properly prepared from the largest, richest, cleanest Madagascar cloves grown!

Rawleigh's ground Ginger and Allspice both had rich, snappy flavor and were "of full strength." Ground from choice, sound, well seasoned ginger roots and allspice.

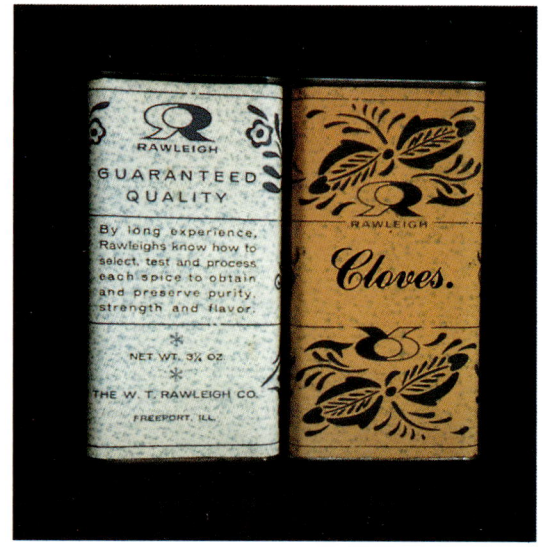

The front and reverse panels of Rawleigh "Cloves" in 3-1/4 ounce containers. $15-$20 ea.

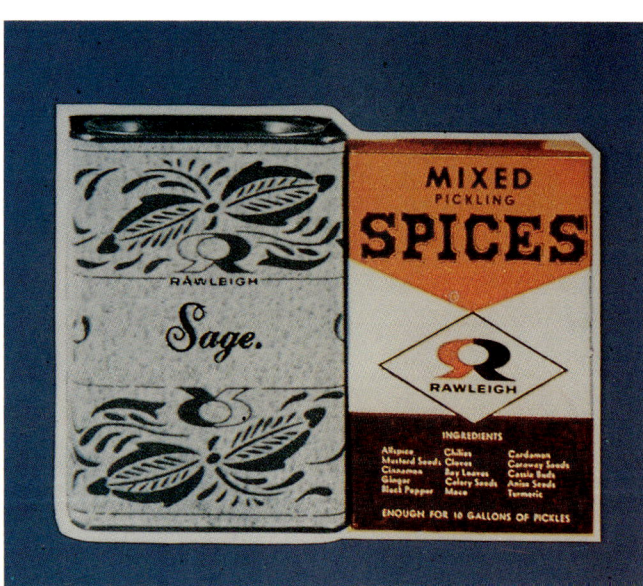

Rawleigh's Sage was "America's most popular herb" and came from Yugoslavia. It was promoted with Rawleigh Mixed Pickling Spices during the 1960s. Rawleigh's Pickling Spices were a blend of 15 different spices which gave a rich flavor to pickles and catsup. $15-$20.

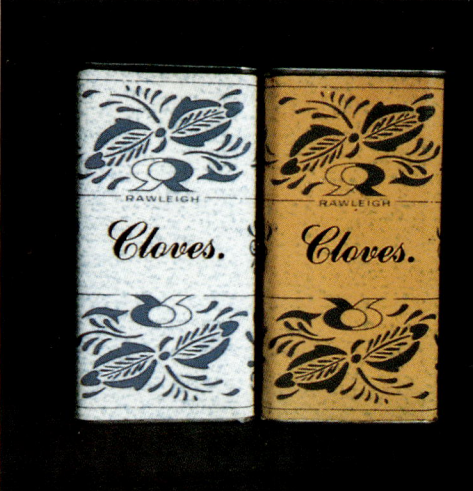

Rawleigh "Cloves." Note the variation in coloring on these unusually designed containers. $15-$20 ea.

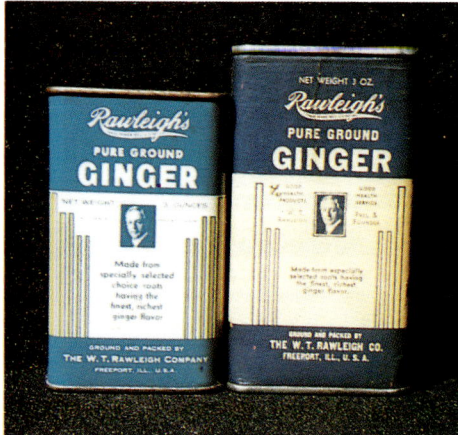

Two variations of sizes for Rawleigh's "Pure Ground Ginger." Ground and Packed by The W.T. Rawleigh Co. Freeport, Ill., U.S.A. Made from especially selected roots having the finest, richest ginger flavor. $15-$20 ea.

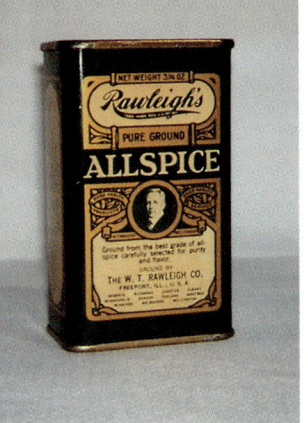

A 3-1/4 ounce metal tin of Rawleigh's pure ground "Allspice." Ground from the best grade of allspice and carefully selected for purity and flavor. Ground by The W.T. Rawleigh Co. Freeport, Ill., U.S.A. Memphis - Richmond - Chester - Albany - Minneapolis - Denver - Oakland - Montreal - Winnipeg - Melbourne - Wellington. By experience, Rawleigh's knew how to select, test, and process each spice to obtain and preserve purity, strength, and flavor. $15-$20.

Unusual Design

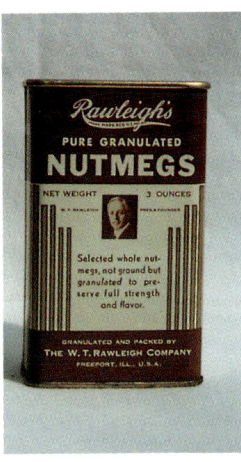

Rawleigh's 3 ounce pure granulated "Nutmegs" — guaranteed wholesome and unadulterated. Sold pure and fresh by Rawleigh dealers direct to consumers. Granulated and packed by The W.T. Rawleigh Company Freeport, Ill., U.S.A. Rawleigh's Nutmeg was prepared from select, oily, rich flavored nutmegs and was ready for use "without troublesome grating, giving the best seasoning satisfaction." $15-$20.

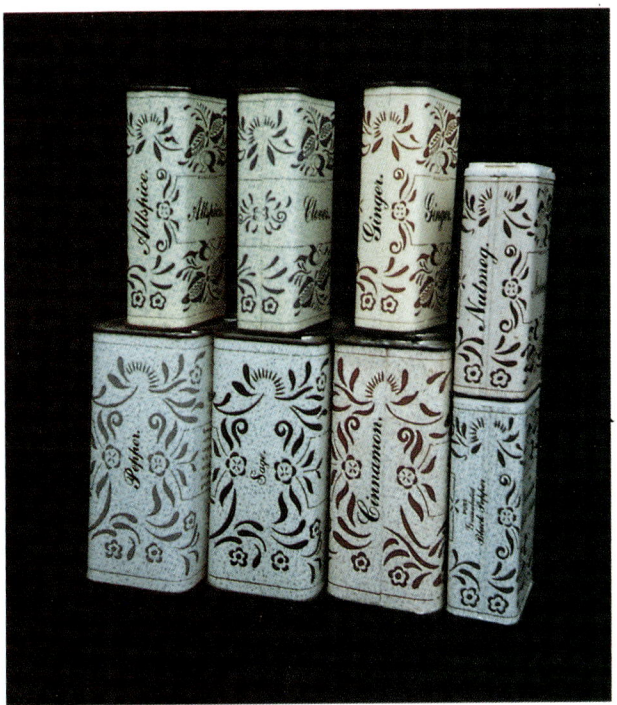

Side views of these unusual decorated containers. The colored design on these containers are found in brown, gray, blue, and teal blue against a solid white background. Recently one was found in green and another in red. Containers vary in packaging markings. THE W.T. RAWLEIGH CO., FREEPORT, ILL., and/or Packed by THE W.T. RAWLEIGH COMPANY Freeport, Illinois 61032.

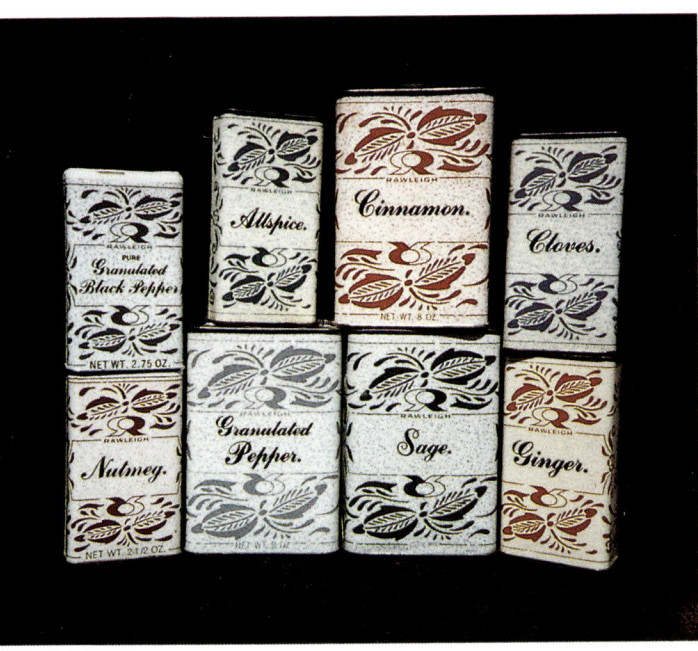

These highly decorated spice containers are gaining a widespread popularity among Rawleigh collectors. These containers are readily available but are escalating in price with demand. Circa 1960s. $15-$20 ea.

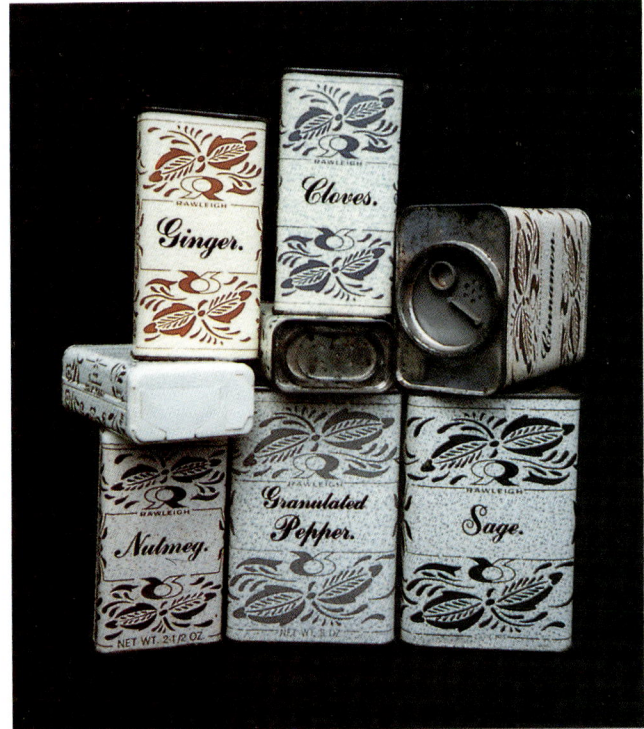

Various metal and/or plastic lids were used to seal these decorated containers' contents. A customer could sift, shake, pour or remove the lid completely for easy use; this also allowed for easier measuring. $15-$20 ea.

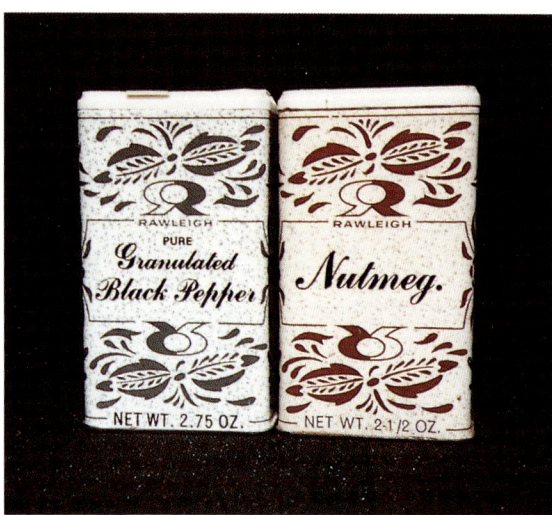

Rawleigh's 2.75 ounce Pure Granulated Black Pepper and 2-1/2 ounce "Nutmeg." The Nutmeg was produced from a carefully selected blend of abundantly oily and aromatic nutmegs, processed to preserve the natural oils which release the pungent, pleasing nutmeg flavor. Both were packed by The W.T. Rawleigh Co. Freeport, Ill. 61032. $15-$20 ea.

Mixed Pickling Spice

Rawleigh's Pickling Spice had 17 selected varieties of whole spices blended for the most delightful flavor in spices.

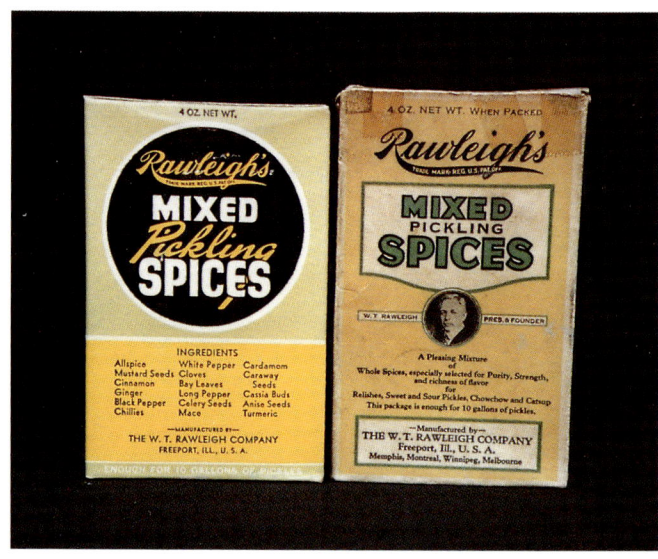

Two different 4 ounce packages for Rawleigh's Mixed Pickling Spices. Manufactured by The W.T. Rawleigh Company Freeport, Ill., U.S.A. Directions were provided for Sweet Mixed Pickles, Tomato Catsup, and Crock Pickles on the reverse sides. The packaging on the right is marked "Manufactured by The W.T. Rawleigh Company Freeport, Ill., U.S.A. Memphis, Montreal, Winnipeg, Melbourne." Both packages had enough spices to prepare 10 gallons of pickles. These cartons have never been opened. $25-$35 ea.

Mustard

Rawleigh's Mustard and Red Pepper had rich, snappy flavor. Both were sold full strength. The Red Pepper was ground from choice, sound, well seasoned ginger roots, pure Jamaica Allspice, and the correct blending of choice varieties of mustard seeds and red peppers.

Rawleigh's Prepared Mustard was made of a combination of clean, high grade mustard seeds, selected especially for their qualities as food condiments. They were blended and especially processed to produce a distinctive richness, mellowness, appetizing tang, and characteristic deliciousness.

Rawleigh's Prepared Mustard made salads, sandwiches, eggs, meats, baked beans, and vegetables more appetizing and taste better.

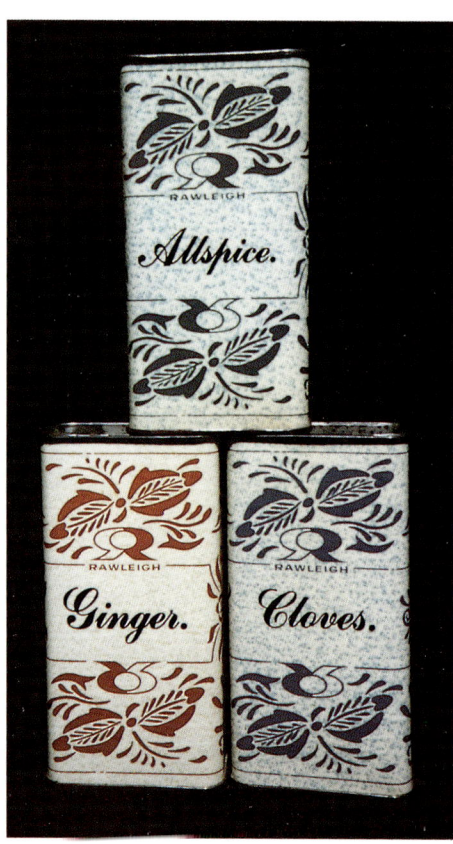

Rawleigh Allspice, Ginger, and Cloves. *Dupler Collection.* $15-$20 ea.

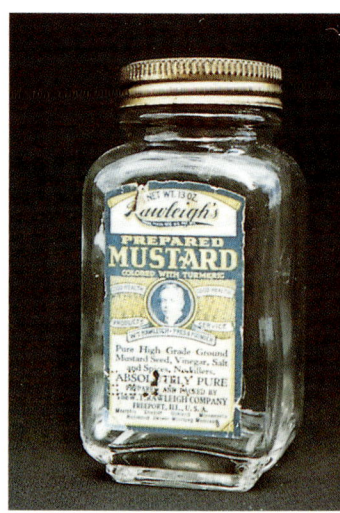

Rawleigh's Prepared Mustard "Colored with Turmeric" was offered in a 13 ounce embossed glass jar with an embossed screw on lid, containing pure high grade ground mustard seed, vinegar, salt, and spices. PREPARED AND PACKED BY The W.T. RAWLEIGH COMPANY FREEPORT, ILL., U.S.A. Memphis Chester Oakland Minneapolis Richmond Denver Winnipeg Montreal. The paper label appears only on the front section; the jar is embossed on the reverse side. $30-$40.

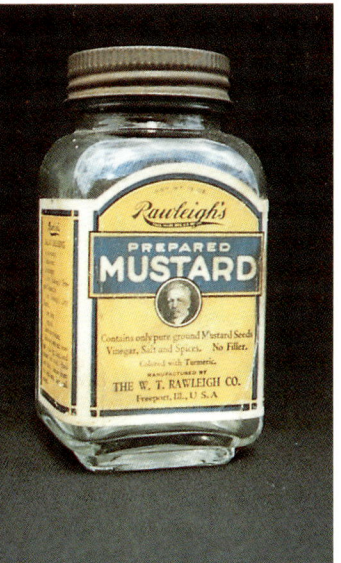

Rawleigh's Prepared Mustard contains only pure ground mustard seeds, vinegar, salt, and spices. MANUFACTURED BY THE W.T. RAWLEIGH CO. Freeport, Ill., U.S.A. The paper label wraps around three sides; recipes were provided on two sides. An embossed glass jar with a screw on lid. $30-$40.

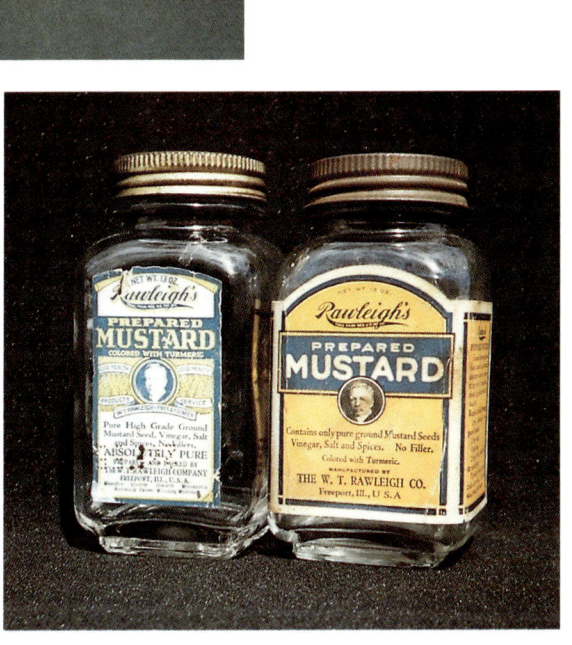

In this original 1927 Rawleigh advertisement, notice the balsa-wood paddle fastened to the neck of the "Prepared Mustard" in the lower right corner.

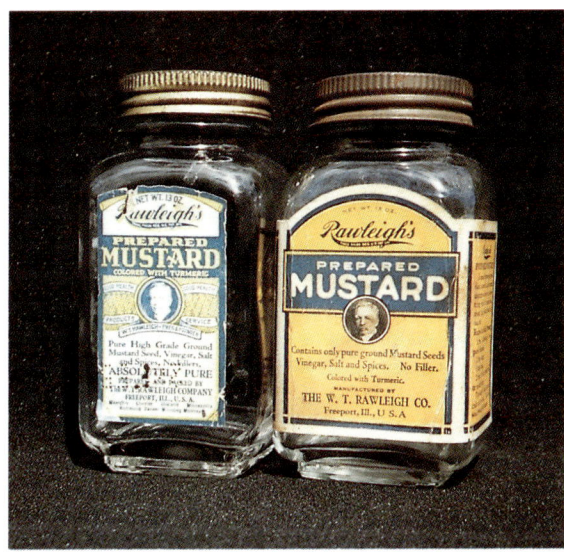

Rawleigh's Prepared Mustard was "absolutely pure," had no filler, and was colored with Turmeric. $30-$40.

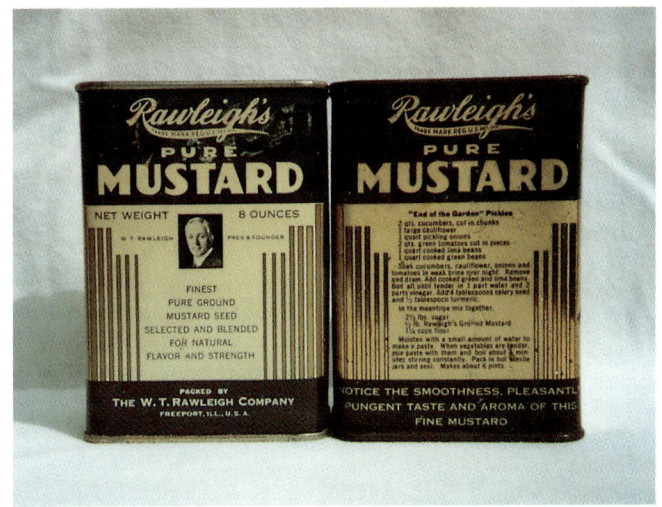

The embossed Rawleigh's balsa-wood paddle. Approximately 4-3/4" this paddle could be used to spread Rawleigh's Prepared Mustard. $50-$60.

The front and reverse panels of Rawleigh's "Pure Mustard" 8 ounce metal containers. "Packed by The W.T. Rawleigh Company Freeport, Ill., U.S.A." On the back panel a recipe for pickles was provide. $15-$20 ea.

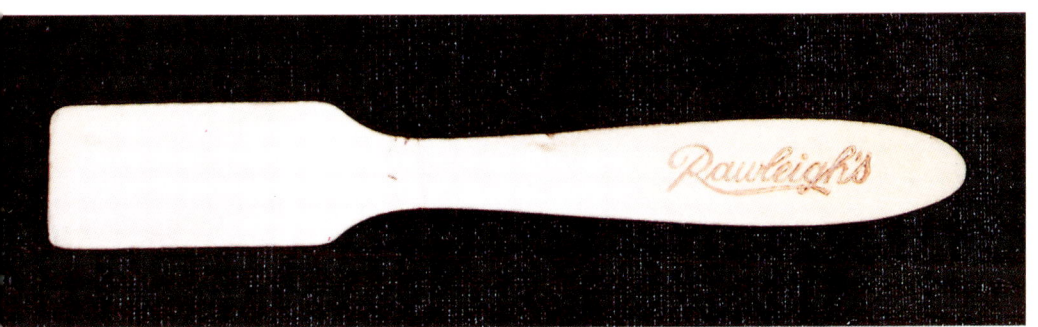

101

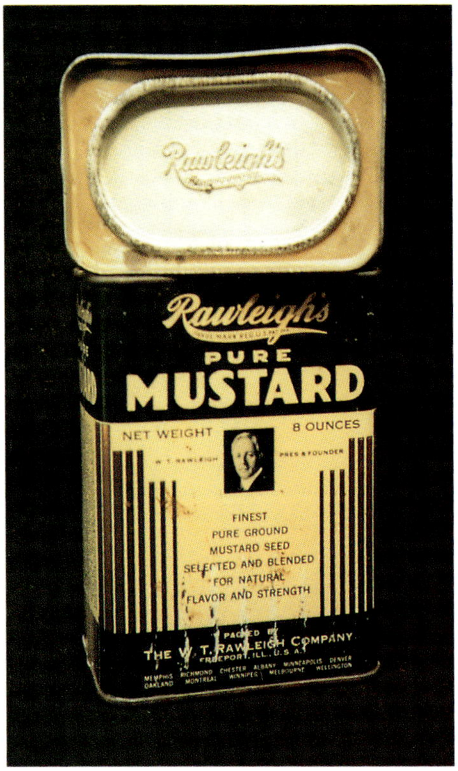

Four New Seasonings

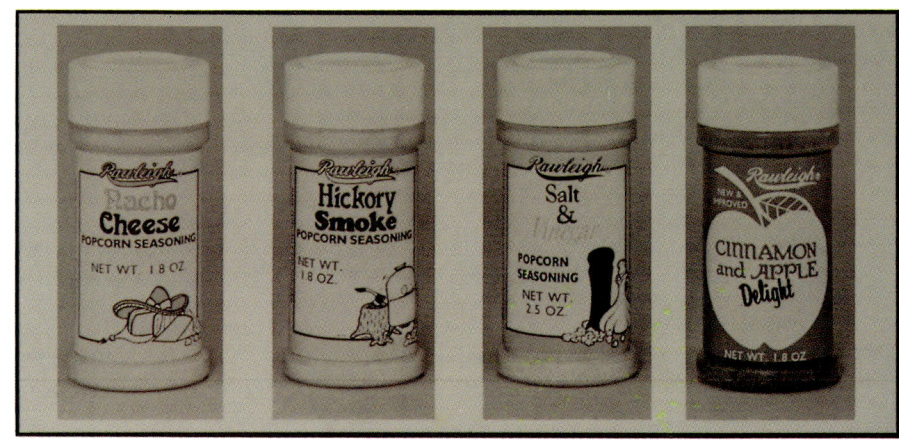

Four new seasonings introduced during the 1980s. Rawleigh Nacho Cheese (Popcorn seasoning), Hickory Smoke (Popcorn seasoning), Salt & Vinegar (Popcorn seasoning), and a new and improved Cinnamon and Apple. *Dupler Collection.* $15-$20 ea.

The embossed snap-on lid on the Rawleigh's "Pure Mustard" 8 ounce metal container. "Packed by The W.T. Rawleigh Company Freeport, Ill., U.S.A. Memphis - Richmond - Chester - Albany - Minneapolis - Denver - Oakland - Montreal - Winnipeg - Melbourne - Wellington." $15-$20.

These gourmet mustards were permanently added to the Rawleigh product line. On the left is "Rawleigh Dusseldorf Gourmet Mustard" and on the right "Rawleigh Spicy Gourmet Mustard," both were popular items. Circa 1980s. $15-$20 ea.

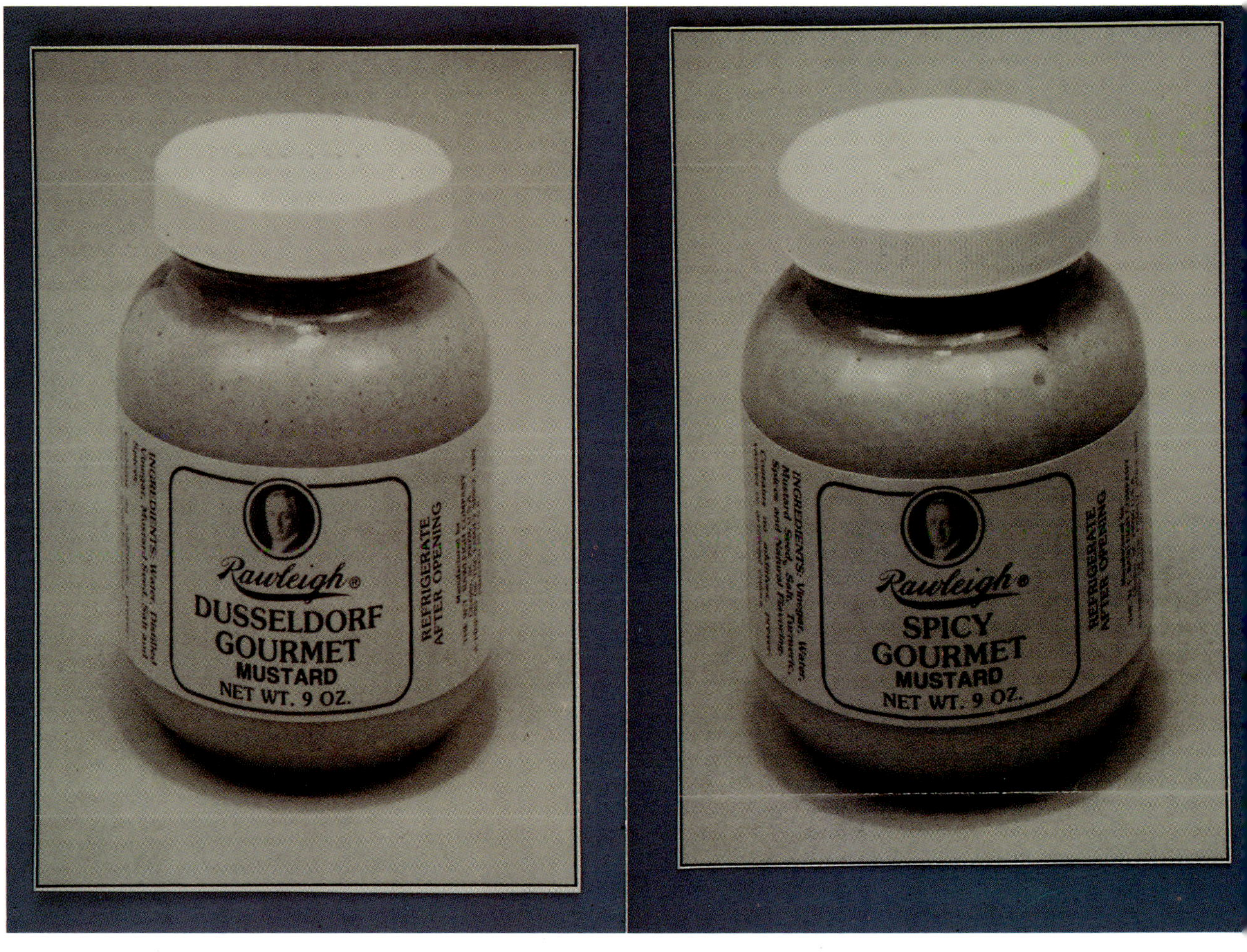

Pepper

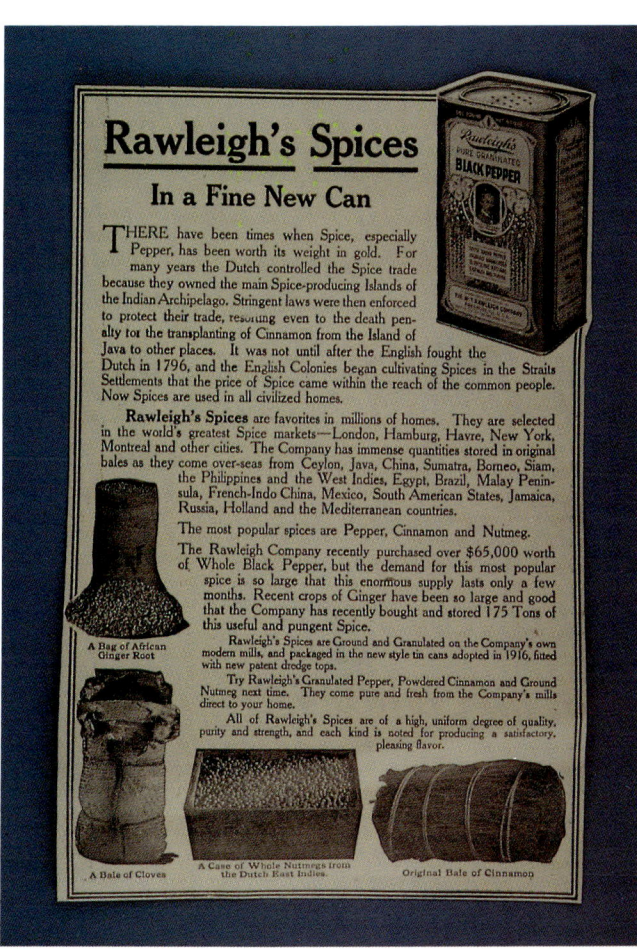

An original page from Rawleigh's 1916 Almanac promoting spices. The advertisement shows the new patent sifter top used exclusively on Rawleigh's spices. To open or close, merely slide the top. $6-$8.

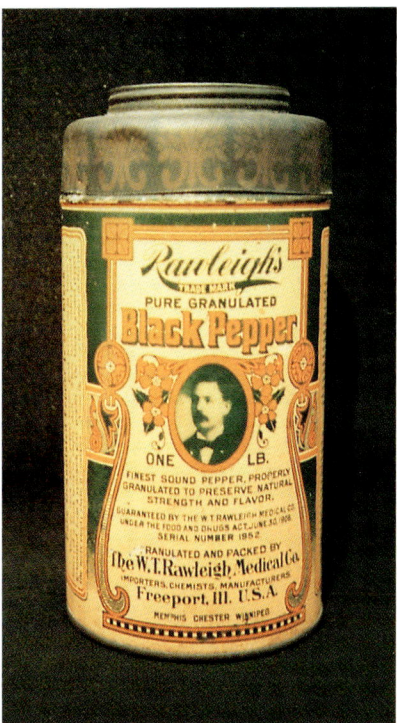

Rawleigh's pure granulated "Black Pepper" in one pound metal container. Granulated and packed by The W.T. Rawleigh Medical Co. Importers, Chemists, Manufacturers. Freeport, Ill. U.S.A. Memphis - Chester - Winnipeg. $80-$100; smaller variation: $50-$75.

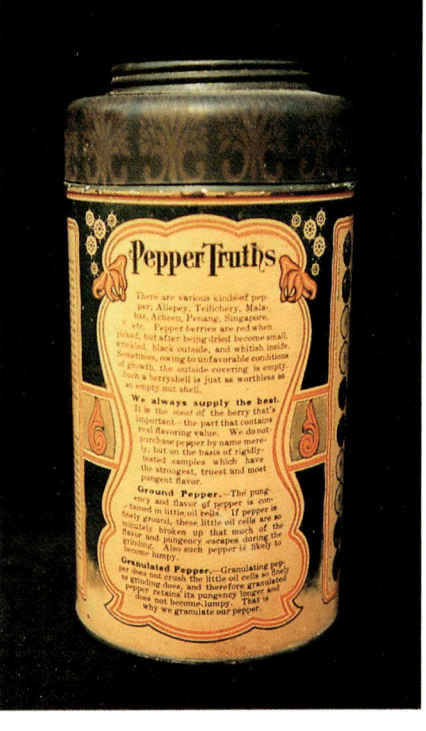

Pepper truths were provide on the reverse side of the granulated "Black Pepper." $80-$100.

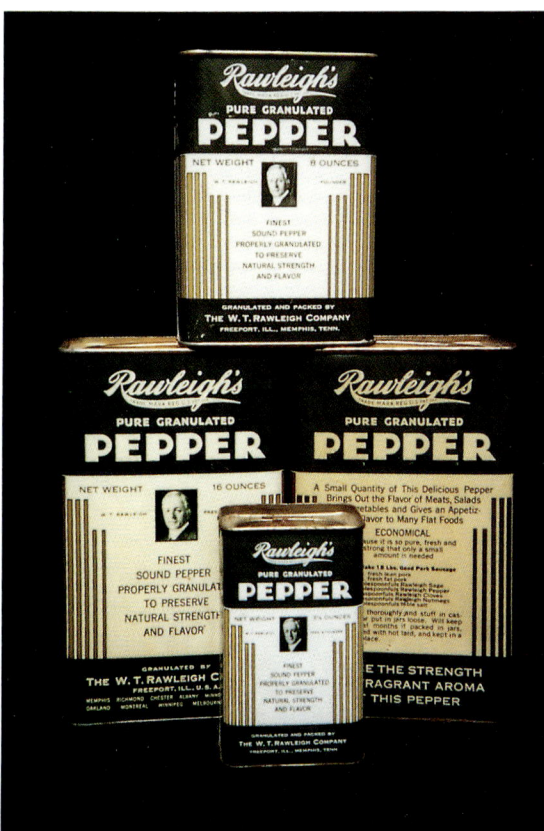

A 3-1/4, 8- and 16 ounce metal Rawleigh's pure granulated "Pepper" containers. Also shown is the reverse panel of a 16 ounce container. *Dupler Collection.* (3-1/4 & 8 oz.) $10-$15 ea.; (16 oz.) $20-$25.

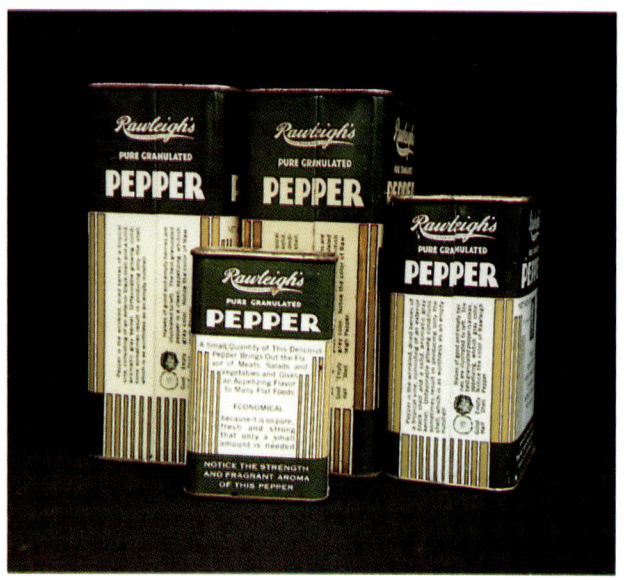

The side and reverse panels of the above pure granulated "Pepper" containers. *Dupler Collection.*

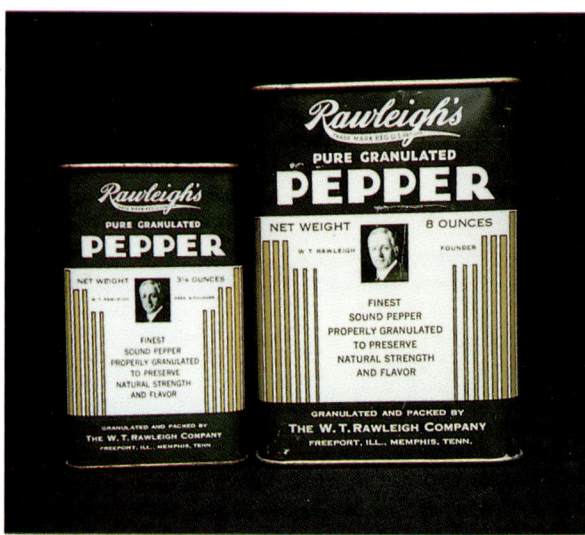

An 3-1/4 and 8 ounce metal container of Rawleigh's pure granulated "Pepper." Granulated and packed by The W.T. Rawleigh Company Freeport, Ill., Memphis, Tenn. *Dupler Collection.* $10-$15 ea.

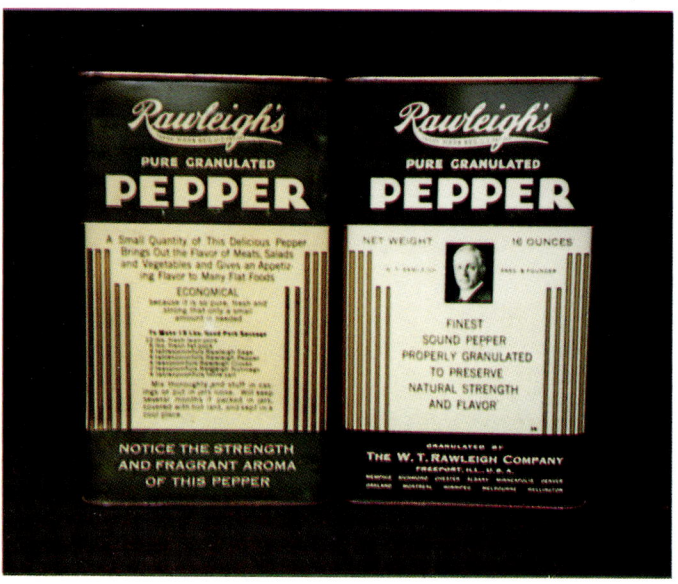

The front and back panels of Rawleigh's 16 ounce pure granulated "Pepper." Granulated by The W.T. Rawleigh Company Freeport, Ill., U.S.A. Memphis - Richmond - Chester - Albany - Minneapolis - Denver - Oakland - Montreal - Winnipeg - Melbourne - Wellington. *Dupler Collection.* $20-$25.

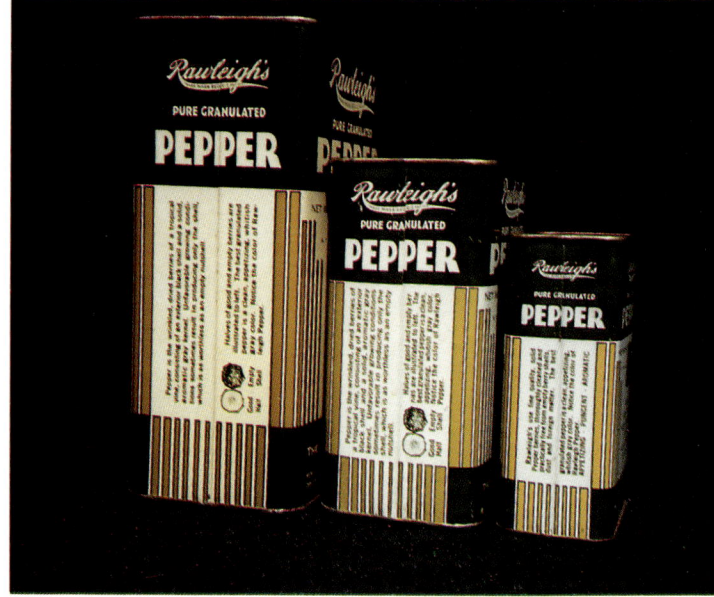

The side panels of Rawleigh's pure granulated Pepper state, "Pepper is the wrinkled, dried berries of a tropical vine, consisting of an exterior black shell and a solid, aromatic gray kernel. Unfavorable growing conditions sometimes result in producing only the shell which is as worthless as an empty nutshell." The company further remarked that the best granulated pepper is a clean, appetizing, whitish gray color. Rawleigh drew attention to the color of their pepper and illustrated the halves of good and empty berries.

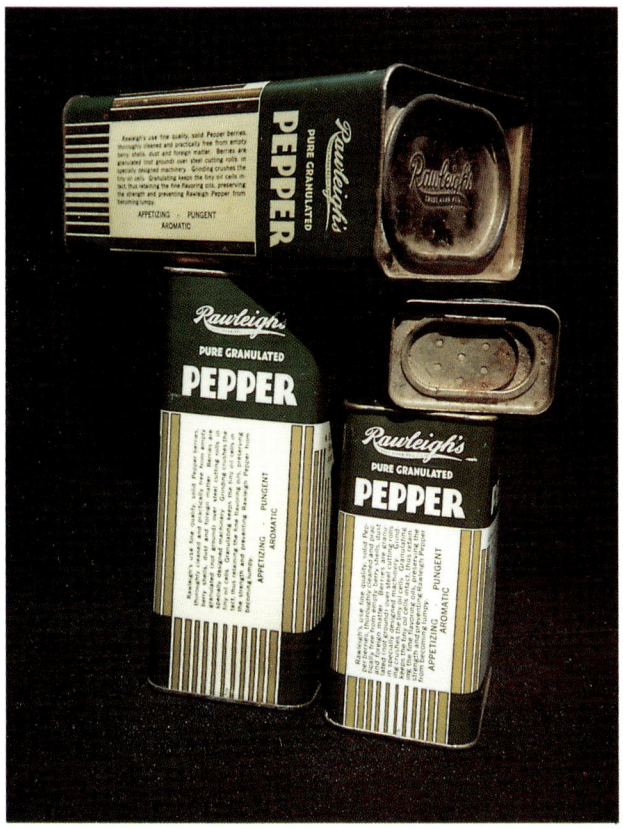

The embossed Rawleigh's pure granulated pepper lid. Note the sifter top used exclusively on Rawleigh's spices. To open or close merely slide the top. *Dupler Collection*.

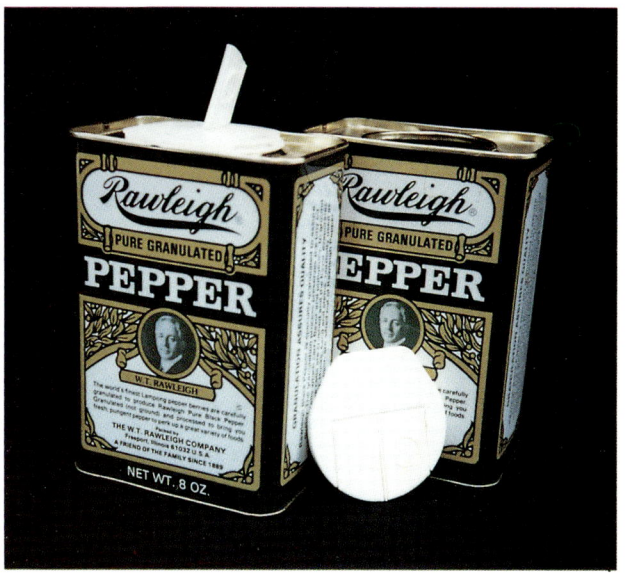

The 8 ounce reproduction tin of Rawleigh Pure Granulated Pepper has a plastic sifter top. In 1986 Rawleigh promoted the pure granulated pepper which featured a 1921 recipe for pork sausage. *Dupler Collection*. $10-$15.

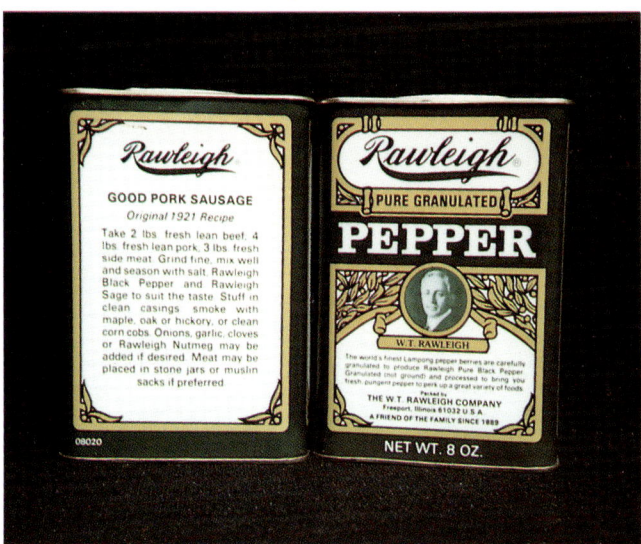

A front and reverse panel of the reproduction of the original black pepper tin used in 1921. Packed by The W.T. Rawleigh Company Freeport, Illinois 61032 U.S.A. Circa mid-1980s. *Dupler Collection*. $10-$15 ea.

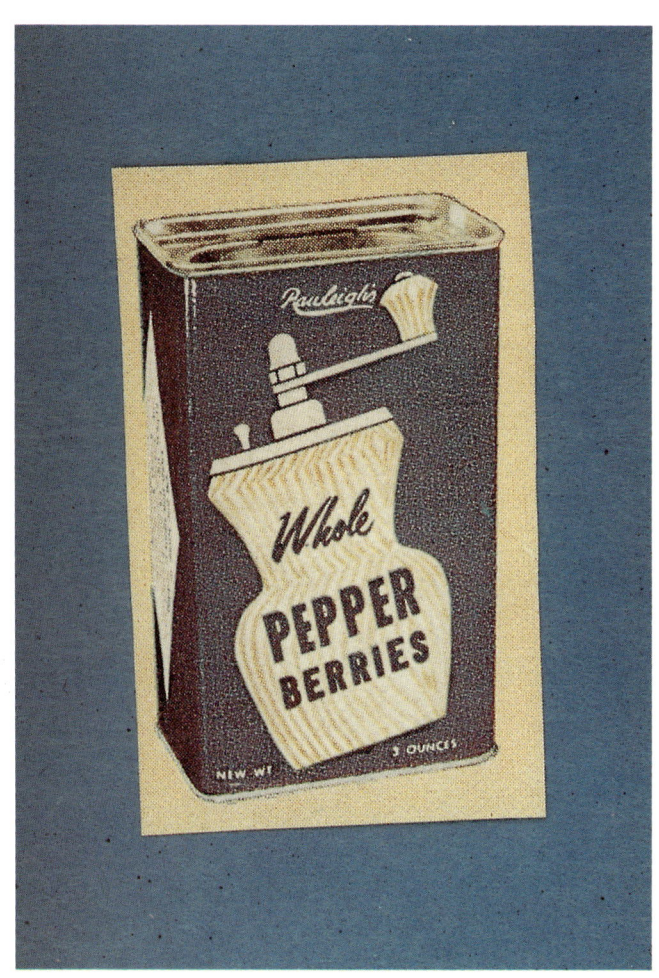

Rawleigh's "Whole Pepper Berries" were available in a 3 ounce container. This product was introduced in 1957. $20-$25.

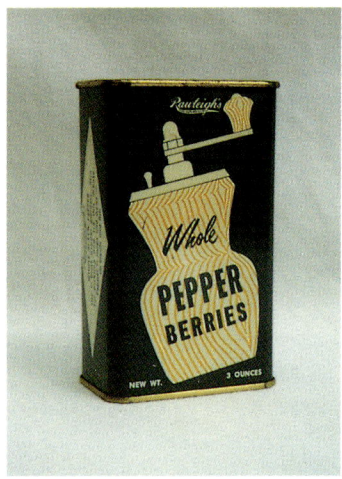

This "Whole Pepper Berries" container is highly sought by collectors and can be somewhat hard to find. $20-$25.

Extracts

Rawleigh Extracts were said to be of an unusual strength. They were advertised as rich, natural, and of lasting flavor.

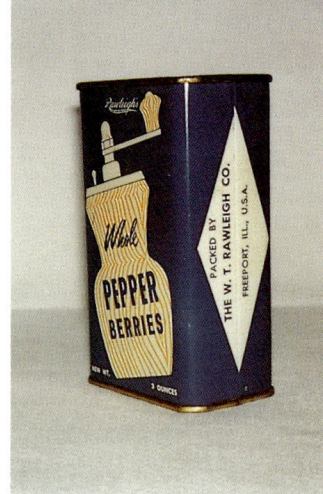

A side panel, "Packed By THE W.T. RAWLEIGH CO. FREEPORT, ILL., U.S.A." On the reverse panel Rawleigh suggested to use this "Whole Black Pepper" in home pepper grinders and/or for pickling and in soups, stews, and on meats and fish. This is a metal container with a snap in and out lid. $20-$25.

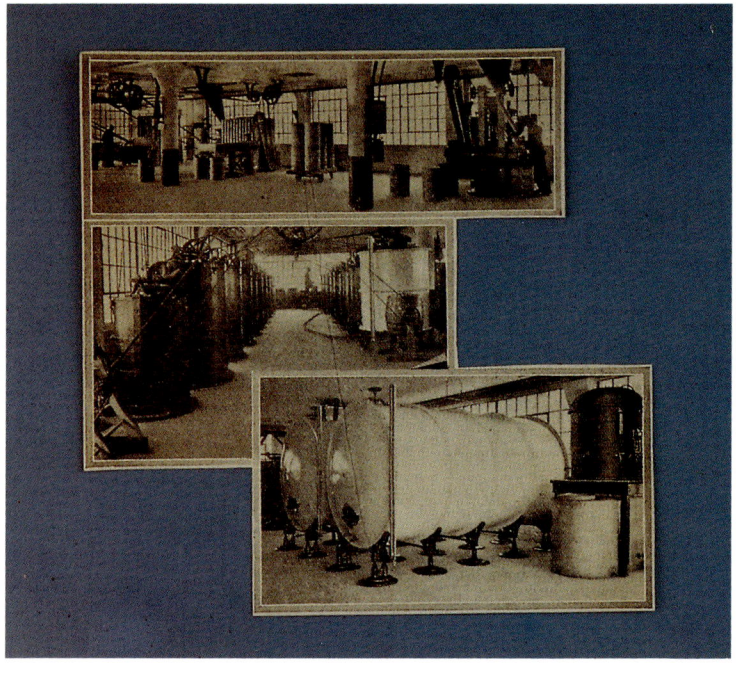

Scenes in Rawleigh's Memphis laboratory showing a small portion of the modern, expensive, up-to-date equipment used in the manufacture of Rawleigh extracts and flavoring, supplied to their southern trade. Circa 1915.

Salad Dressing Mix

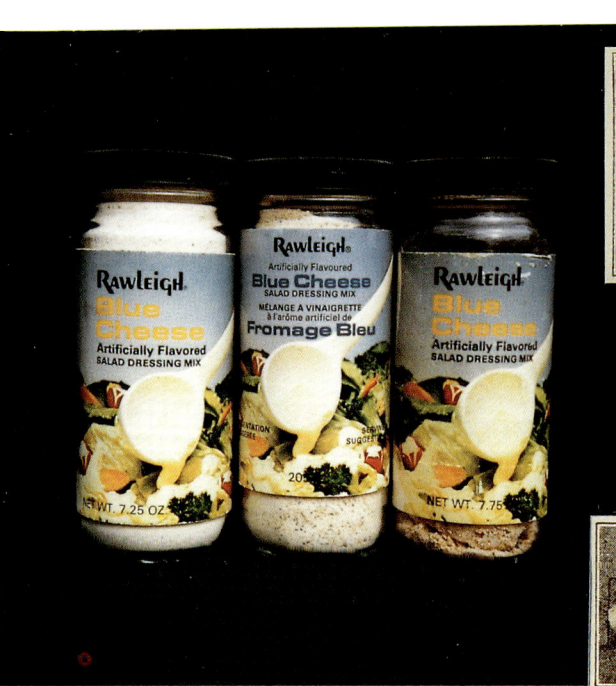

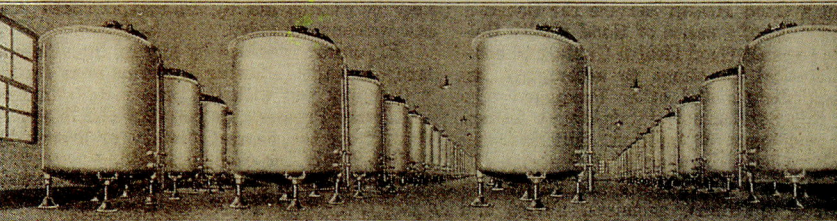

Steel, glass-lined tanks in which Rawleigh Cough Syrup and other liquid medicines, Fruit Drinks, Sweet Clover, and Extracts were mixed. Each tank had a capacity of 600 gallons. At the Freeport facilities over 60 of them were in regular use. Circa 1932.

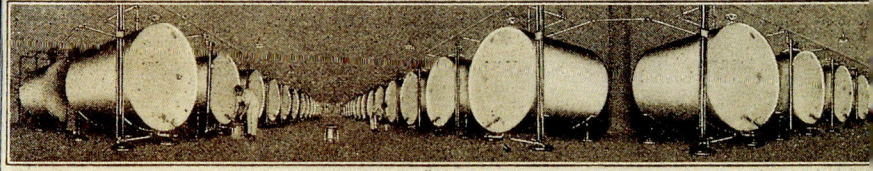

Rawleigh Blue Cheese Artificially Flavored Salad Dressing Mix. Manufactured by THE W.T. RAWLEIGH COMPANY Freeport, Illinois 61032. The middle container is marked "Mfd. by/Fab. per W.T. Rawleigh Co., Freeport, IL. U.S.A. W.T. Rawleigh Co. LTD. St. Laurent, Que. $10-$15 ea.

Some of the more than 100 glass-lined steel tanks with capacities of 1250 to 4000 gallons where most Rawleigh liquid preparations were aged for many weeks or months. Circa 1932.

Vanilla Compound

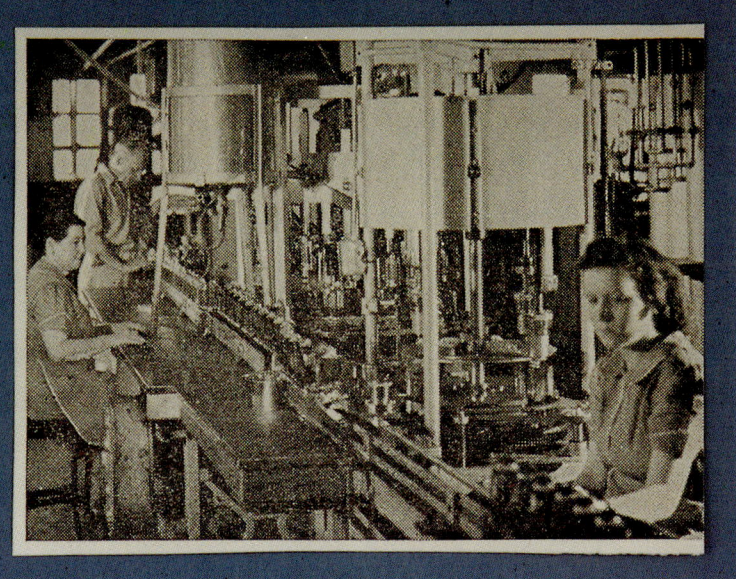

An example of the many thousands of dollars worth of modern machinery and equipment used in the Rawleigh factories in the United States, Canada, Australia, and New Zealand. Rawleigh spared no reasonable expense.

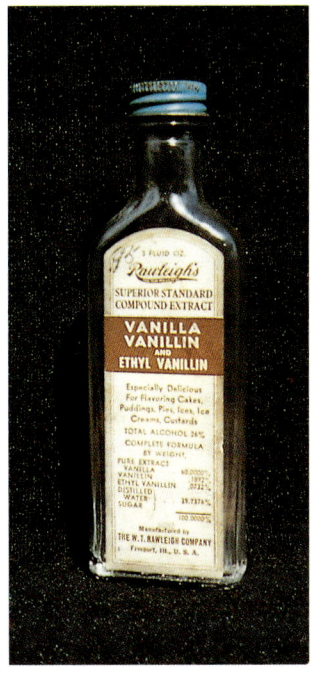

Rawleigh's Vanilla, Vanillin, and Ethyl Vanillin: a 3 ounce glass bottle with metal blue cap. Manufactured by The W.T. Rawleigh Company Freeport, Ill., U.S.A. *Dupler Collection.* $10-$15.

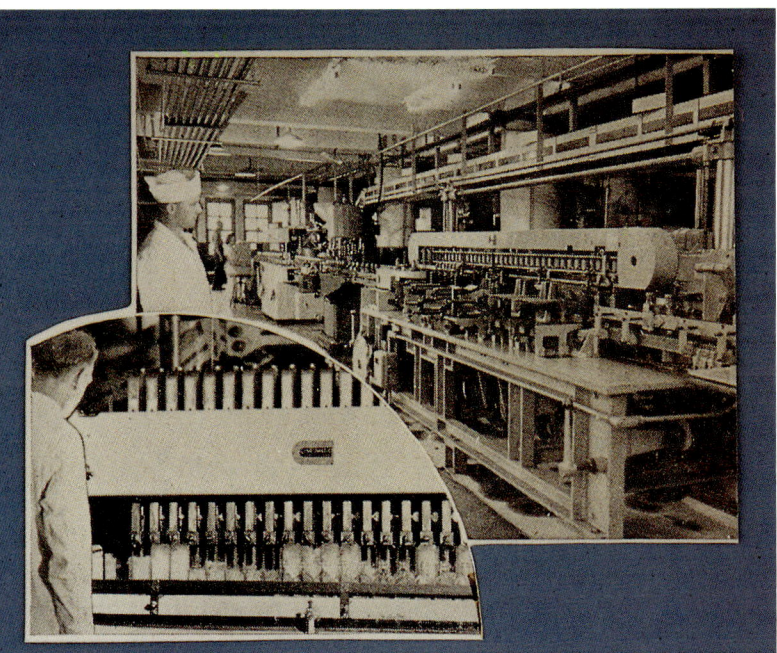

The new bottling equipment that cleaned, filled, capped and labeled bottles automatically up to 120 a minute. The top picture shows a complete line section with the insert providing a close-up view of bottles being filled twenty at a time at the rate of 96 bottles a minute with Rawleigh's Lemon Extract. Circa 1949.

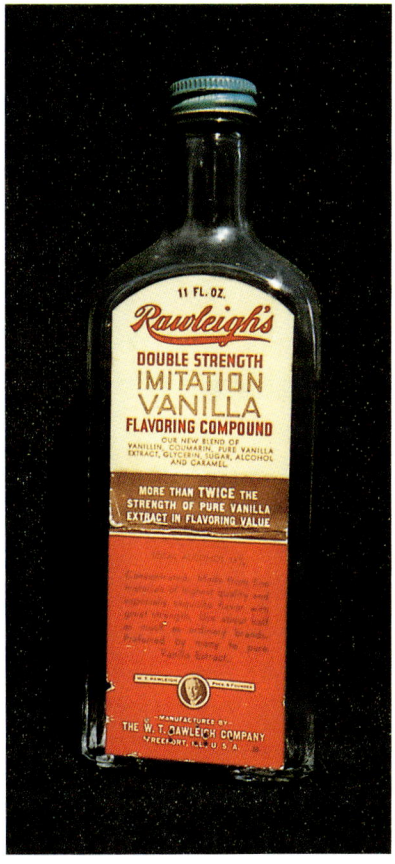

Rawleigh's Double Strength Imitation Vanilla Flavoring Compound, an 11 ounce glass bottle with a metal blue cap. Rawleigh used this blue metal cap on various products. This cap is embossed with their famous name. Manufactured by The W.T. Rawleigh Company Freeport, Ill., U.S.A. *Dupler Collection.* $10-$15.

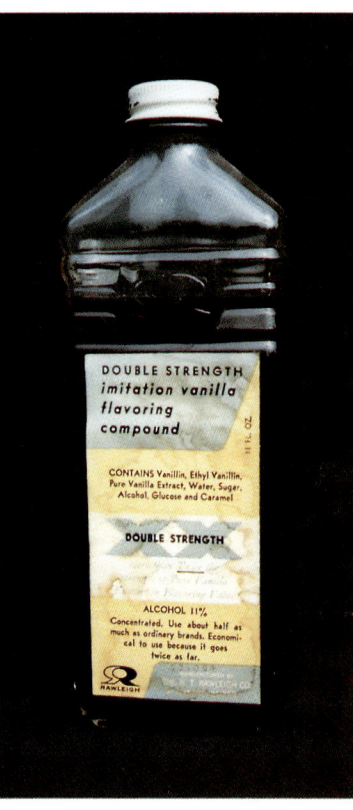

Rawleigh Double Strength Imitation Vanilla Flavoring Compound, an 11 ounce glass bottle with a metal cap. Manufactured by The W.T. Rawleigh Company Freeport, Ill., U.S.A. *Dupler Collection.* $10-$15.

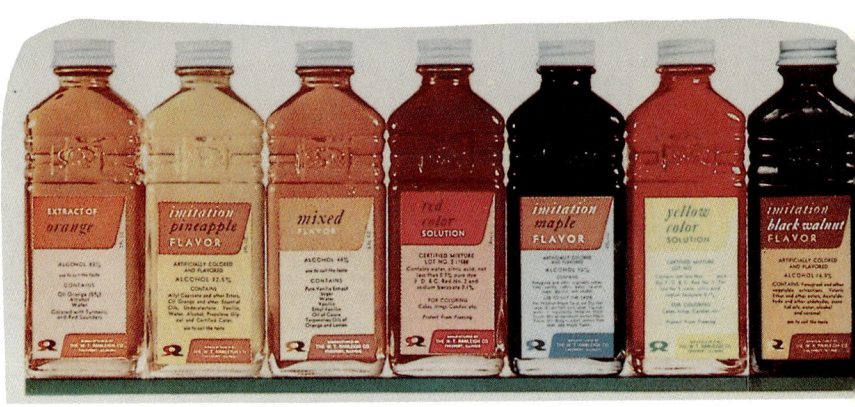

An original advertisement that read, "Using these fine flavors to vary your favorite foods." Rawleigh promoted the Orange Extract, Imitation Pineapple Flavor, Mixed Flavor, Red Color Solution, Imitation Maple Flavor, Yellow Color Solution, and Imitation Black Walnut Flavor. These bottles are readily available and presently are inexpensive. Circa 1960s. $6-$8 ea.

Rawleigh's Mixed Flavor was a blend of pure extracts of vanilla, lemon, orange, and Cassia providing a "delightful variety in desserts." Rawleigh's Orange Extract was the highest quality natural flavor made from the finest oil of the orange and was of full standard strength.

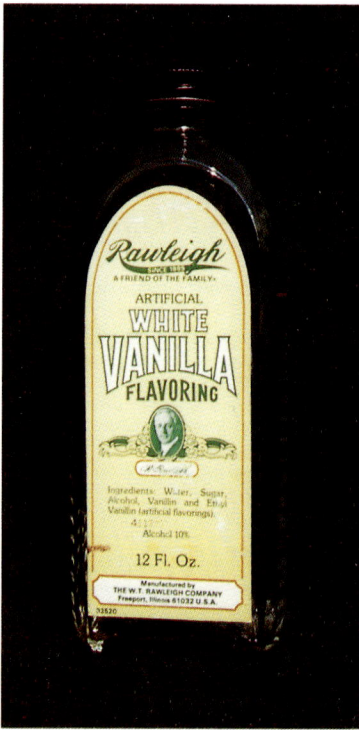

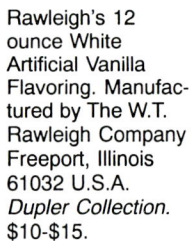

Rawleigh's 12 ounce White Artificial Vanilla Flavoring. Manufactured by The W.T. Rawleigh Company Freeport, Illinois 61032 U.S.A. *Dupler Collection.* $10-$15.

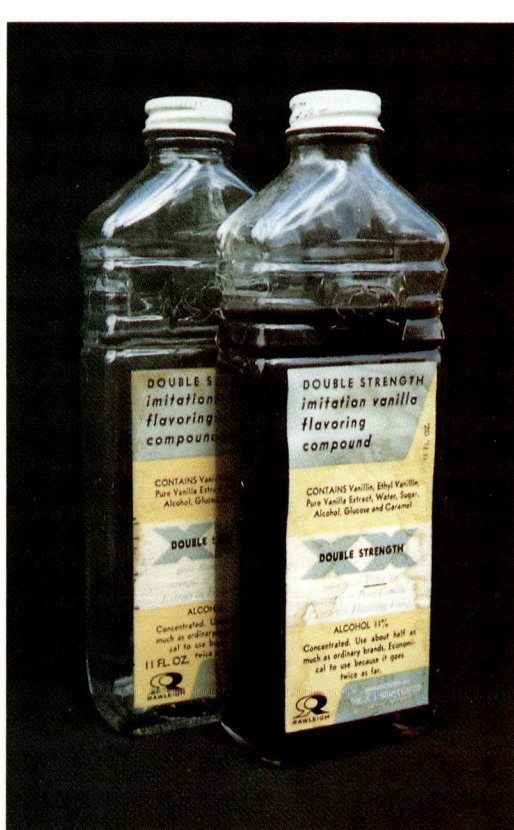

Two 11 ounce bottles of Rawleigh Double Strength Imitation Vanilla Flavoring Compound. These were blue ribbon winners; professional cooks and new brides praised Rawleigh's Vanilla for the full rich body that no other vanilla had. *Dupler Collection.* $10-$15 ea.

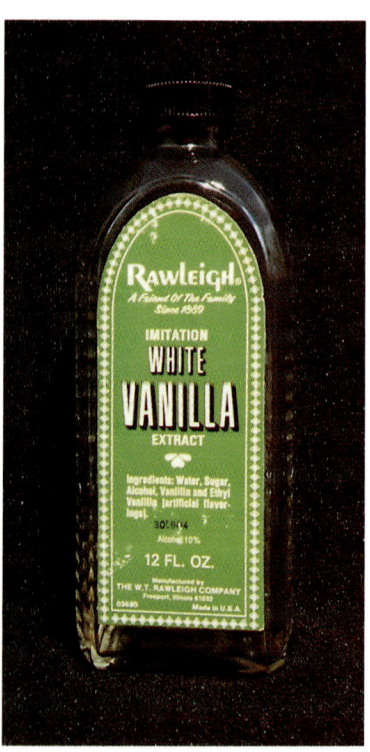

Rawleigh White Artificial Vanilla Extract, a 12 ounce glass bottle with a metal cap. Manufactured by The W.T. Rawleigh Company Freeport, Illinois 61032 U.S.A. *Dupler Collection.* $10-$15.

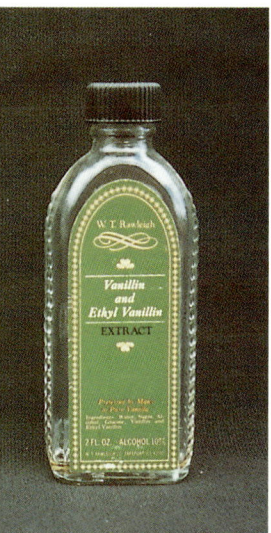

W.T. Rawleigh Vanillin and Ethyl Vanillin Extract, a 2 ounce glass bottle with a plastic cap. W.T. Rawleigh Co., Freeport, Ill 61032. $10-$15.

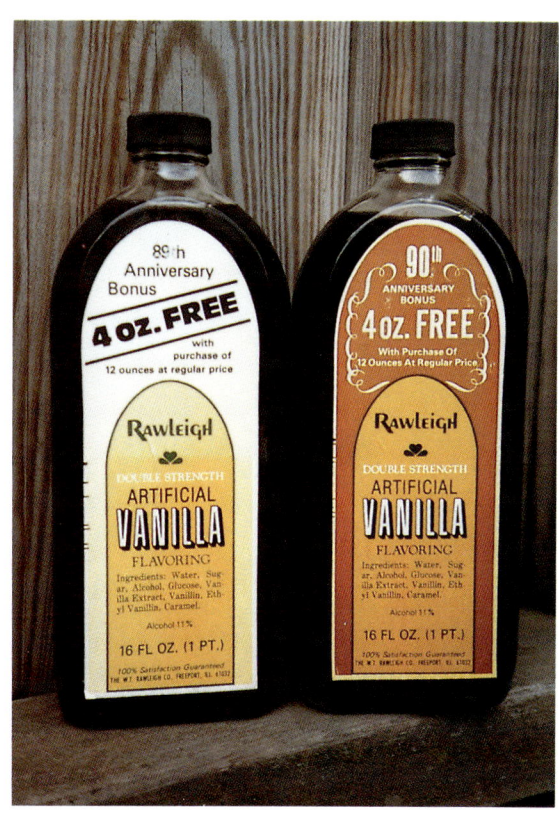

Rawleigh's 89th (1978) and 90th (1979) Anniversary Bonus "Double Strength Artificial Vanilla Flavoring." The 4 ounce bottle was "FREE With Purchase of a 12 ounce At Regular Price." The W.T. Rawleigh Co., Freeport, Ill. 61032 *Bushue Collection.* $20-$25 ea.

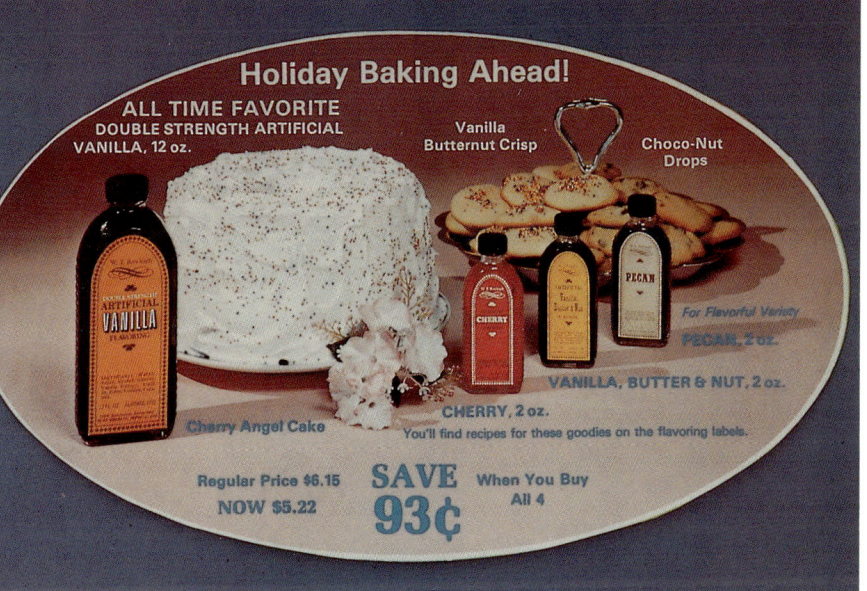

In 1976 this "Holiday Baking Ahead!" advertisement appeared in a Rawleigh publication.

Butter & Nut Flavoring

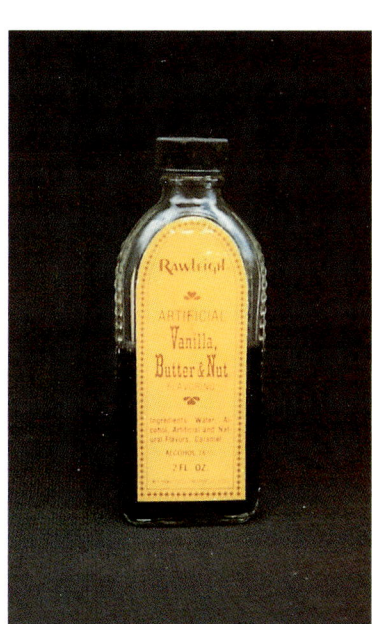

Rawleigh Artificial Vanilla, Butter & Nut Flavoring, 2 ounce glass bottle with a plastic cap. W.T. Rawleigh Co., Freeport, Ill 61032. *Dupler Collection.* $10-$15.

Lemon Extract

Rawleigh's Lemon Extract was made from the finest oil of lemon and gave a natural fruity flavor because of its superior quality and full standard strength.

Walnut and Maple Flavors

Rawleigh Walnut and Maple Flavors were synthetically made. A syrup rivaling true maple could be made at low cost by adding Rawleigh Maple Flavoring to sugar syrup. These flavors were popular in cakes, icings, ice creams, and candies.

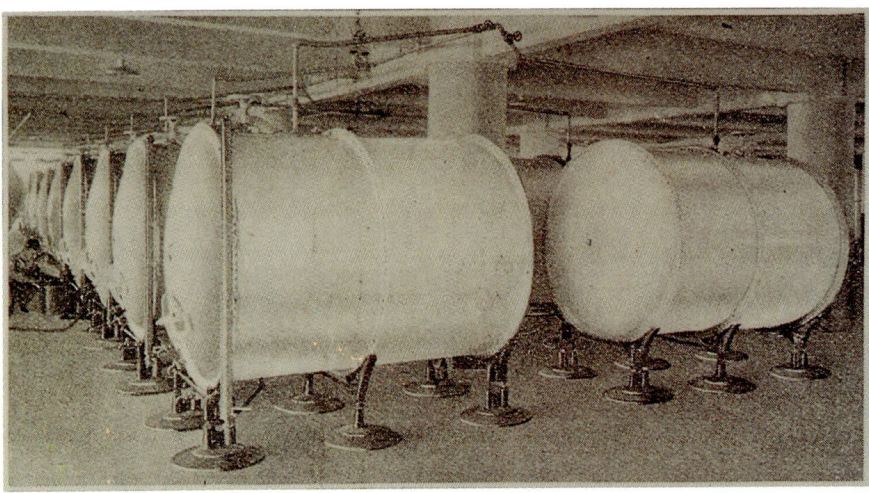

This photograph displays copper containers of pure oil of lemon and was printed in 1916. This was only a portion of a Rawleigh shipment imported from Sicily and the oils of lemon and orange were valued at over $35,000 dollars.

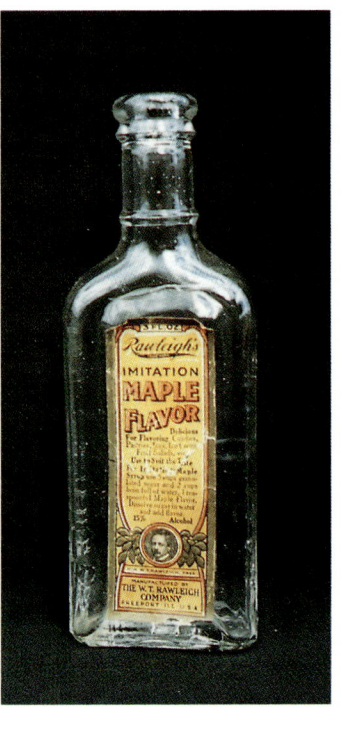

Rawleigh's Imitation Maple Flavor. Manufactured by The W.T. Rawleigh Co. Freeport, Ill. U.S.A. *Dupler Collection.* $10-$15.

Almond, Wintergreen, and Peppermint

High quality extracts were made from natural oils of almond, wintergreen, and double distilled American peppermint oil. These extracts were used for flavoring cakes, desserts, ice creams, candies, and icings. Wintergreen and peppermint also had their medicinal uses.

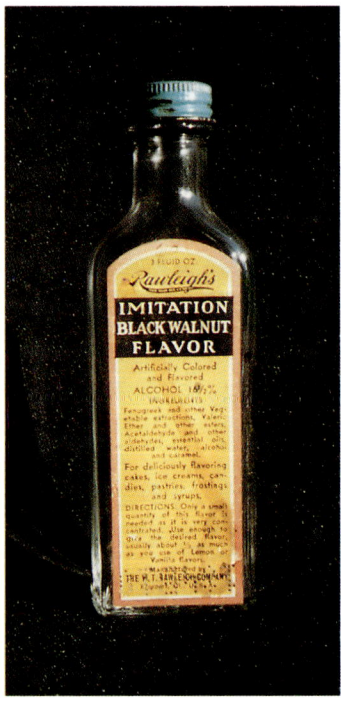

Rawleigh's Imitation Black Walnut Flavor. Manufactured By The W.T. Rawleigh Company Freeport, IL. U.S.A. *Dupler Collection.* $10-$15.

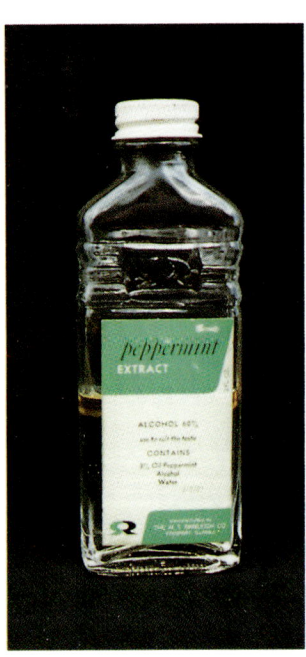

Peppermint Extract packaged in a 3 ounce glass bottle with a metal cap. Manufactured by The W.T. Rawleigh Co. Freeport, Illinois. *Dupler Collection.* $10-$15.

Strawberry, Pineapple, and Banana

Rawleigh's Strawberry, Pineapple, and Banana flavors were synthetically made to give a fruity taste and added variety to cakes, desserts, and ice cream. These popular flavors were concentrated, economical, and satisfying.

Miscellaneous

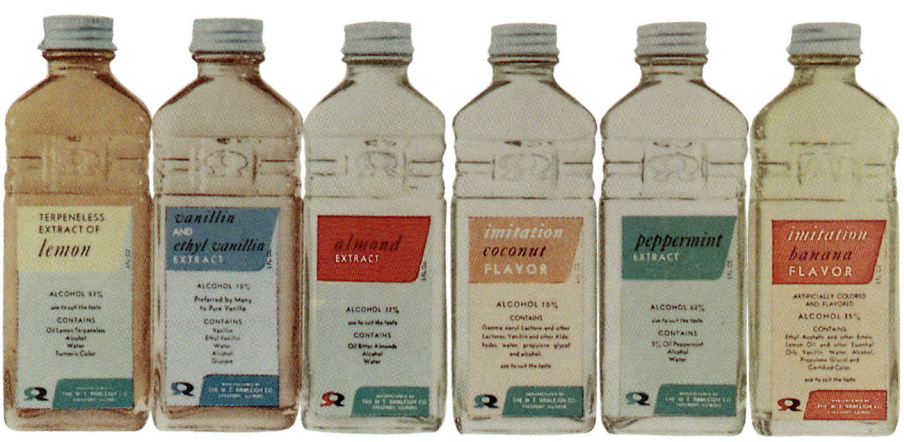

"Use these fine flavors to vary your favorite foods." Rawleigh promoted the above Lemon, Vanillin & Ethyl Vanillin, Almond, Coconut, Peppermint and Banana flavoring during the 1960s.

Red and Yellow Color Solutions

Rawleigh's Color Solutions were safe, certified colors for attractively tinting of cakes, icings, candies, sherbets, jellies, desserts, or beverages.

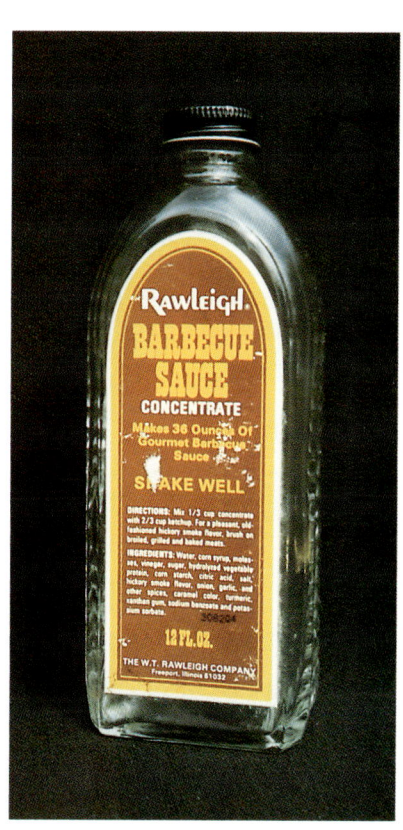

A 12 fluid ounce Rawleigh Concentrate Barbecue Sauce bottle. The W.T. Rawleigh Company Freeport, Illinois 61032. *Dupler Collection.* $10-$15.

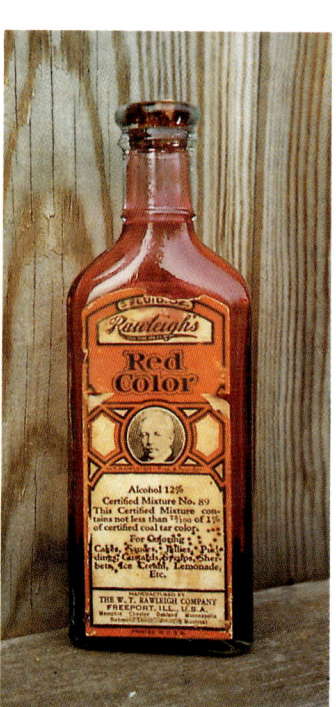

A 5 fluid ounce Rawleigh's Red Color. Manufactured By The W.T. Rawleigh Company Freeport, Ill., U.S.A. Memphis - Chester - Oakland - Minneapolis - Richmond - London - Winnipeg - Montreal. $20-$25.

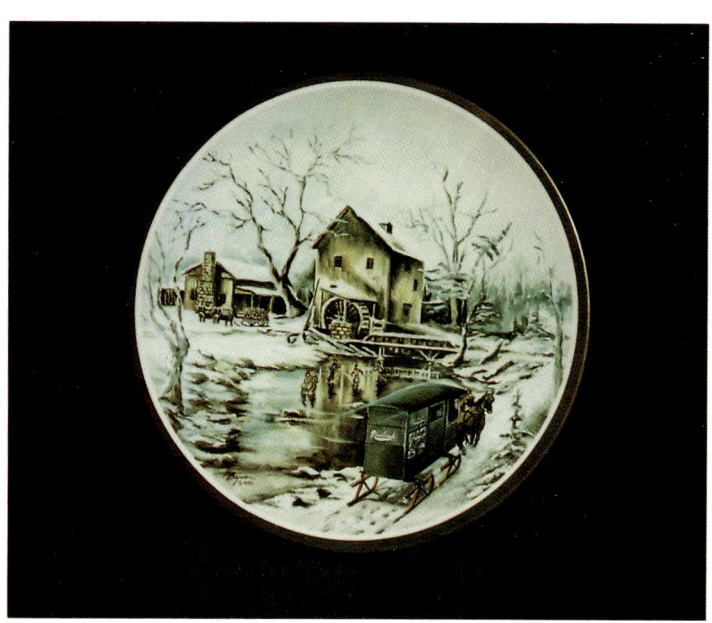

The illustration on the 1985 Rawleigh Collector's Fruit Cake tin is a reproduction from an original oil painting which was commissioned by The W.T. Rawleigh Company, Freeport, Illinois. The fruit cake that came inside was made with Rawleigh products: Double Strength Vanilla, Butter Rum Flavoring, Orange Extract, Lemon Extract, Butter Flavoring, Almond Extract, Cinnamon, Nutmeg, Ground Cloves, and Allspice. $20-$25.

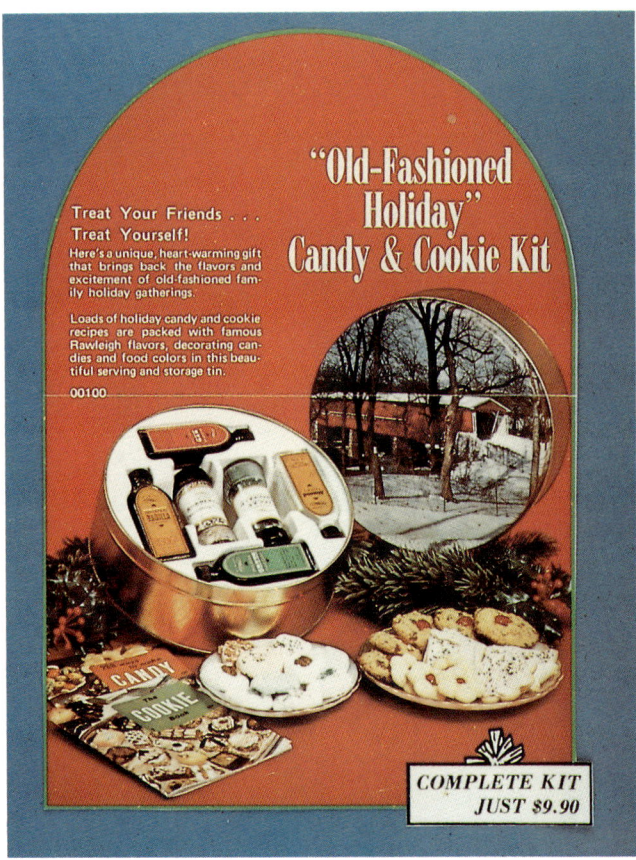

An original 1970s Rawleigh advertisement for an "Old Fashioned Holiday" Candy & Cookie Kit. $20-$25 complete.

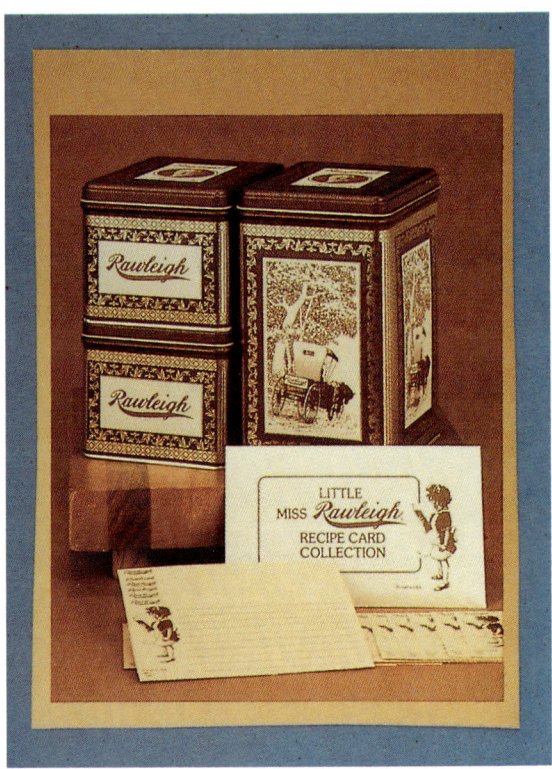

An original 1986 advertisement for Rawleigh's limited edition heritage canisters. Little Miss Rawleigh Recipe Cards were available in packs of 25. Each card depicted "Little Miss Rawleigh" with a cookbook and a spoon. Lines were provided on the front so favorite recipes could be printed.

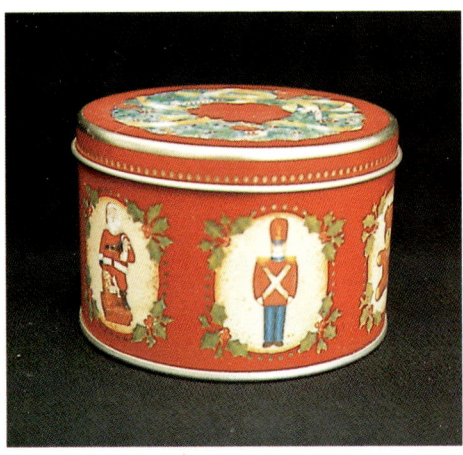

The metal container held 12 ounces of "Rawleigh's Old-Fashioned Christmas Candy." Distributed by The W.T. Rawleigh Co., Freeport, IL. 61032 USA. *Bushue Collection.* $20-$25.

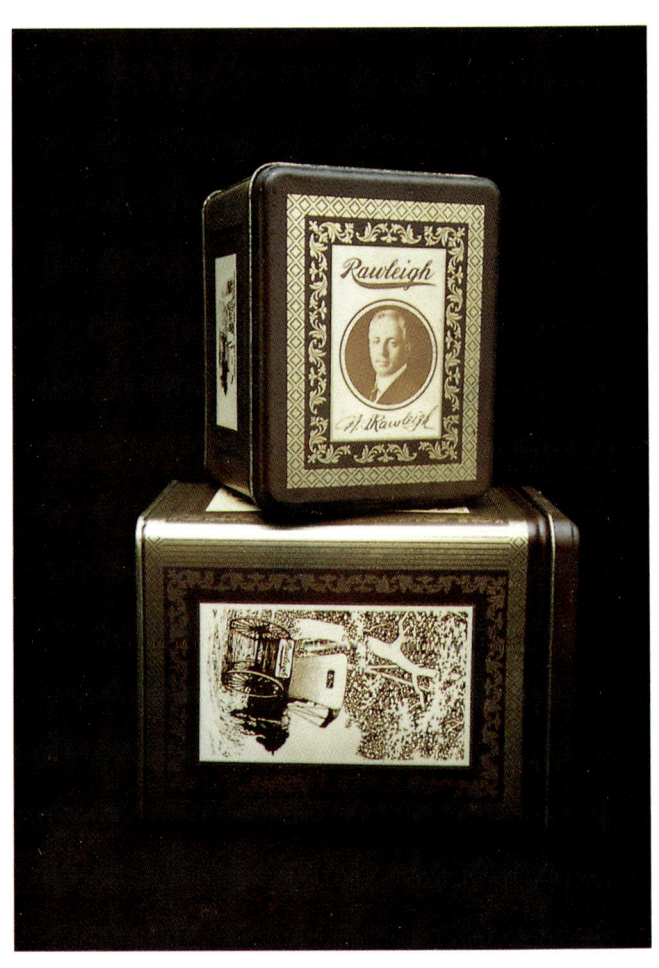

The Rawleigh canisters were offered in a SMALL size 4-3/4" x 3-3/4" x 3-1/4" and LARGE size 4-3/4" x 3-3/4" x 6". W.T. Rawleigh's photograph and the famous Rawleigh trademark appears on these limited edition heritage canisters. $10-$20 ea.

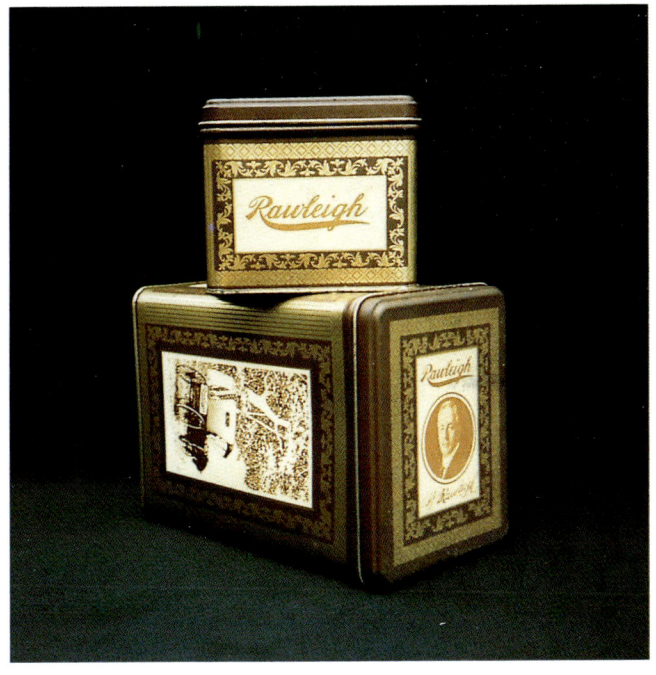

These canisters were ideal for storage or decoration. As these were limited editions, they may require time in locating. $10-$20 ea.

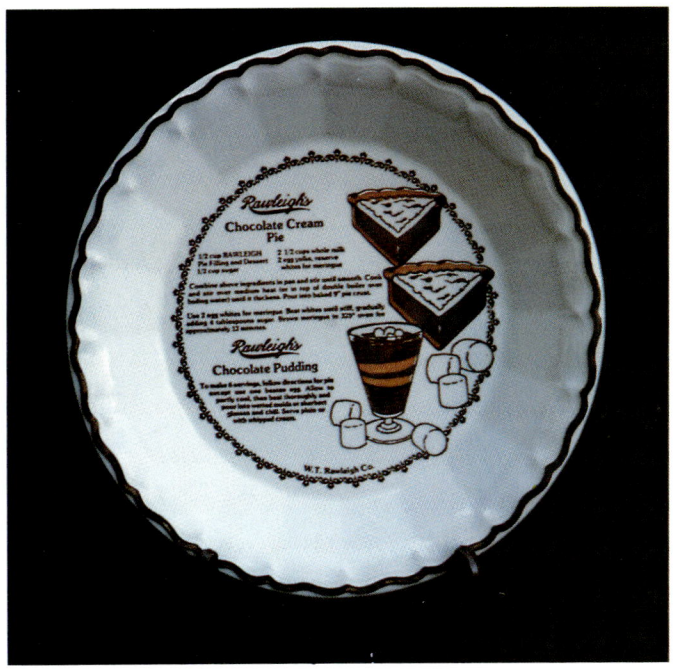

A 10-1/2" diameter Rawleigh's Chocolate Pie Baker. Circa 1984. $20-$30.

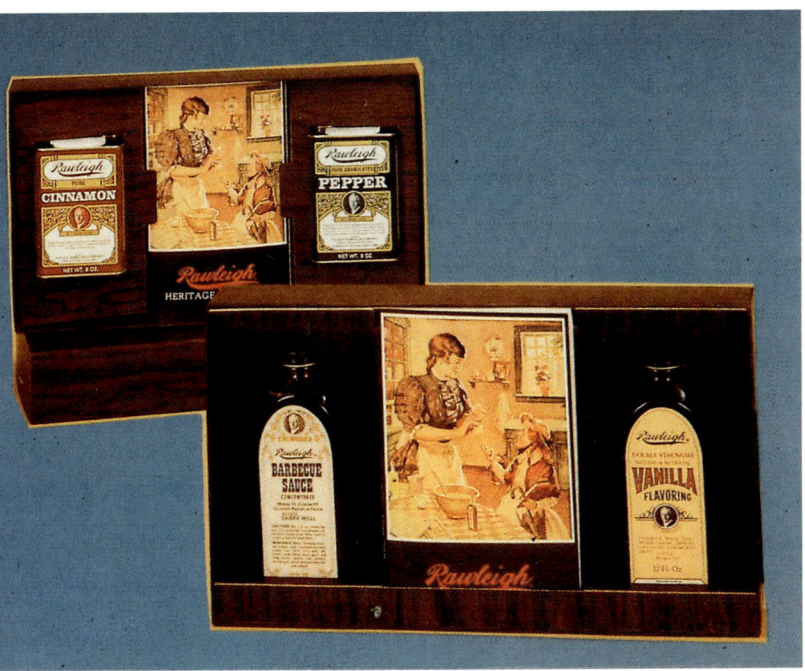

In 1986 customers could select from one of the Rawleigh Gift Sets shown here. Rawleigh Gift Set with 8 ounces of Black Pepper and Cinnamon, plus the Heritage Cookbook or a Rawleigh Gift Set with 12 ounce bottles of Rawleigh's famous Vanilla and Barbecue Sauce Concentrate, and the Heritage Cookbook. Either of these sets were perfect gifts for any occasion. The Heritage Cookbook was also available separately.

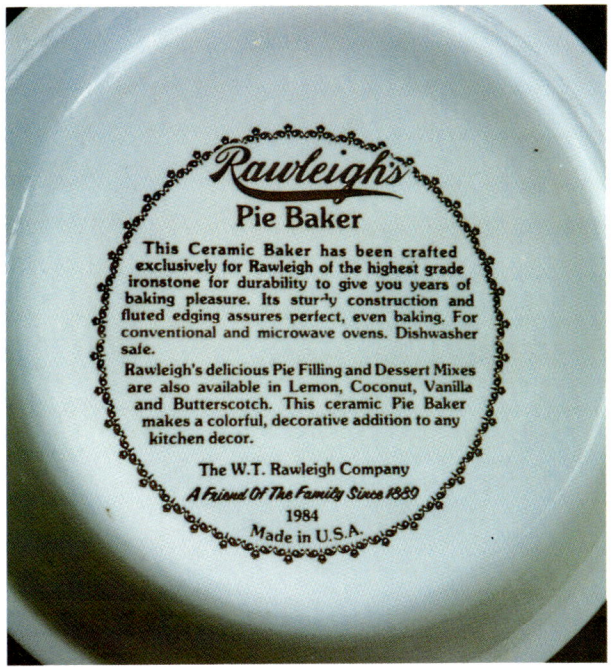

The reverse side of Rawleigh's Chocolate Pie Baker. $20-$30.

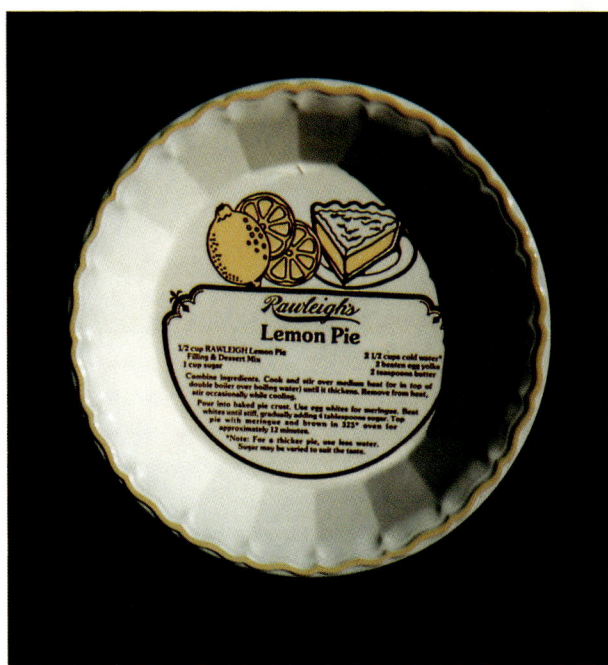

A 10-1/2" diameter Rawleigh's Lemon Pie Baker. In 1986 three collectible pie bakers were available. Chocolate, Lemon, and Coconut, each baker featured Rawleigh's award winning pie recipes. These pie bakers were microwave oven and dishwasher safe. $20-$30 ea.

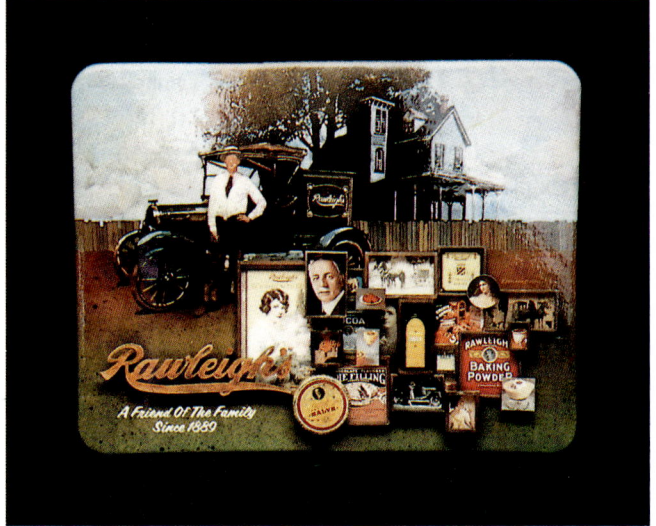

Rawleigh's combination wall plaque and table hot pad "Hot Plaque".™ This pad (measuring approximately 8-1/2" x 6-1/2") has a special heat resistant plastic finish that will withstand heat up to 500 degrees. Makes a perfect table protecting pad for hot dishes from the oven or stove. The plastic finish also resists grease, dirt, etc. Genuine cork back. $15-$20.

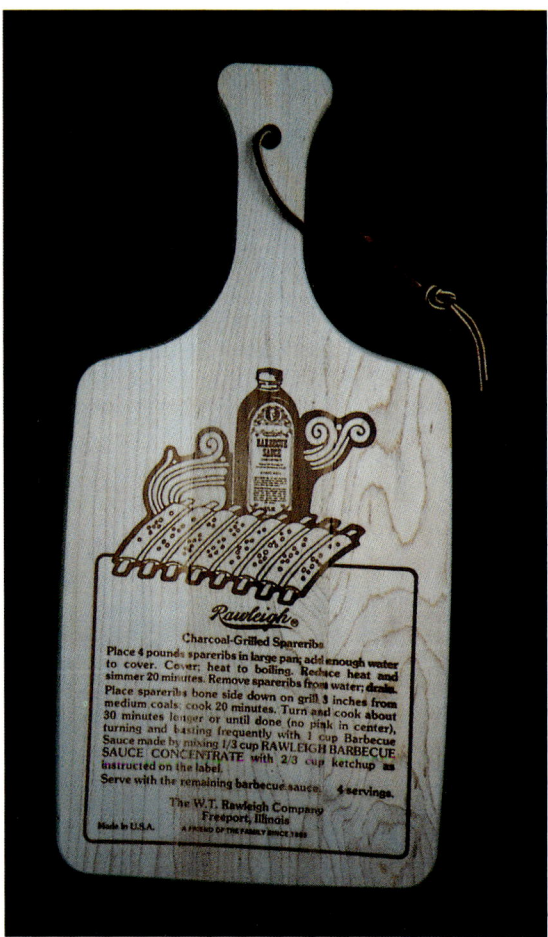

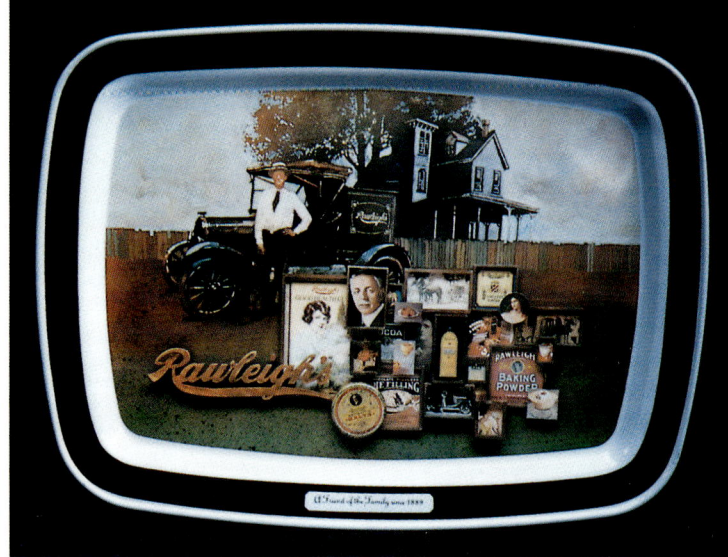

Rawleigh's metal serving tray. The photograph from the wall plaque and table hot pad is repeated on this 14-3/4" x 11" tray. "A Friend of the Family since 1889." $40-$50.

The Rawleigh cutting board added charm to any kitchen decor and served as a versatile kitchen utensil. On the front side was a recipe for bar-b-que spareribs. $20-$30.

In 1986, three racks were promoted in Rawleigh's catalog. A flavoring rack held eight 2 ounce containers of Rawleigh flavors and extracts in a traditional single tier rack. Two spice racks were also available. A single tier held 8 containers and a double tier held 16 spice and seasoning containers. The spice racks could not hold large onion flakes or large steak seasoning containers. Each rack was marked "Rawleigh®" across the top section. $50-$75 ea.

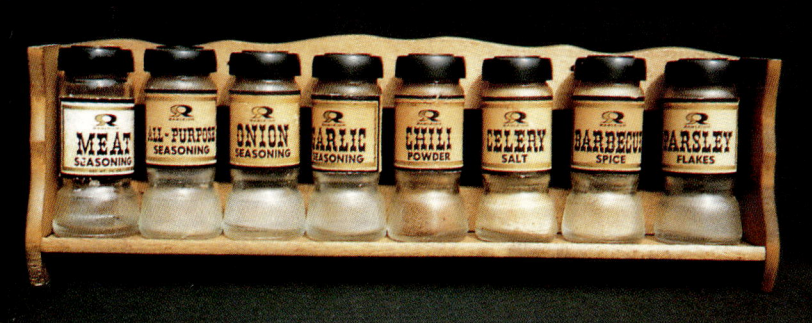

Rawleigh's eight bottle spice rack. No indication of the famous Rawleigh trademark appears on the wooden rack. $40-$50 complete.

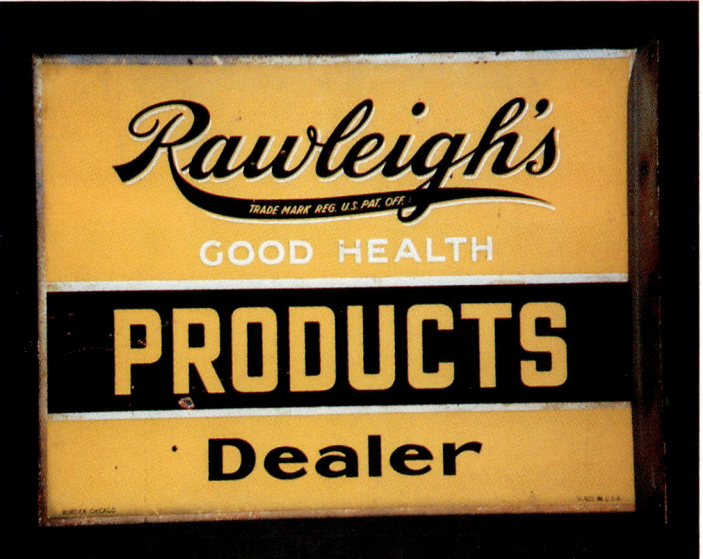

"Rawleigh's Good Health PRODUCTS Dealer" sign. This enamel 18-1/4" x 13-1/2" sign hung outside a residence indicating a dealer resided inside and that Rawleigh products were available. Shown elsewhere in this publication is an 84th Anniversary sign that could be placed inside a dealers car window. $100-$150.

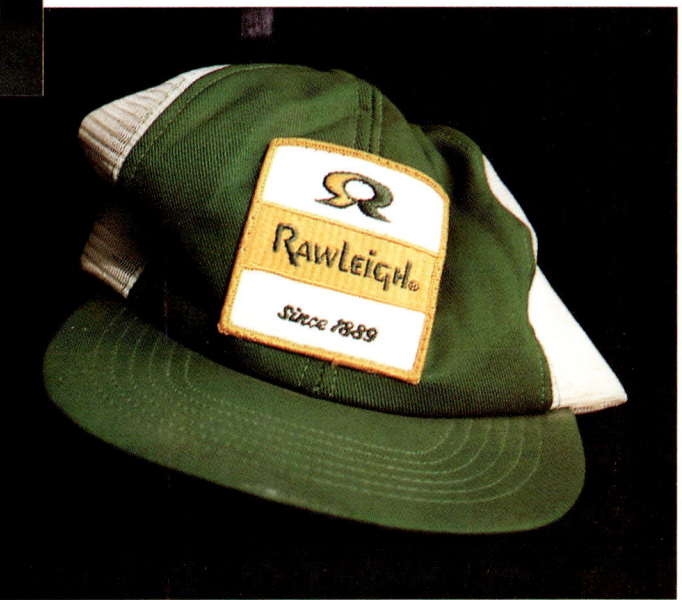

"Rawleigh® Since 1889" baseball hat. *Bushue Collection.* $20-$25.

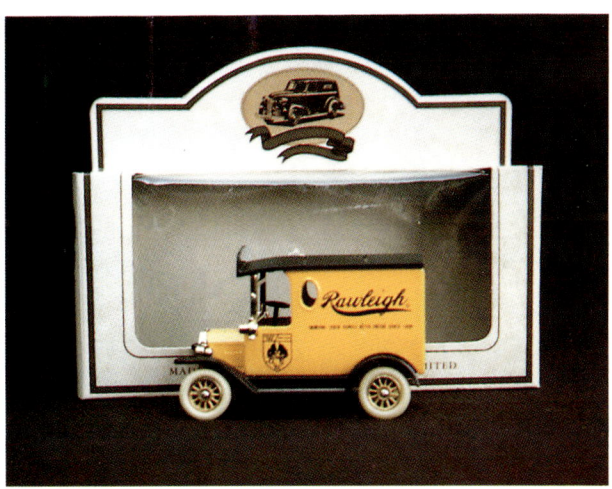

The die-cast metal replica of the Rawleigh truck was "Made in England by Lledo (London) Limited. *Bushue Collection.* $30-$40.

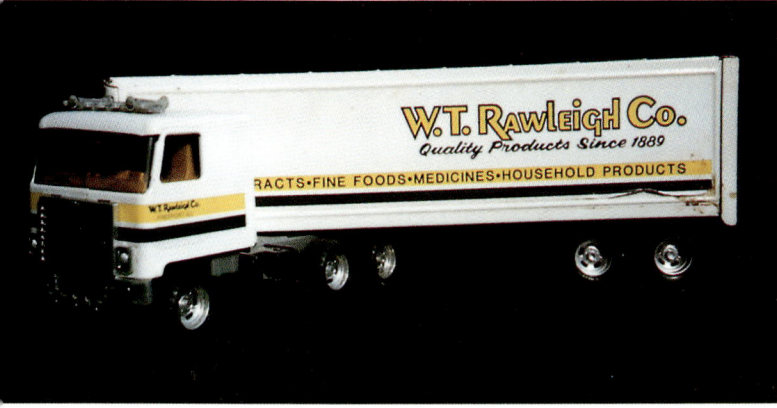

A reproduction of the Rawleigh semi tractor-trailer that delivered many orders across America. The trailer rear doors swing open on this rugged steel truck. Offered in December 1981, there was a limited quantity of this sturdy truck. This truck is highly sought by both Rawleigh and toy collectors. Be prepared, this truck is very expensive because of the limited quantity available. *Bushue Collection.* $125-$150.

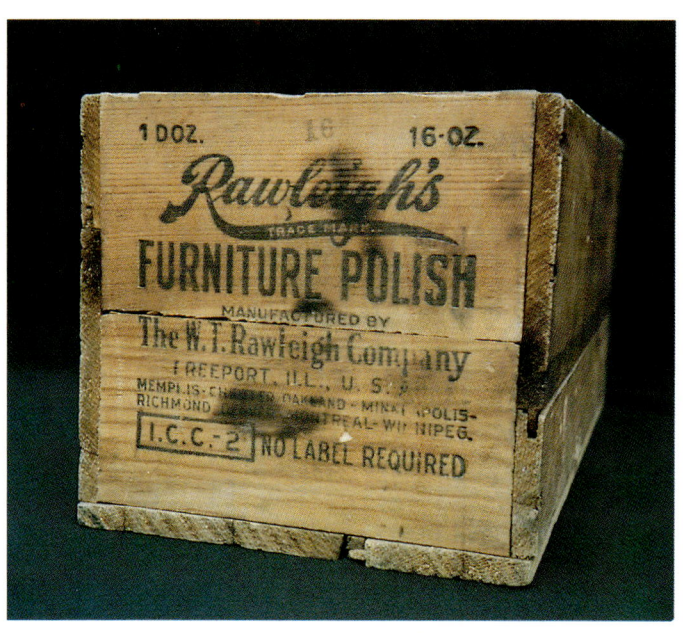

This wooden Rawleigh's Furniture Polish crate held one dozen 16 ounce containers of polish. Manufactured by The W.T. Rawleigh Company Freeport, Ill., U.S.A. $80-$100.

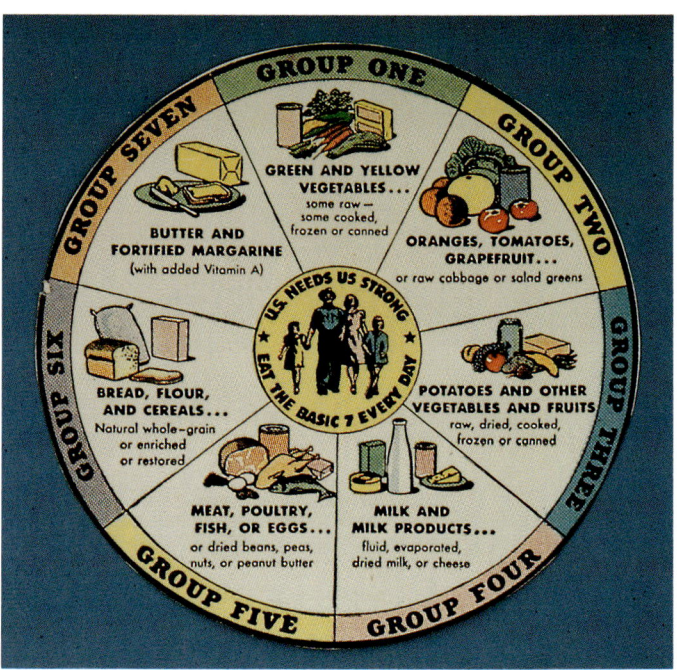

In 1946, Rawleigh published a health chart to help plan well-balanced meals. The suggestion was made that everyone should eat some food from each of the seven groups shown on the chart each day.

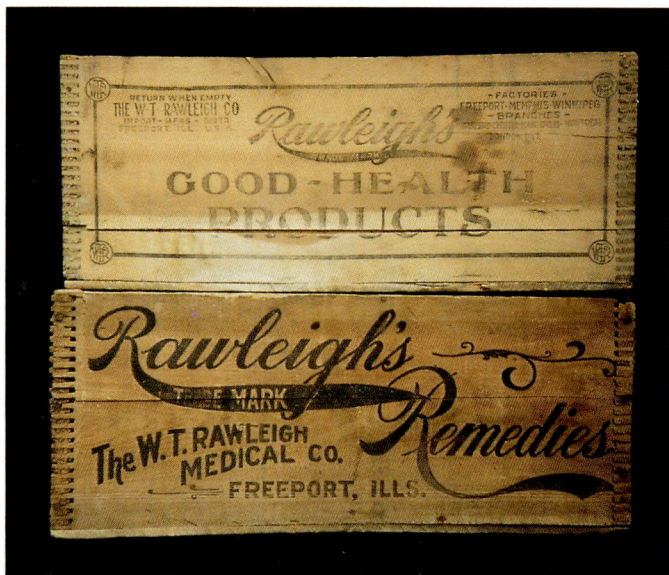

Two different Rawleigh packaging crates. The W.T. Rawleigh Medical Co. crate (bottom) is shown elsewhere in this publication. These wooden crates are escalating in price and demand. $100-$150 ea.

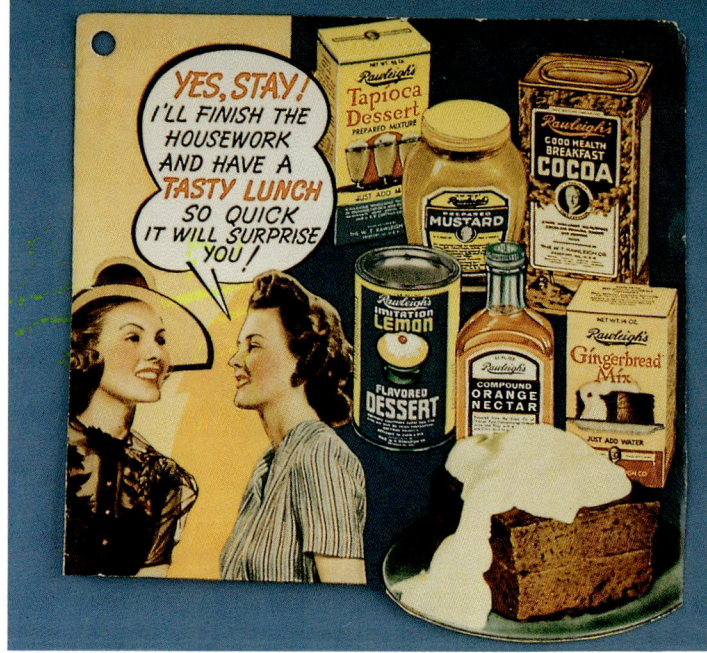

In 1941 Rawleigh promoted the products shown in this original advertisement. Many of these products appear throughout this publication.

Care of Your Products

It is wise to remember that Rawleigh products in mint condition bring a higher price in the secondary market than those of poor condition. Purchase only items in mint quality condition unless you run across an item in lesser condition that you feel that you can not live without.

Do not apply water to your metal products (or submerge them); this will cause rusting to begin or to continue. To keep your metal products in excellent condition, it is suggested that you apply a light coat of good car wax to the surface of each item. Using a cotton ball or Q-tip, apply the wax in small sections, but never apply pressure. Repeat the process until the surface has been covered — this creates a protection against the elements that might otherwise damage your products. Wipe residue off with a soft cloth. It may be wise to first experiment on a worthless tin. Remember, practice makes perfect!

On metal products with severely rusted areas, apply a light coat of WD-40, available at most hardware stores. Using a Q-tip, gently apply WD-40 to the effected area of the product. Wipe the residue off with a soft cloth. Repeat this process as often as needed.

Keep an eye on your products for any indication that they have been invaded by insects. You may not know what lives in (or is growing beneath the lids of) your products. Never consume an old product and keep old products out of the reach of small children.

Any Rawleigh bottle that has a cloudy coating on an inner or outer surface may be submerged in a product called "LIME-A-WAY."® An interior filmy coating may also be removed by filling the bottle and dissolving an effervescent denture tablet inside. Be extremely careful with these products and keep them away from children and from your eyes.

To use "LIME-A-WAY,"® place the cloudy bottle into a shallow pan and cover it with "LIME-A-WAY."® It is wise to leave the bottle submerged for six to eight weeks. Check occasionally and add more liquid if needed. This product can also be poured directly into the cloudy bottle, shaken, and placed out of the way for some time. Check the bottle occasionally and, once again, if liquid seems low, add more. NEVER submerge bottles or jars with paper labels as this will remove and/or cause harm to those labels.

It is not uncommon for collectors of advertising products to seal them for protection. Often an inexpensive substitute of plastic or Saran wrap is used. I am totally against this practice. Placing products inside plastic bags or wrapping them in any of the various products that are readily available could be dangerous to your items. If moisture gets into this wrap/plastic covering, your product is ill-fated. Seek professional assistance in caring for any product, either metal or cardboard. There are firms that will professionally wrap advertisement articles and products. Use your better judgment!

Condition Factor

Rawleigh products in mint condition are those free from rust, scratches, or blemishes, and which still retain 100% of the original wrapper, label, and/or carton. Lids must be intact and free of any blemish. Only those products in mint condition receive the highest prices. Full containers are much more desirable those that are empty.

Products from the early era of the Rawleigh Medical Company are highly sought. Often referred to as rare tins, these items are worth more than common pieces of later years.

Designs currently popular are those that bear the "La Jaynees" or "Florencia" brand name and many of the cosmetics and toiletries lines. Talcum powder containers are highly collectible and escalating in price.

Intricate design, shape, labels, coloring, and unusual sizes help to increase value and demand. Rawleigh packaging did not undergo changes often. The product always remained the same. Remember collecting is an INVESTMENT!

Sometimes the condition factor does not play an important part with those early products. I have seen early Rawleigh products in poor condition demand higher prices than those of later years and those of better condition.

Price is what you as a collector find necessary to pay or are willing to pay. What is high to one person may be low to another and vice versa. Prices differ in different regions of the country.

The outward aspect of a Rawleigh cardboard containers is important. Look for containers that are not crushed, torn, ragged in appearance, or on which the cover has faded. Cardboard containers in damaged condition are reduced in value to much the same extent as damaged metal or tin.

Rawleigh's wooden shipping or packaging crates are highly sought. Seldom have I seen any of those in poor condition. Often the original wooden lid is missing; this is not uncommon. Watch for lids that have been professionally replaced.

Chapter 6.
COSMETICS, TOILETRIES, AND WORK SAVERS

Cosmetics and Toiletries

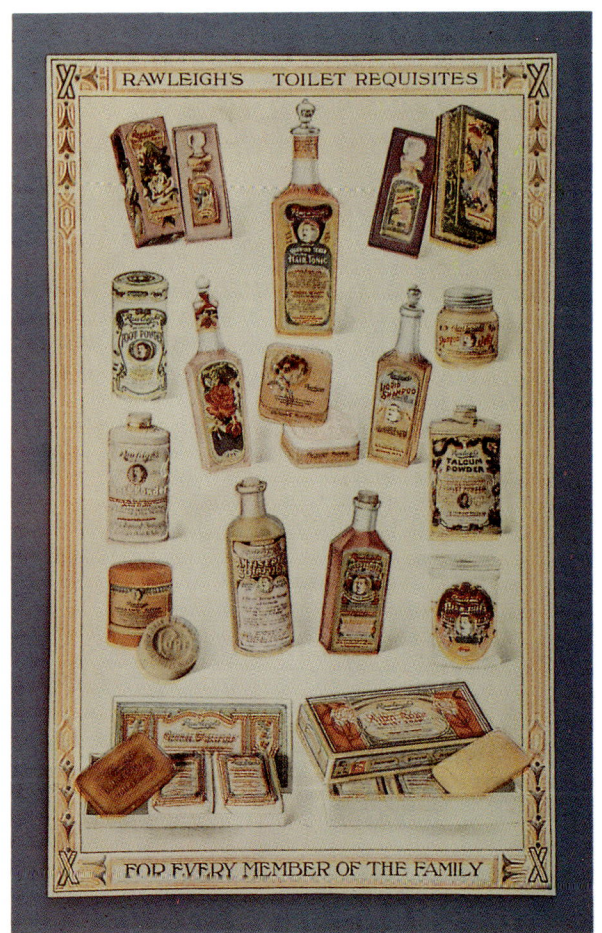

An original 1915 advertisement for "Rawleigh's Toilet Requisites For Every Member Of The Family." This original printing is somewhat blurred.

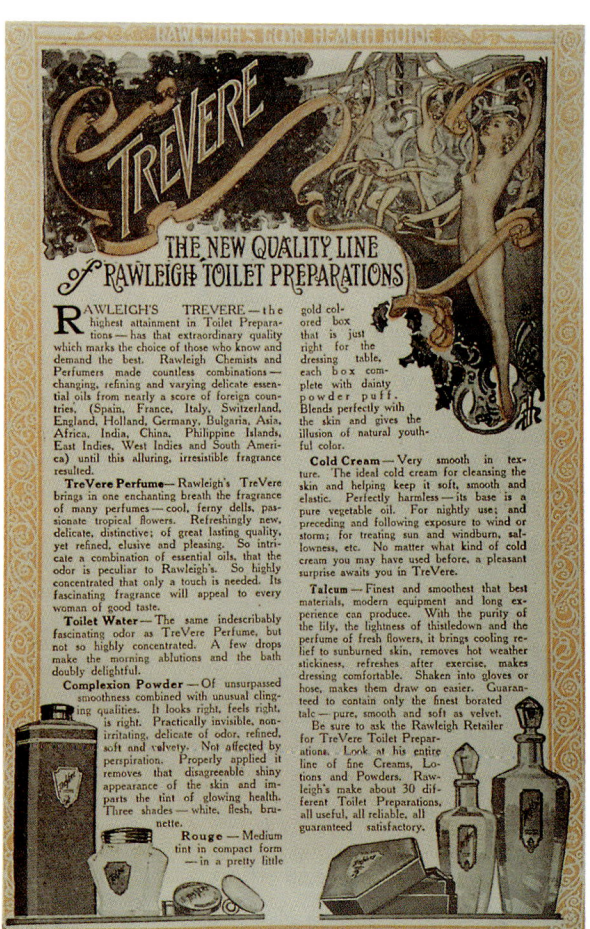

An original 1917 advertisement for "Rawleigh's Scientific Toilet Necessities." These products will require time in locating and will be expensive. $150-$200 ea.

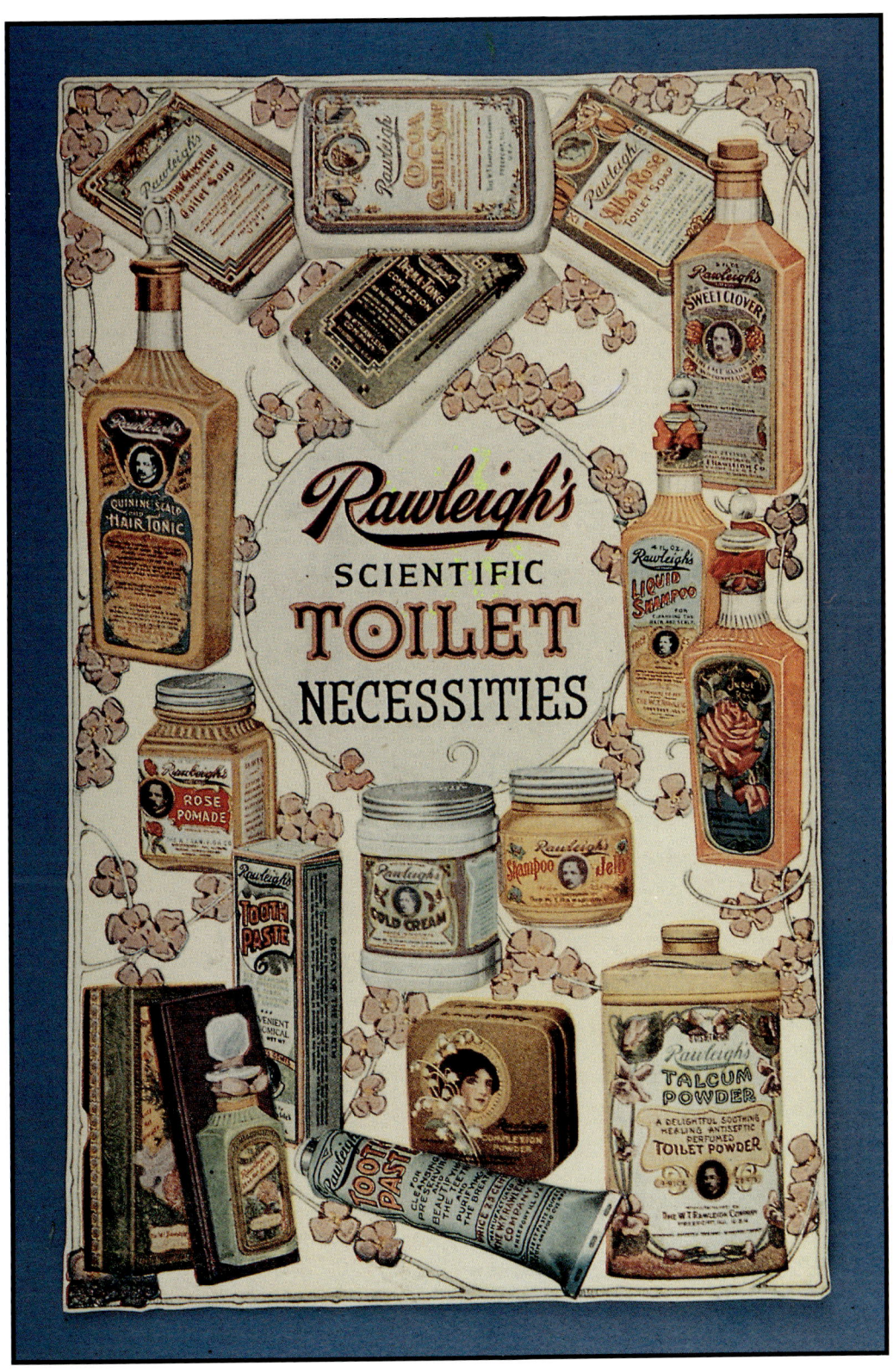

An original 1922 advertisement for "TREVERE The New Quality Line of Rawleigh Toilet Preparations." Talcum and perfume containers are highly sought by collectors and have escalated in the secondary market. $200-$250 ea.

La Jaynees

In 1929, "La Jaynees" creations were of uniform artistic style. They were designed for those who wished to have real elegance and the harmony of distinctive effect in the things that every woman regarded as necessities in the care of her skin and complexion and for enhancing her beauty and comfort. Improvements in Rawleigh's "La Jaynees" line of cosmetic art included Poudre, Poudre Toiletter, Talc, Cream, Lipstick, Rouge, Compacts, Face Lotion, Perfume, and Toilet Water. For men, there was Shaving Cream and After-Shaving Lotion, and Dental Cream — and there was Soap for everyone. Rawleigh's "La Jaynees" line was introduced in 1928.

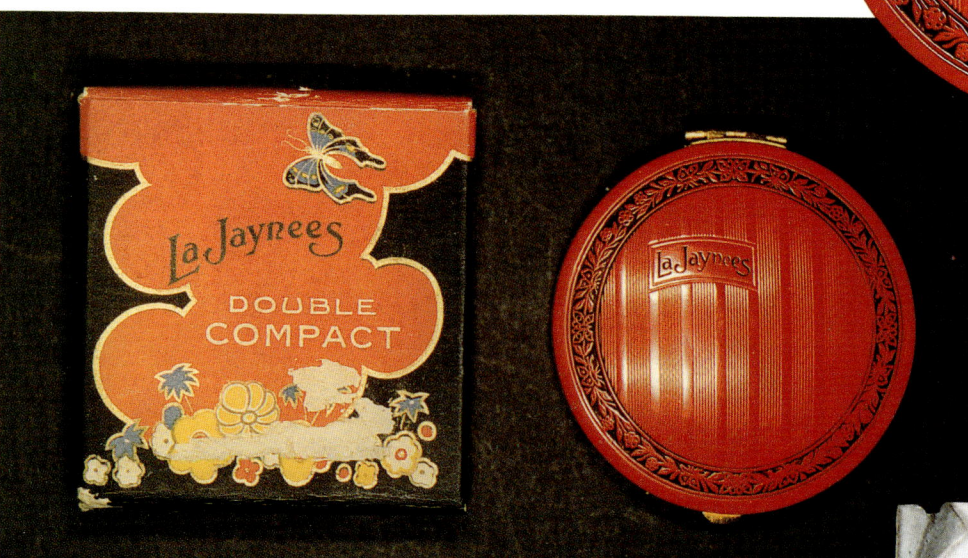

The double compact offered powder on one side, rouge on the opposite side, and a handy mirror, all in one. This "La Jaynees" compact has never been used. A paper insert reads "La Jaynees The Spirit of Springtime and Youth, Rawleigh's Freeport, Ill." $100-$125.

The "La Jaynees" Double Compact with the original carton. The compact is marked "Rawleigh's Freeport, Ill" and the carton is marked on the reverse side, "Rawleigh's Freeport, Ill. U.S.A." Original packaging increases value and collectors pay extra for items that are MIB (mint in box). $100-$125 complete.

This cardboard carton held one dozen tubes of "La Jaynees" lipsticks. Circa 1929. $120-$180 complete.

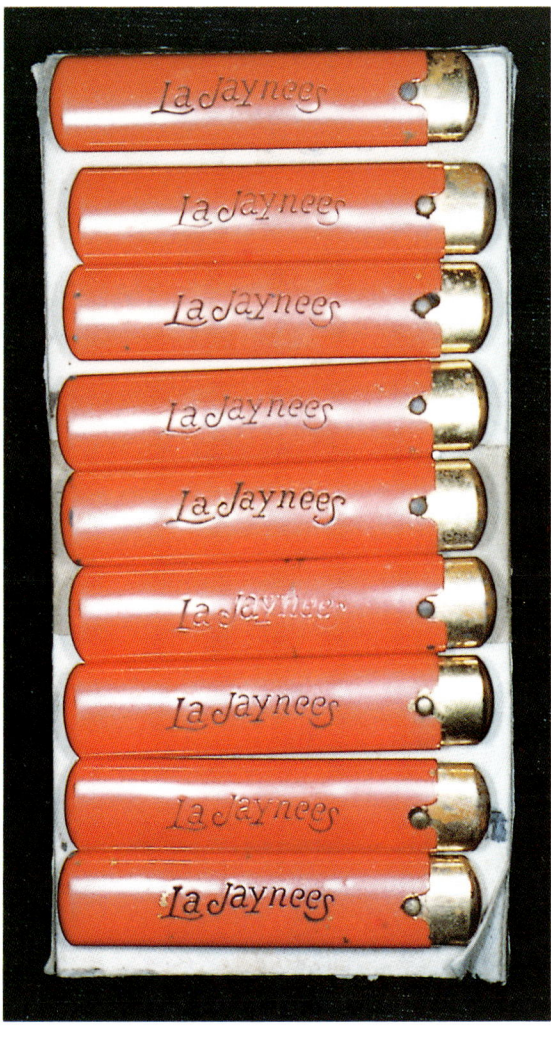

Nine tubes of "La Jaynees" lipstick that have never been used. Collectors believe these were samples given away to prospective customers. $10-$15 ea.

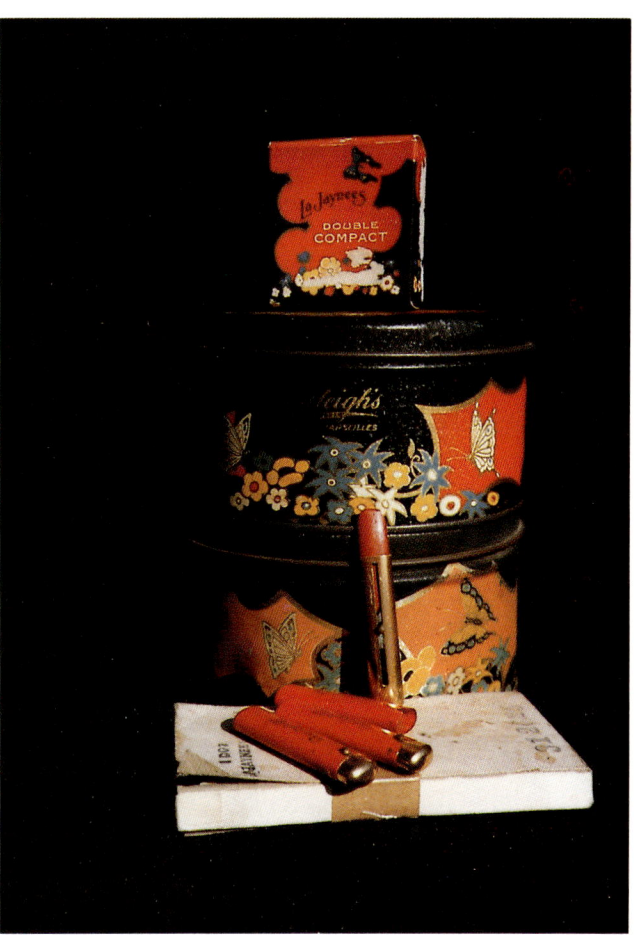

"La Jaynes" lipstick, the "Double Compact," and two tins of "La Jaynees Poudre Toilette." Cosmetic preparations are highly collectible and escalating in price. Lipstick, $10-$15 ea. Compact, $100-$125. Poudre tin, $40-$50 ea.

"La Jaynees" lipstick with original "Handle with Care!" paper work. Each tube is marked "La Jaynees" and on the reverse side "Rawleigh's Freeport, Ill." $10-$15 ea.

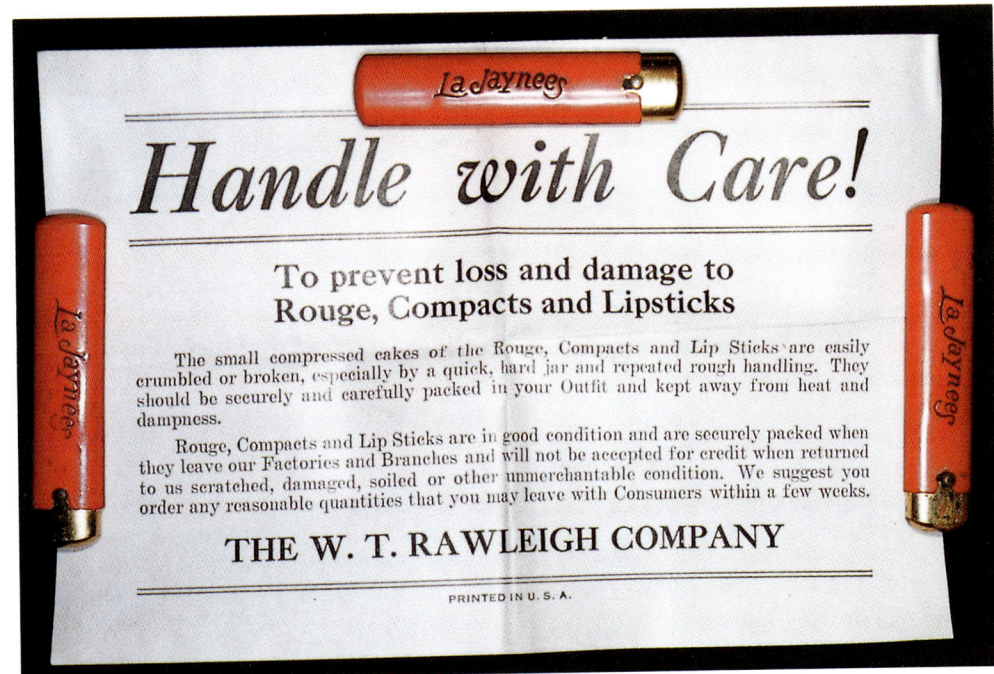

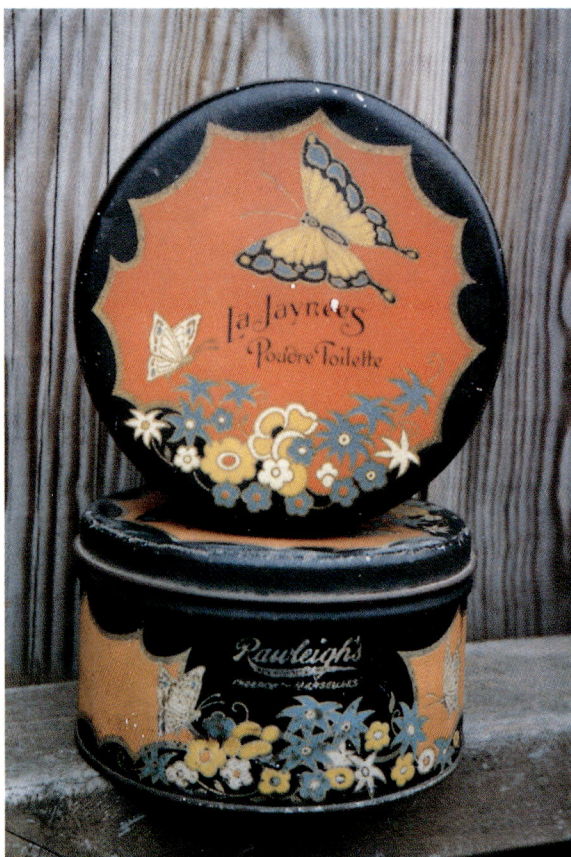

"La Jaynees Poudre Toilette." These are metal containers with Snap-On lids, each container is approximately 5" in diameter and 2-1/2" high. The side of each container is marked "Rawleigh's Freeport - Marseilles." *Dupler Collection.* $40-$50 ea.

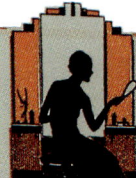

An original promotion for Rawleigh "Cosmetics & Toiletries." Note the "La Jaynees" cosmetic preparations. Circa 1935.

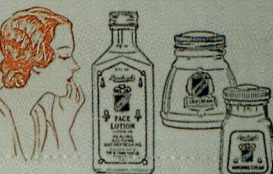

An original 1941 advertisement of "La Jaynees" and other Rawleigh bath products. "La Jaynees" preparations appeared periodically in Rawleigh publications.

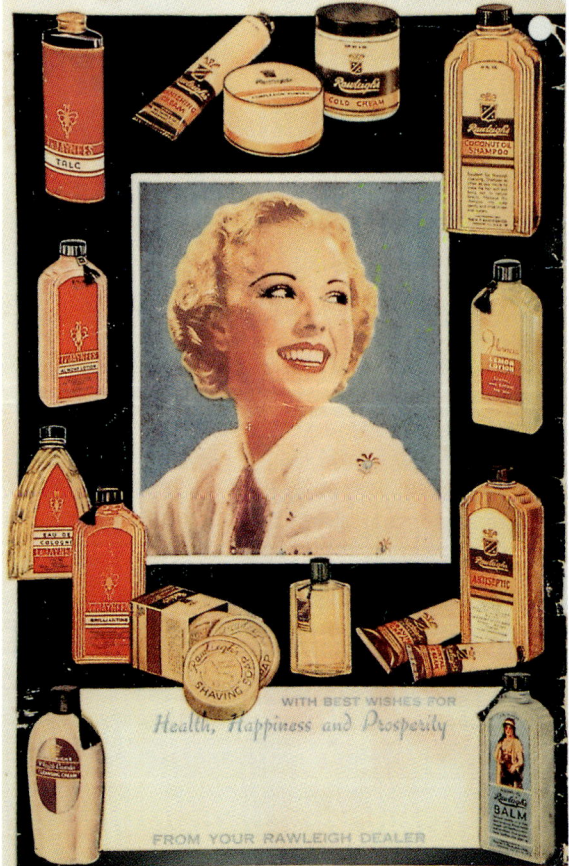

Rawleigh's newest line of toiletries — the Florencia. Introduced in 1932, "sweet memories of a thousand spring times were suggested by the romantic old-world fragrance of this new product." Available in talc, complexion powder, poudre toilette, cold and cleansing creams, lemon lotion, and cream, perfume, and bath salts.

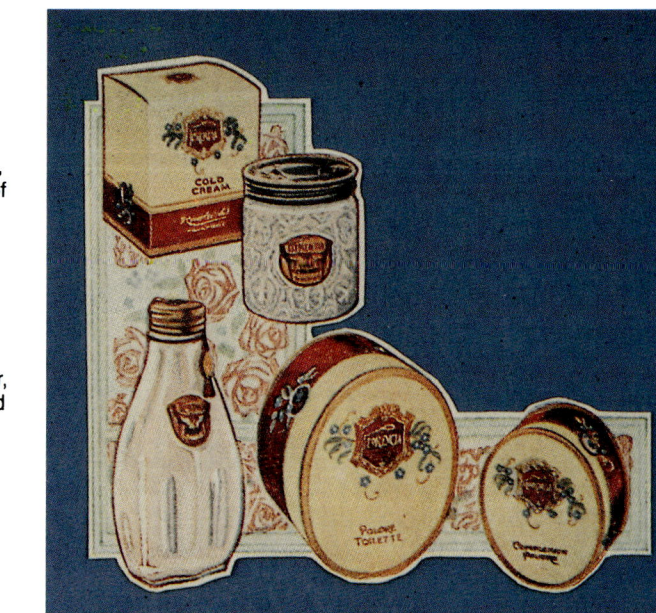

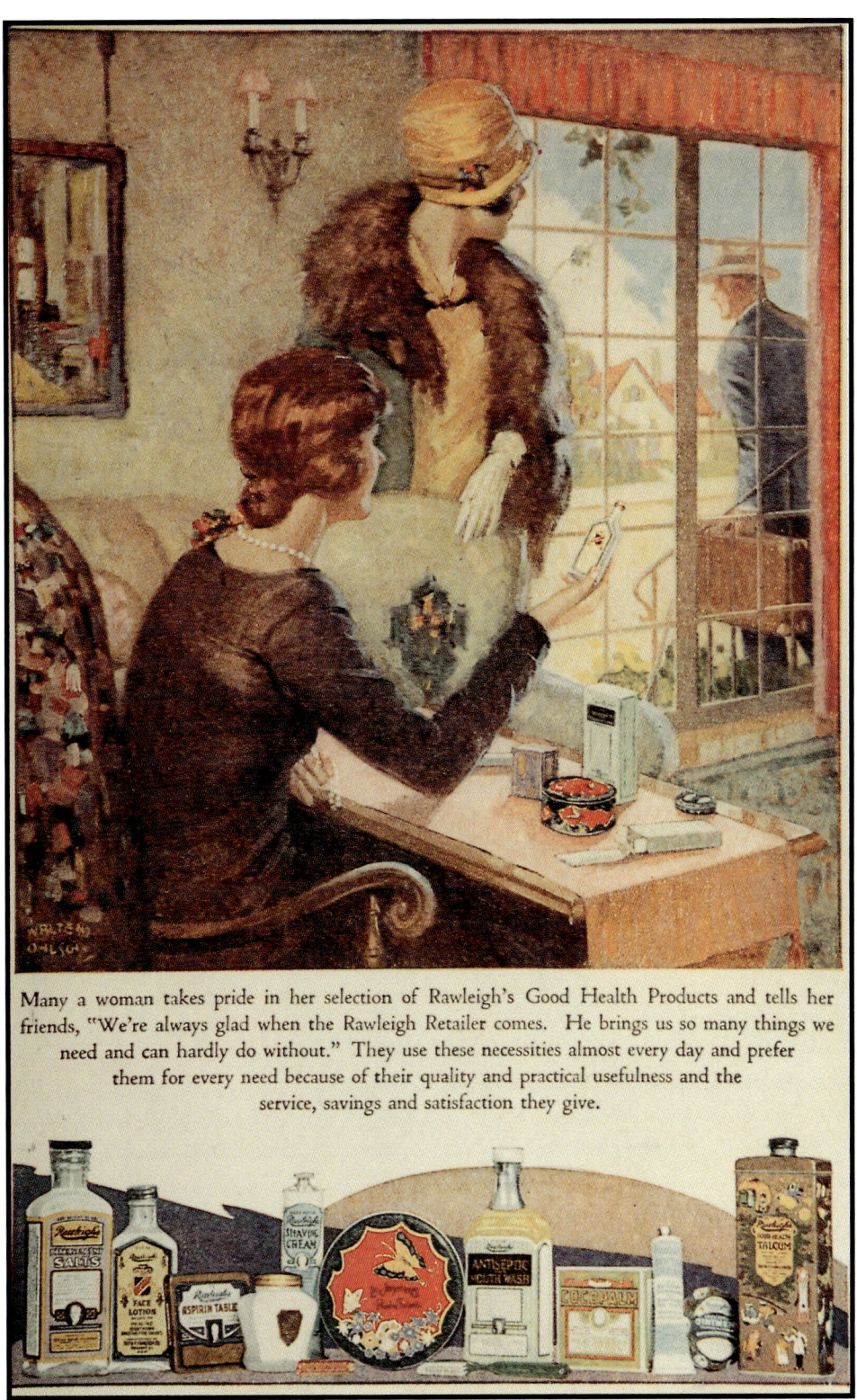

These women were satisfied with their "Rawleigh's Good Health Products" in 1929. Note the "La Jaynees Poudre Toilette" and other Rawleigh necessities shown at the base of the advertisement. Many of these products appear throughout this publication.

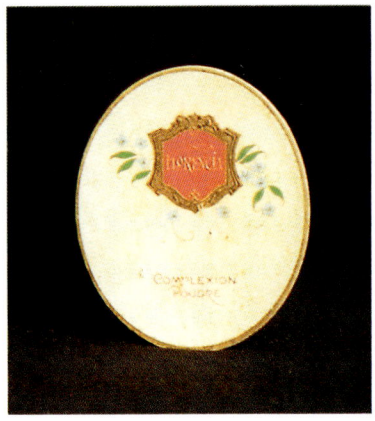

"Florencia Complexion Poudre Brunette." This was an exquisitely dainty powder of surpassing quality to heighten and maintain natural freshness and charm. It intimately blends and clings and has a sweet, refreshing fragrance and imparts a glow of modest vivacity and an enduring winsomeness. Marked "Rawleigh FREEPORT, ILL. U.S.A." $40-$50.

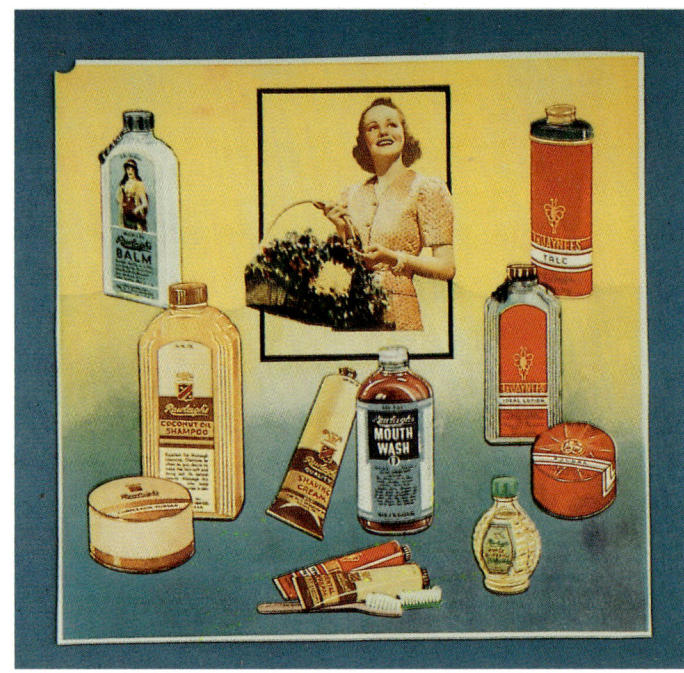

An original Rawleigh's 1946 advertisement for a selection of popular Rawleigh products.

Secrets of Loveliness

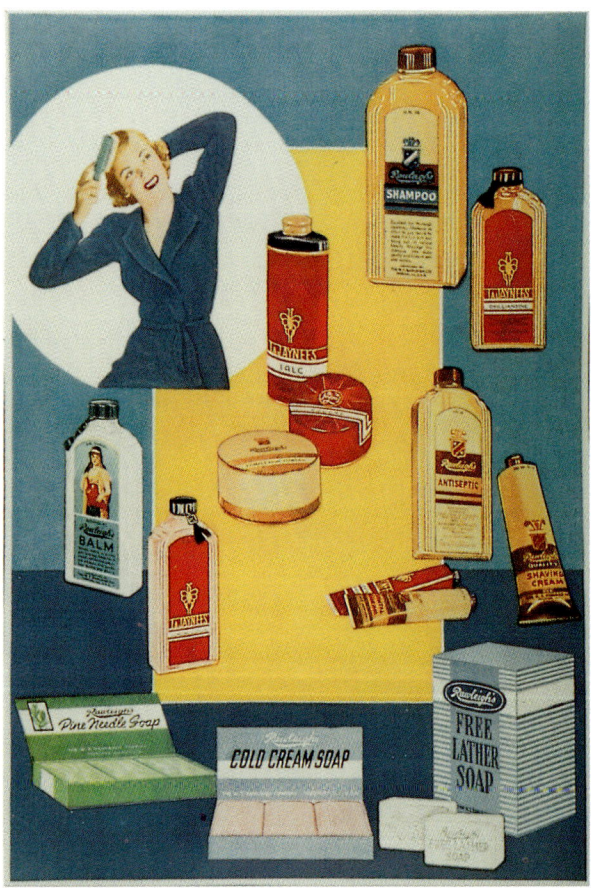

In 1944 "La Jaynees" products were promoted with Rawleigh soaps, creams, shampoo, and balm. The bottle of Rawleigh's BALM, shown on the left and the selection of Rawleigh's soap shown at the bottom are highly sought by collectors of cosmetic preparations. A word of warning, soap cartons MUST contain the original Rawleigh soap to be of any value.

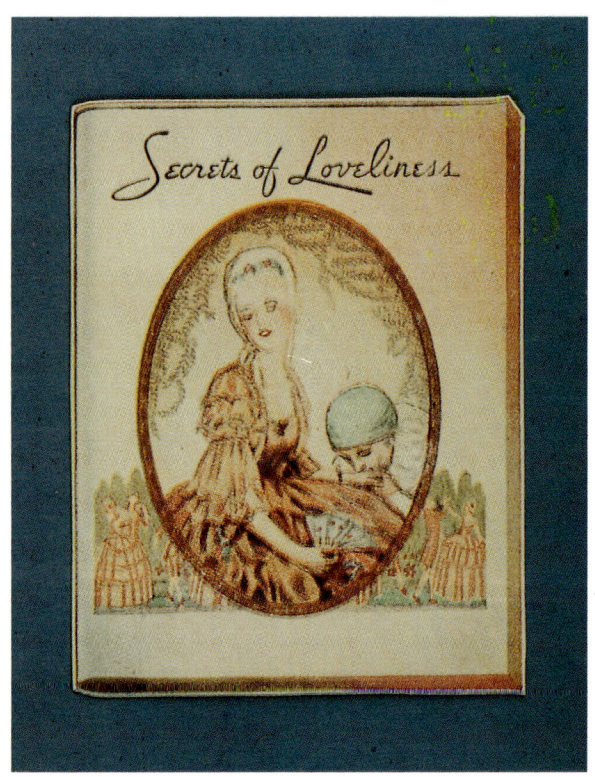

"Secrets of Loveliness," a complimentary copy of this guide was available in 1933 from a Rawleigh dealer. This guide provided information on how to keep a youthful complexion, proper ways to apply powder and rouge, and also contained helpful ways to enhance and preserve ones charm. $20-$25.

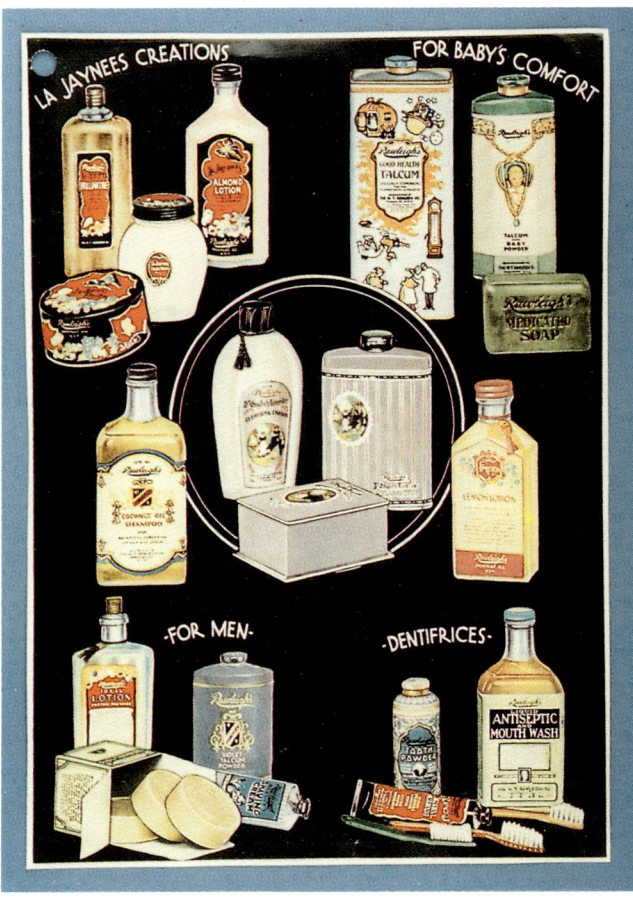

The original advertisement for La Jaynees creations, for baby's comfort, men, and dentifrice's appeared in a 1938 Rawleigh's publication. Many of these products are featured throughout this publication; others are either lost to time or sources were not available at the time of this writing.

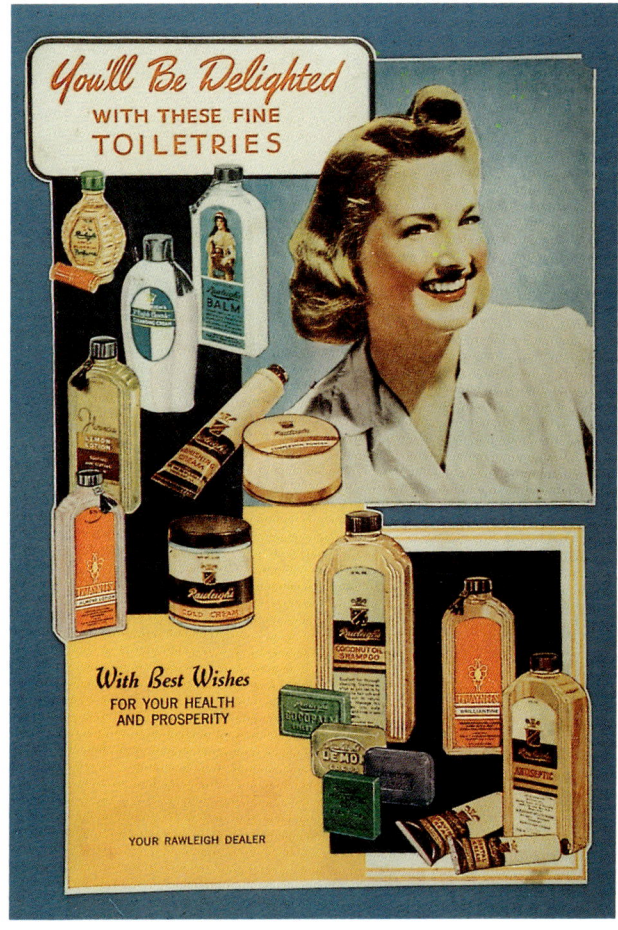

"You'll Be Delighted with these fine toiletries" appeared in Rawleigh's 1942 "Good Health Guide Almanac Cook Book."

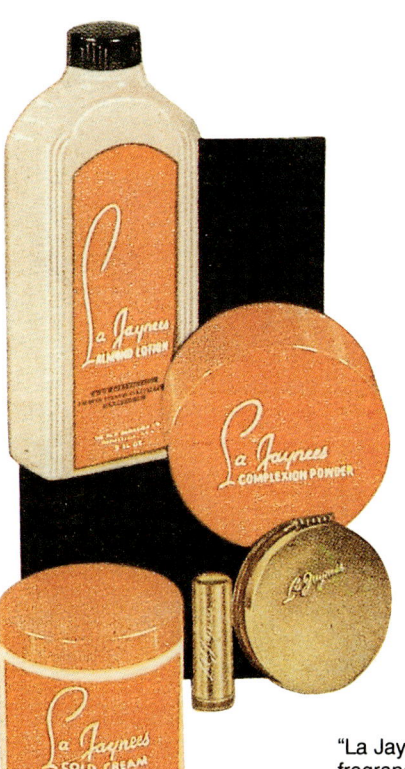

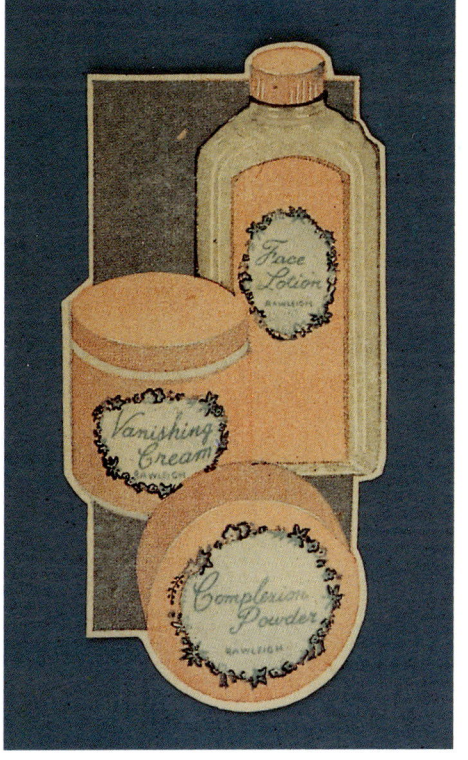

An original advertisement for Rawleigh Face Lotion, Vanishing Cream, and Complexion Powder. Circa 1948. $10-$20 ea.

"La Jaynees" products added a brilliant style and uniform harmonizing fragrance with the spirit of youth. Circa 1948.

125

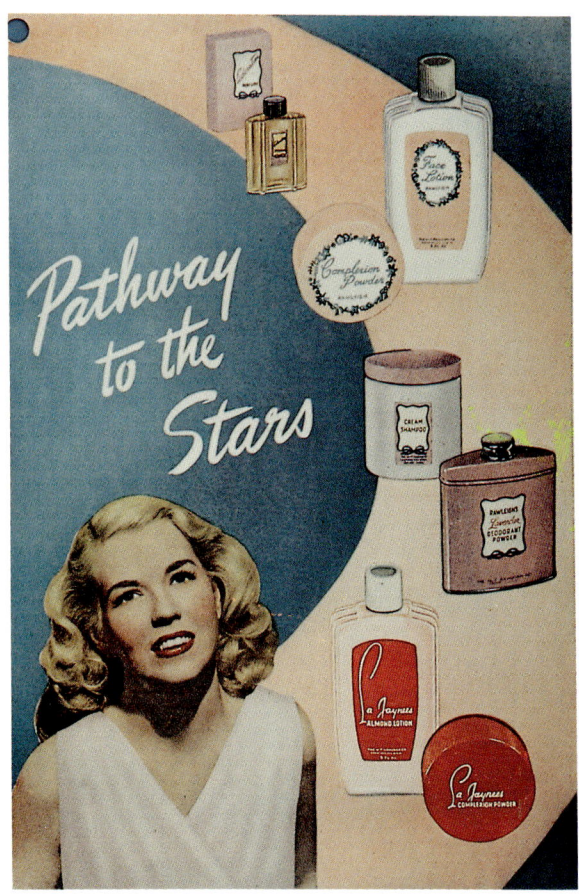

An original advertisement "Pathway to the Stars." Rawleigh's promoted perfume, face lotion, complexion powder, shampoo, deodorant powder, La Jaynees Almond Lotion, and La Jaynees Complexion Powder. Circa 1949. $10-$20 ea.

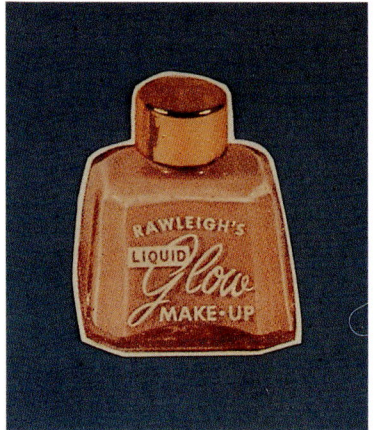

In 1958 "Ask your Rawleigh dealer to show you these and his other beauty aids." Rawleigh's Liquid Glow Make-Up was so natural that no one could tell you had used it.

In 1958 "Rawleigh's Powder Pack" was immensely popular.

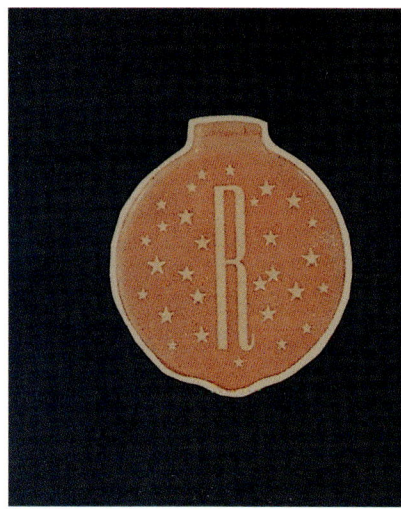

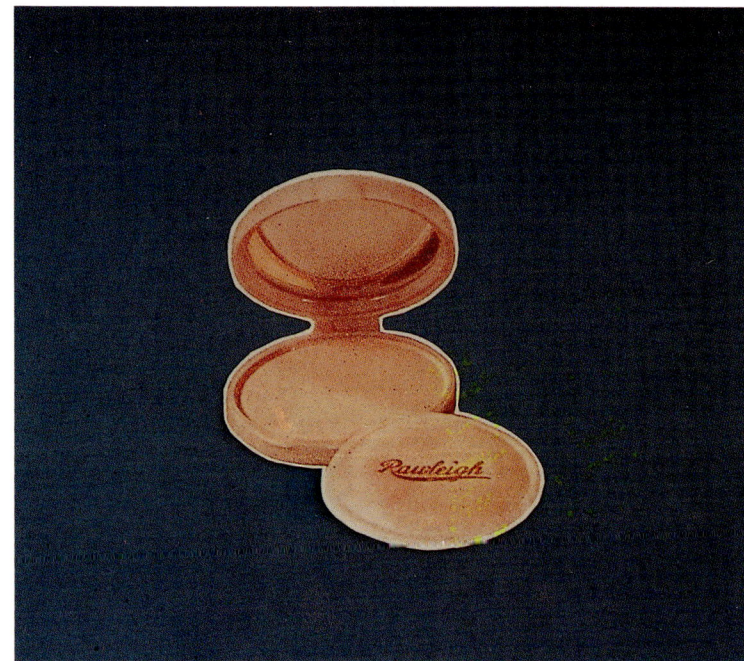

An open Rawleigh Powder Pack. The foundation and powder-in-one contained lanolin.

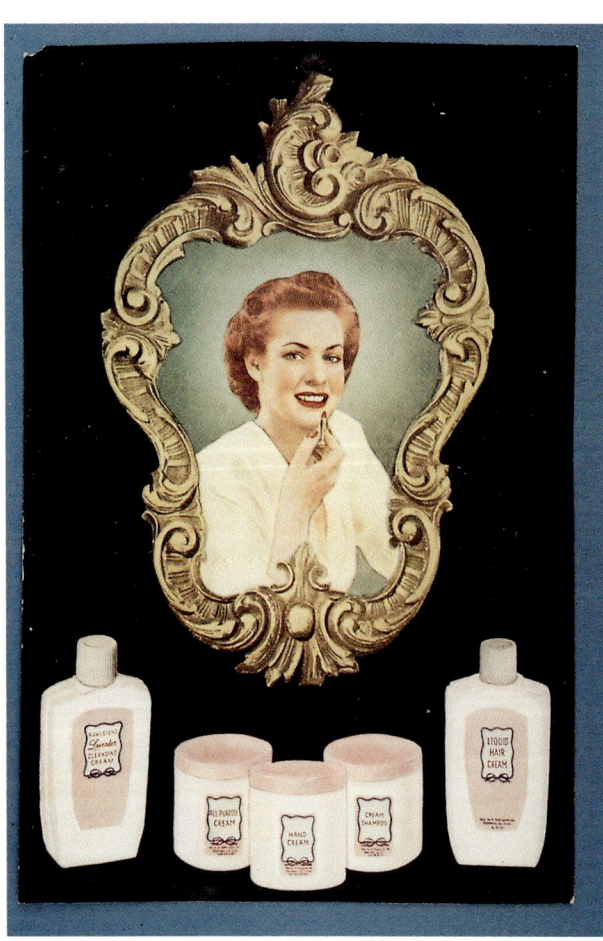

Rawleigh's Lavender Cleansing Cream, All Purpose Cream, Hand Cream, Cream Shampoo, and Liquid Hair Cream were promoted in 1951. $10-$20 ea.

Talcum

Rawleigh's Talcum was of unusual quality — made of the best materials by exacting processes which ensured exceptionally fine, soft powder. Four kinds were available — Violet, Pan Jang, Talcum, and Baby Powder. Offered in handsome sifter-top cans. Extra large size and unusually good values.

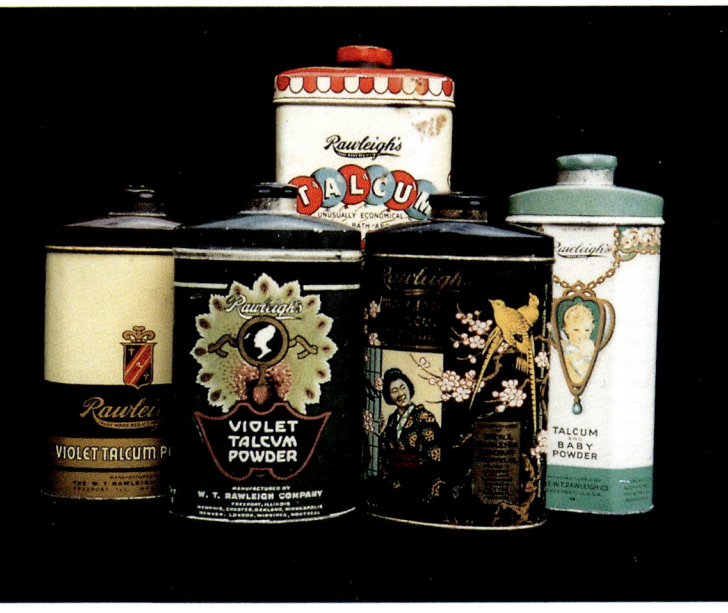

Rawleigh Talcum Powder containers are among the most sought after advertisement items for Rawleigh collectors. Any of these containers (and those shown on the following pages) are rapidly escalating in price.

"Try these New Products" appeared in a 1948 Rawleigh publication.

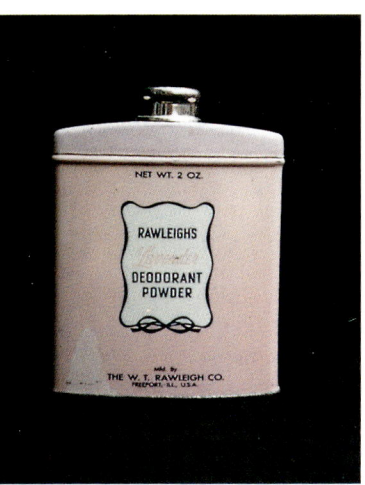

Rawleigh's Lavender Deodorant Powder. This metal 2 ounce deodorant powder was "Mfd. By The W.T. Rawleigh Co. Freeport, Ill., U.S.A. *See* original 1948 advertisement shown previously. *Shepard Collection.* $50-$60.

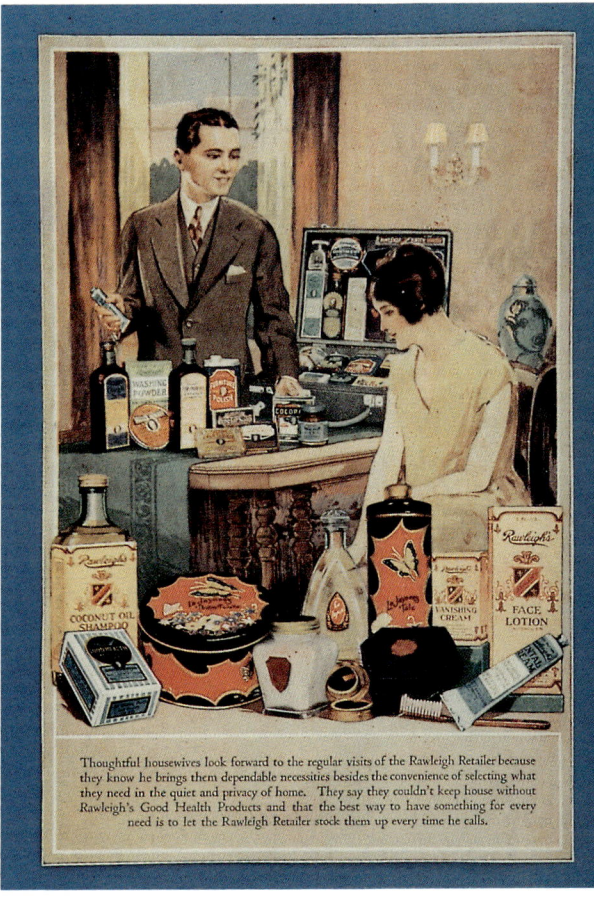

An original Rawleigh's advertisement from a 1928 Rawleigh's Good Health Guide publication. Dependable necessities were delivered by the Rawleigh retailer.

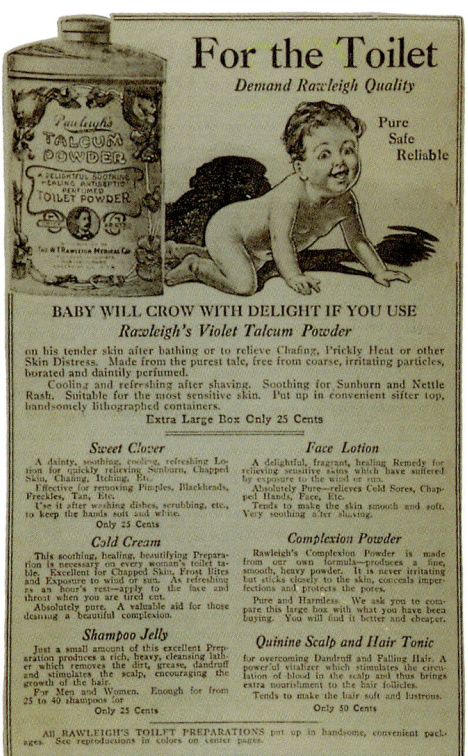

An original 1916 "For the Toilet" advertisement. See the note at the bottom of the advertisement, "ALL RAWLEIGH'S TOILET PREPARATIONS put up in handsome, convenient packages. See reproductions in colors on center pages." This center page appears elsewhere in this chapter.

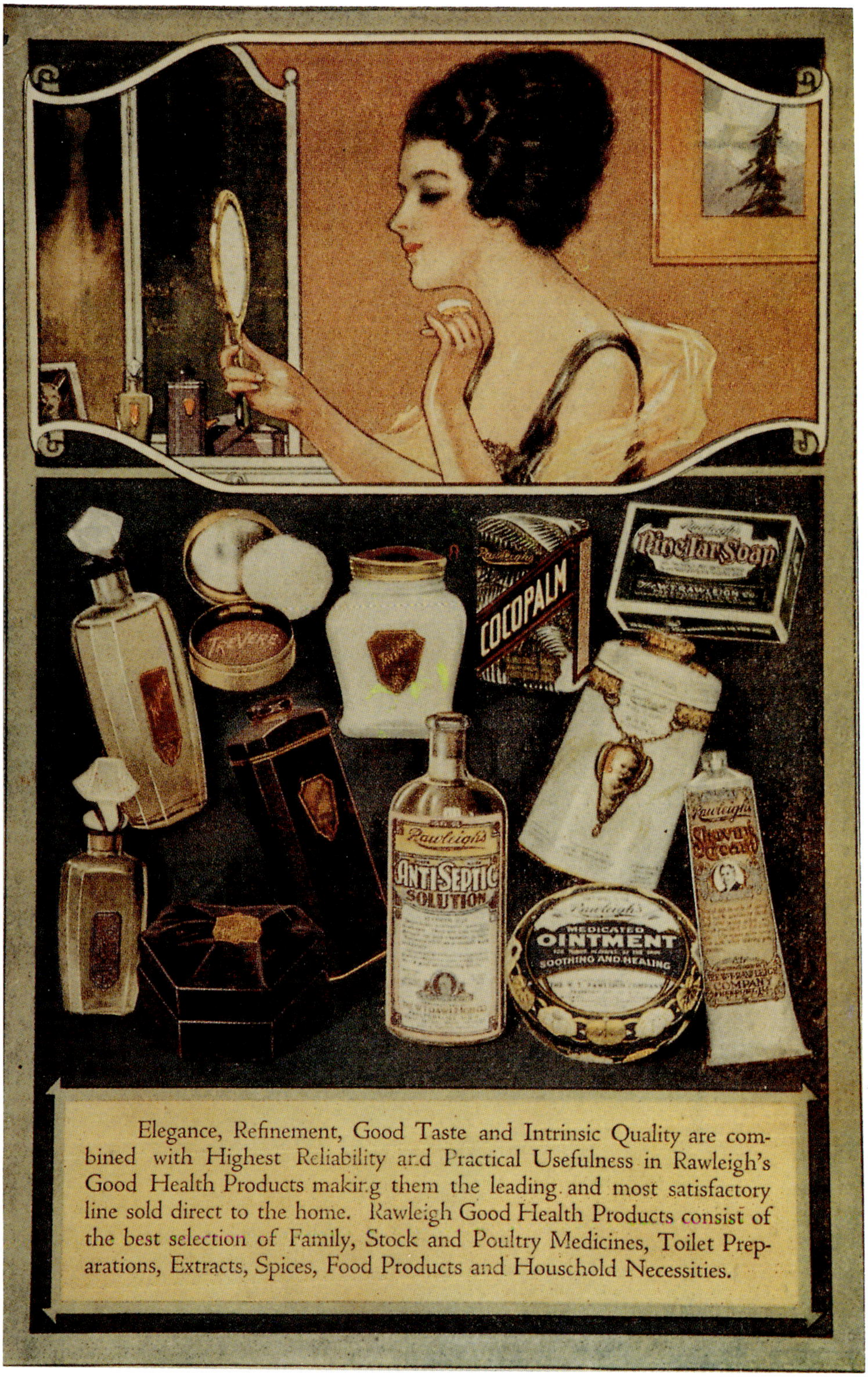

An original Rawleigh's advertisement from a 1923 Good Health Guide publication. Older products are in greater demand and will be more expensive.

The Good Health Fairies

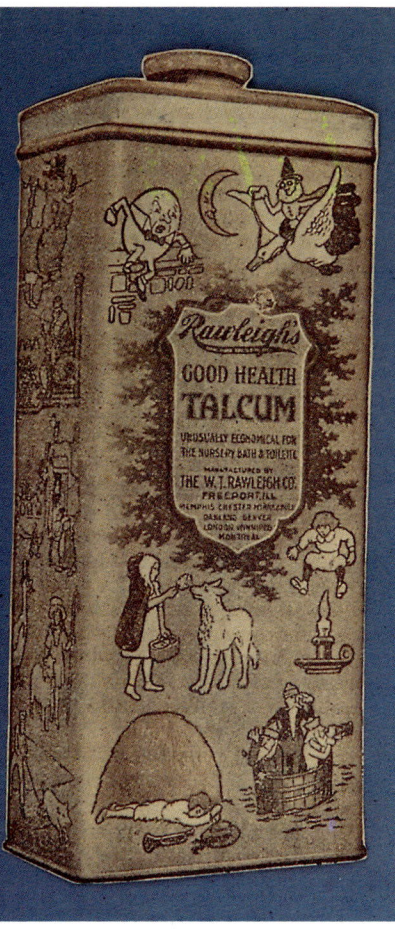

"Rawleigh's Good Health Talcum" promoted in 1925. This talcum can be found in either a cardboard or metal container. A brochure accompanied the above "Rawleigh's Good Health Talcum." Nursery rhymes were printed on the publication which children read and then found the picture on the can for each rhyme. $125-$150.

In 1925 Rawleigh promoted this Talcum by printing the following advertisement ($75-$100 for this original advertisement):

Jean and John were twins, and such nice twins too. But they had one fault which was big and bad enough to almost spoil their lives. For they didn't want to eat what their wise mother knew was the food they should eat, to always be strong and well. Jean and John thought they didn't like these foods and they wanted sweet puddings, pies, cakes, meat and candy all the time, and even coffee instead of milk.

One night just as they sat down to dinner their father smiled and said, "Well, what do you suppose I saw on the way home tonight?" Mother couldn't guess, but Jean guessed a little kitten and John guessed a big dog. "No," said father, "But I saw big signs saying a big circus is coming soon and I guess you kiddies are old enough to go this year."

"Oh," gasped the twins, for they knew what a circus was. They had seen a parade last year and think of going inside that big white tent where all the animals are!

Just then Mother passed them their supper; a nice baked potato, green spinach, a lovely custard, baked apple, and a glass of milk. As usual Jean and John frowned and commenced to grumble. They wouldn't drink milk, they hated spinach and all vegetables; were tired of custards and wanted fried potatoes, apple pie and cake. Their mother looked at them gravely and then said slowly, "Well, daddy — if Jean and John won't eat what they should without grumbling, they just can't go to the circus at all." And Father said, "Well, Mother, you are right. But I shall be very sorry if they can't go."

Jean and John looked at each other in amazement. Then they both began to eat without a word. But that night after they had been put to bed and everything was dark, Jean said, "Wouldn't it be terrible not to go to the circus? Whatever shall we do?" "Humph; I guess we'll have to eat," said John from his little bed. They lay there quite a while in silence, each thinking about it, when presently a beautiful lady seemed to come into the room. She was so lovely and kind she didn't scare them at all. "Come, Jean and John, with me," she said. "I am Good Health and I want to show you something."

They climbed out of their beds and she took them both by the hand and they went away. They seemed to travel through space quite a while and then the lady entered a house. "I want you to know some of my friends," said she, "For whoever knows Good Health well, must know these people too," and she introduced them to a big kind man called Strength, another called Bravery, and still another called Success. And then two beautiful ladies she called Pleasure and Contentment came in. After talking with them a little, she said, "My friends and I want to show you two little villages of fairy folk, and then let you choose which fairies you'd rather have work for you."

Jean and John clapped their hands with joy for they loved to read about fairies and were so anxious to see some. The first village, though, they didn't like very well. The little fairies looked all brown and cross and some were ugly and deformed. They acted surly, but seemed to know Jean and John.

"Who are they?" cried the children. "These are the food fairies in pies, cakes, sweets, candies and unwholesome foods," replied Good Health. "There are a lot of them, but they don't make children happy. They spoil their lives by making them puny, weak, sickly, cross and crippled, so they can't enjoy life. They work for children whose mothers don't know what is good for their children to eat, and for children who won't eat what they should when they are fortunate enough to have a mother who knows."

"We don't believe we like them very well," said the children guiltily.

"All right, we'll go on," said Good Health.

The next little town was much nicer. All the little fairies were dressed in pretty bright colors. They were gay and nimble, cheerful, busy and happy.

"These are nice fairies," said Jean, "Who are they?"

"I'll let them tell you," and so Good Health clapped her hands and a lot of fairies came running. "This is Jean and John," said Good Health, "Tell them who you are,"

"We know Jean and John's mother," cried all the fairies delightfully. Then one in bright red said, "I am the fairy Iron in Spinach, red apples and all fruits and vegetables, who makes your cheeks rosy and your blood good." "And I am the Lime in milk and cereals who makes your bones strong so you can run and play and your teeth good to chew with," said a white one.

"All I am the Vitamin fairy," and one in green, "I live in milk, butter, fruits, and vegetables too, and I make you grow big like your father and mother."

"And I give you lots of strength and energy and I live in cereals, eggs, custards, baked potatoes and the like," said another.

And thus they went on, each telling what he did for children until Jean and John were thoroughly ashamed of themselves.

"Oh, Good Health," they cried, "We want these nice fairies to work for us too." "All right," said she, "But you must eat what mother wants you to eat so that these fairies can give you Good Health and all these friends. Then you will be strong and brave, happy, contented and successful."

Then they all smiled and left Jean and John.

The next morning when mother brought their cereal, Jean said as she ate it greedily, "I can almost see the fairies in it, can't you?" And John said, "Yes, I wonder if elephants, lions and tigers eat this to get strong too." They both smiled happily and being twins, they didn't seem to think it strange that they both had the same dream.

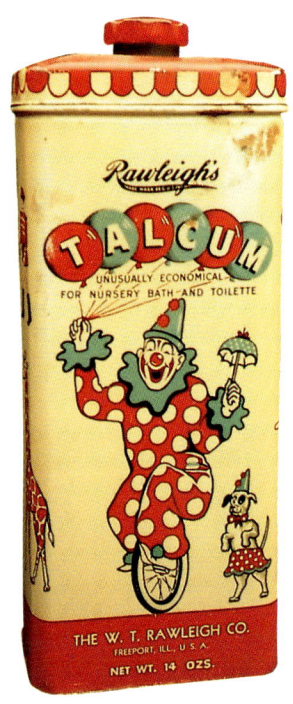

Rawleigh's 14 ounce Talcum, "unusually economical for nursery bath and toilette." The W.T. Rawleigh Co. Freeport, Ill., U.S.A. $100-$125.

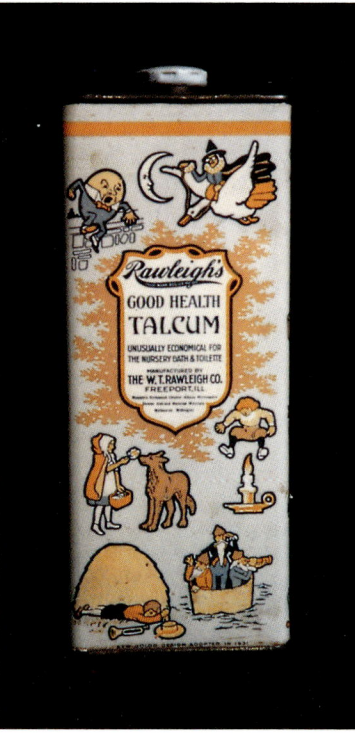

A metal "Rawleigh's Good Health Talcum." Manufactured By The W.T. Rawleigh Co. Freeport, Ill. Memphis - Richmond - Chester - Albany - Minneapolis - Denver - Oakland - Montreal - Winnipeg - Melbourne - Wellington. This container is marked at the base "New Color Design Adopted in 1931." $125-$150.

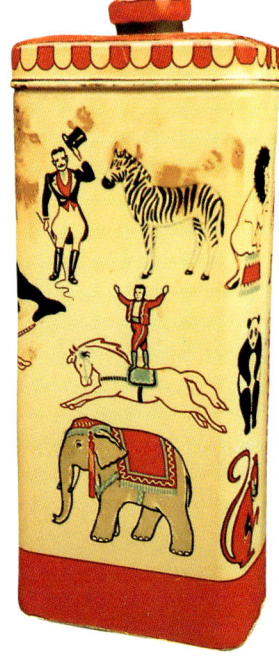

Circus animals, clowns, and feats of physical skills are depicted on the Rawleigh's Talcum. $100-$125.

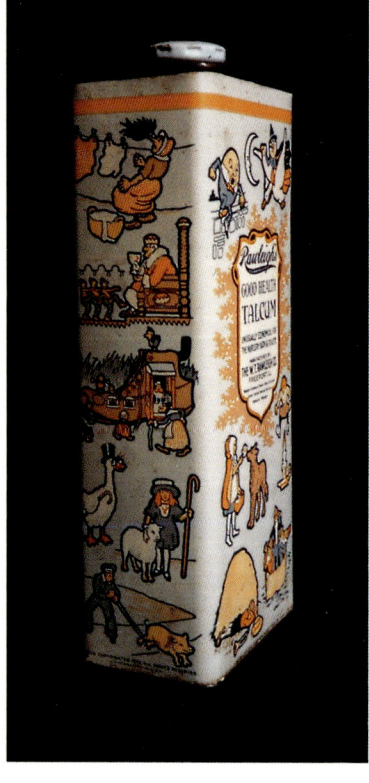

Nursery rhyme characters appear on the surface of this "Rawleigh's Good Health Talcum." $125-$150.

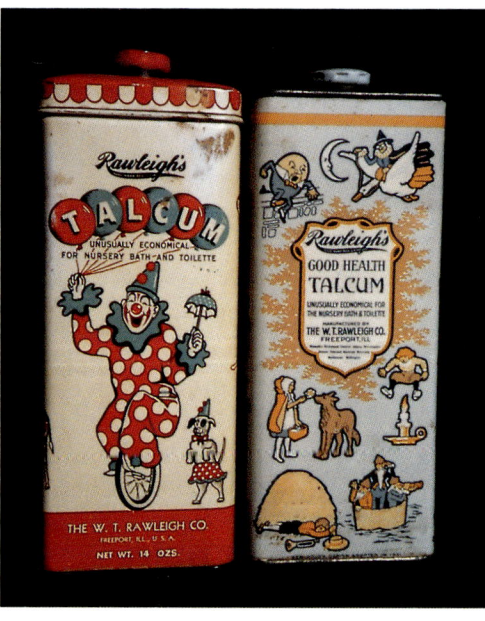

Two of the most sought after Rawleigh Talcum containers. These containers are gradually escalating in price.

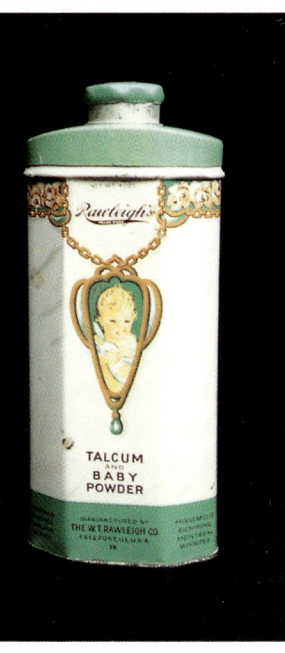

Rawleigh's 4 ounce Talcum and Baby Powder. Metal sifter-top tin. Manufactured By W.T. Rawleigh Company Freeport, Ill. U.S.A. - Memphis - Chester - Oakland - Denver - Minneapolis - Richmond - Montreal - Winnipeg. $125-$150.

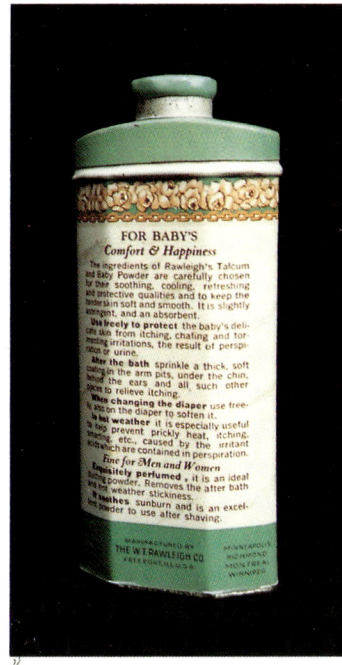

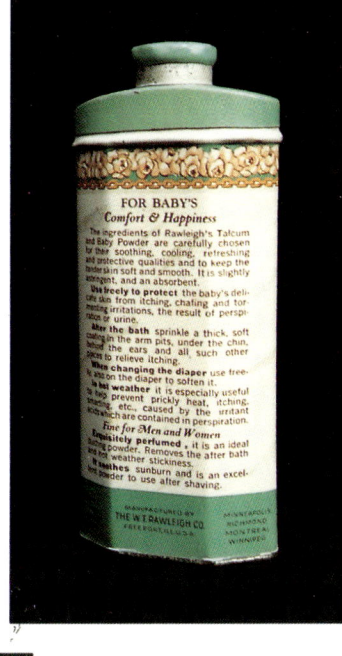

Rawleigh's 5 ounce Violet Talcum Powder. Manufactured by The W.T. Rawleigh Company Freeport, Ill., Memphis, Tenn. Metal sifter-top tin. This talcum is shown later in this chapter with additional Rawleigh products. $75-$100.

Rawleigh's Talcum and Baby Powder, for baby's comfort and happiness. Directions were provided on the reverse side for use in protection, after bath and while changing diapers. This talcum was fine for men and women too. $125-$150.

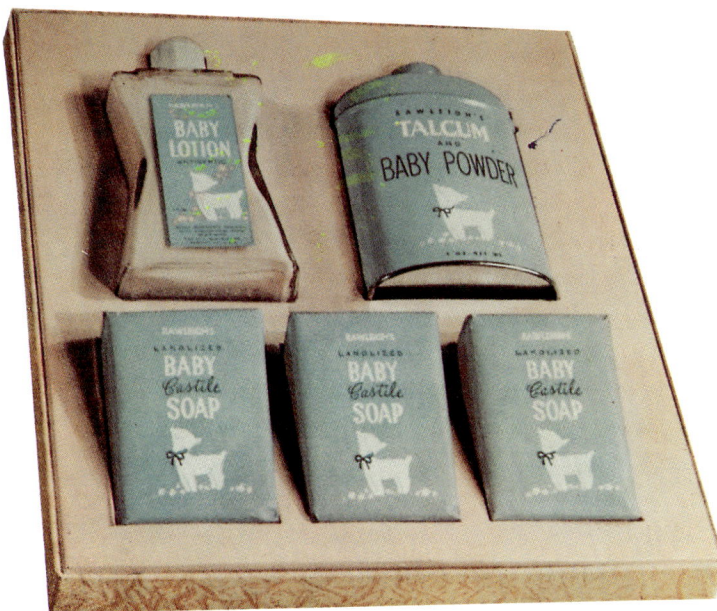

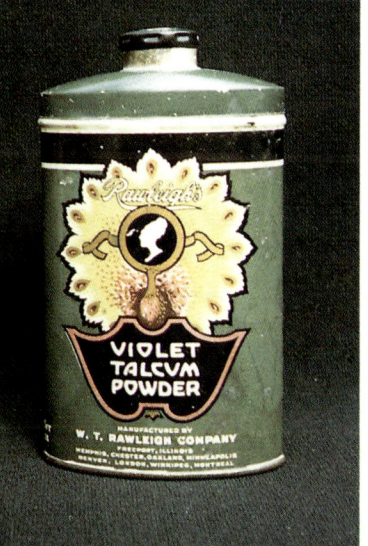

In 1958 mothers appreciated the Rawleigh gift set shown here. The set included baby lotion, three bars of castile soap, talcum and baby powder. $75-$100 complete.

Rawleigh's 8 ounce Violet Talcum Powder. Metal sifter-top tin. Manufactured By W.T. Rawleigh Company Freeport, Illinois - Memphis - Chester - Oakland - Minneapolis - Denver - London - Winnipeg - Montreal. $95-$120 ea.

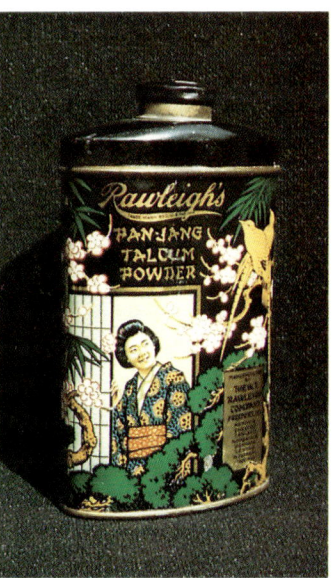

Rawleigh's Pan-Jang Talcum Powder with an Oriental scene. Metal sifter-top tin. Manufactured By W.T. Rawleigh Company Freeport, Illinois - Memphis - Chester - Oakland - Minneapolis - Richmond - Denver - Montreal - Winnipeg. $95-$120.

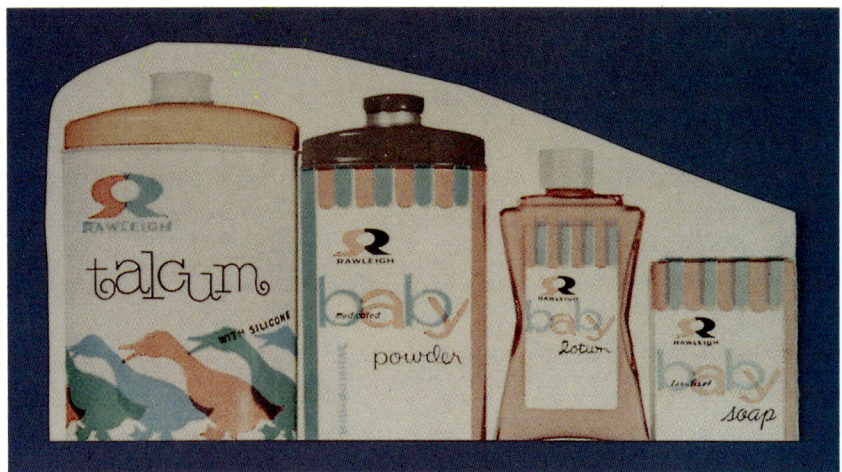

During the 1960s, Rawleigh promoted a 19 ounce Nursery Talcum with silicone, 6 ounce medicated baby powder with silicone, a 4 ounce baby antiseptic lotion, and lanolized baby castile soap. These containers were decorated in attractive pink and blue. $20-$30 ea.

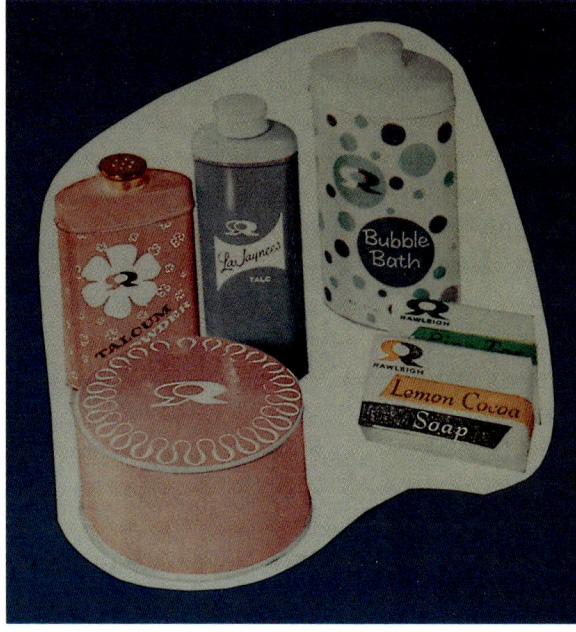

During the 1960s, Rawleigh promoted the 4 ounce Rawleigh talcum powder, 6 ounce dusting powder, 4 ounce La Jaynees talcum powder, 9 ounce bubble bath and lemon cocoa soap. La Jaynees was still popular in the 1960s in an attractive blue container.

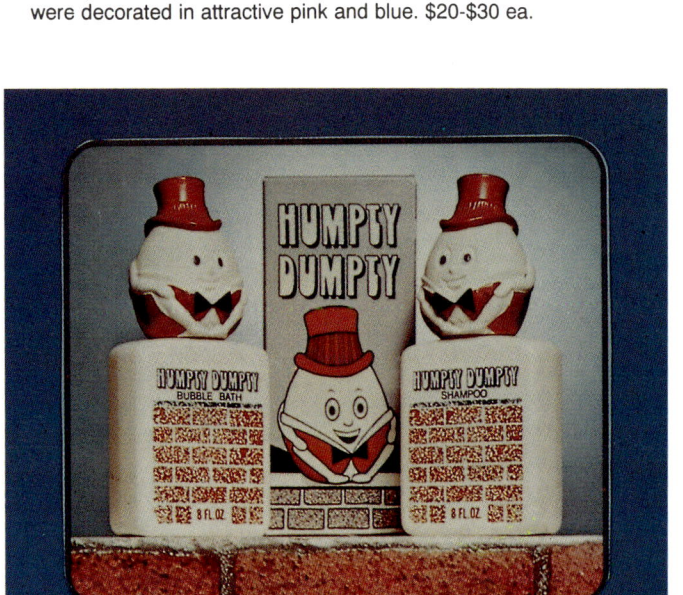

Humpty Dumpty Shampoo, 8 ounce, and 8 ounce Bubble Bath. This all-time favorite nursery rhyme character sits atop these highly collectible bath time products. $30-$40 ea.

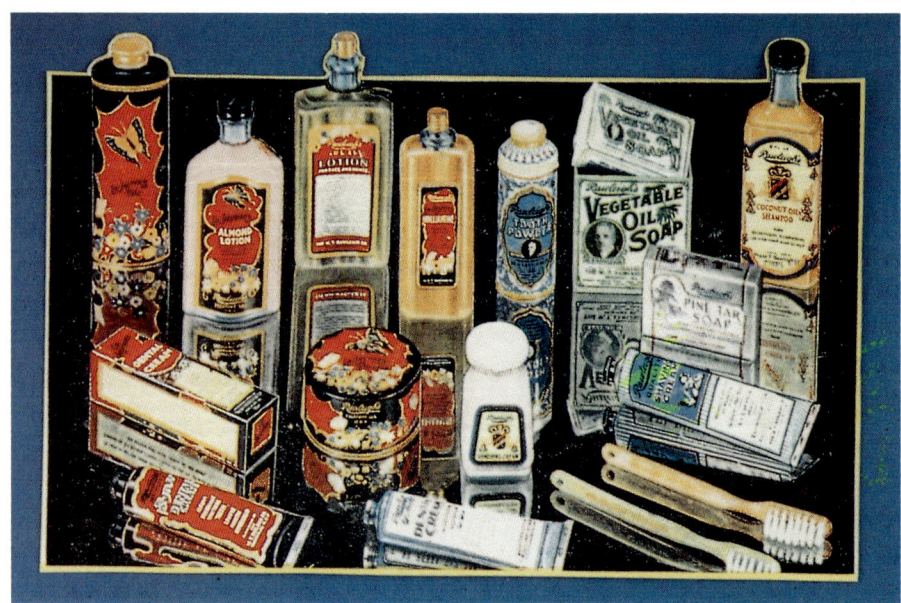

An original 1937 "For Health and Beauty" advertisement for Rawleigh's La Jaynees products, shampoo, soaps, lotions, creams, tooth brushes, and powders. Note the highly decorated Rawleigh's Tooth Powder container (blue/white/yellow) top right, next to Vegetable Oil Soap.

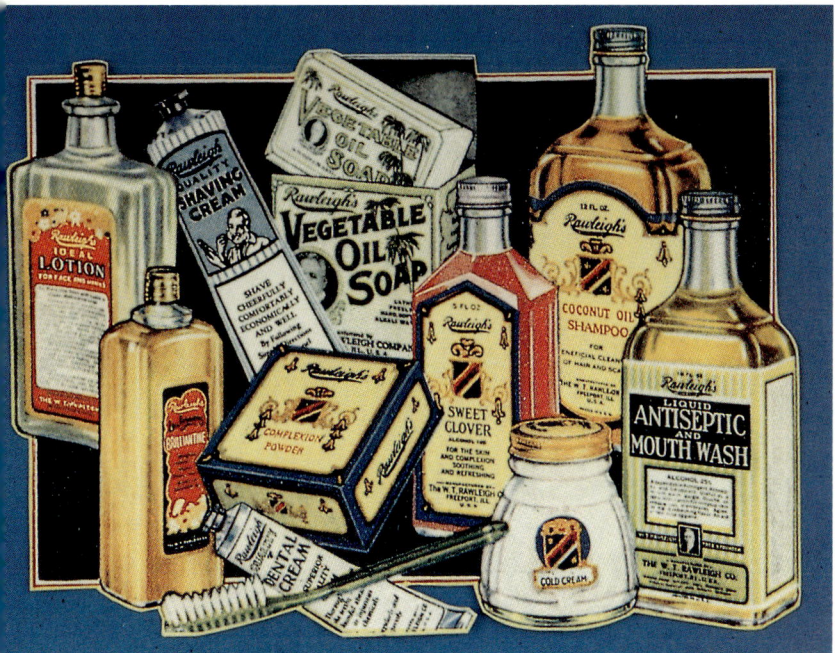

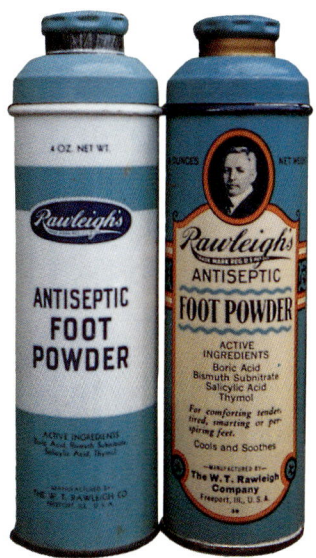

Two different Rawleigh's Antiseptic Foot Powder containers. Manufactured by The W.T. Rawleigh Company Freeport, Ill., U.S.A. Metal sifter-top tin. $50-$75 ea.

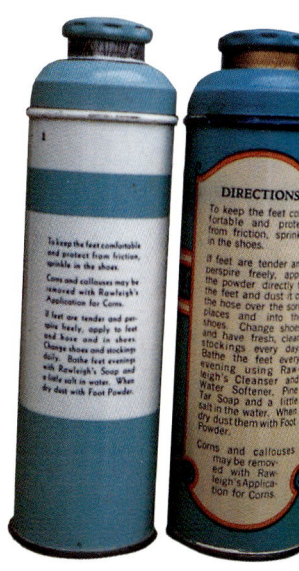

This is a 1935 original advertisement for Rawleigh products. Rawleigh's Ideal Lotion, Shaving Cream, Vegetable Oil Soap, Coconut Oil Shampoo, Sweet Clover, Complexion Powder, Cold Cream, La Jaynees, Dental Cream, and Antiseptic and Mouth Wash. Many of these products appeared regularly in Rawleigh publications.

The reverse side where DIRECTIONS were provide on Rawleigh's 4 ounce. Antiseptic Foot Powder containers. $50-$75 ea.

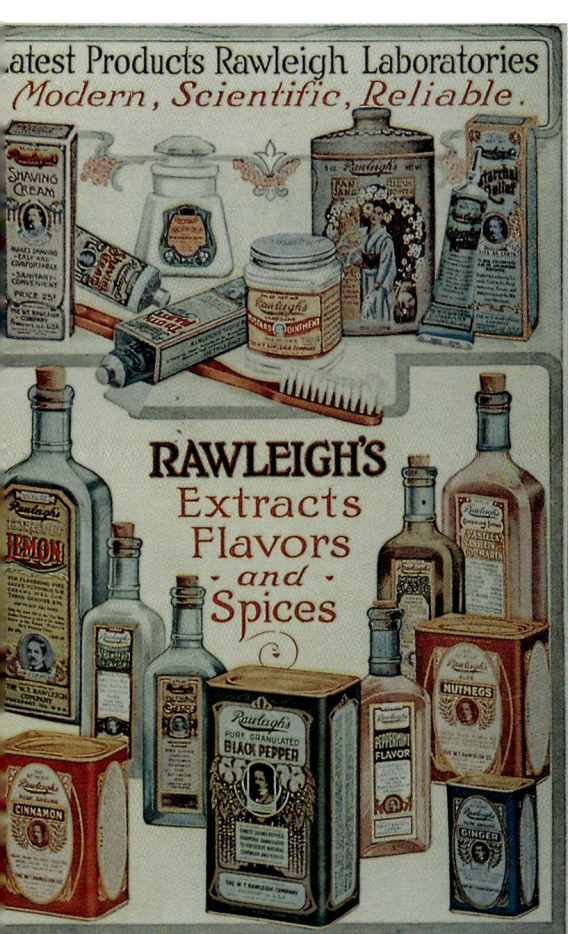

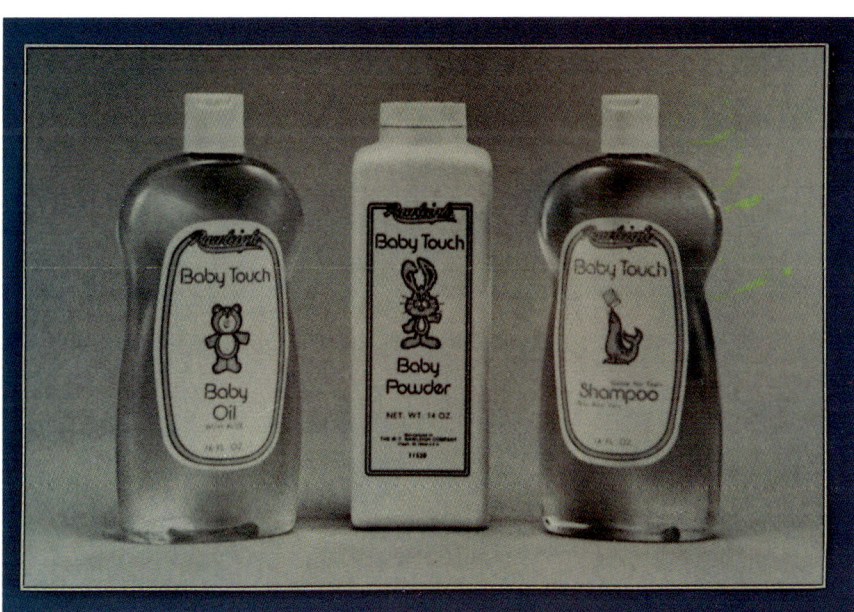

The W.T. Rawleigh Co. was proud to introduce a complete new line of baby care products. Baby Touch Baby Oil with Aloe Vera (16 ounce), Baby Touch Baby Powder (14 ounce), and Baby Touch Shampoo with Aloe Vera (16 ounce). Circa 1980s. $10-$20 ea.

In 1917, Rawleigh promoted the latest selection of toiletries, extracts and spices. These products were excellent in quality, strength, and purity.

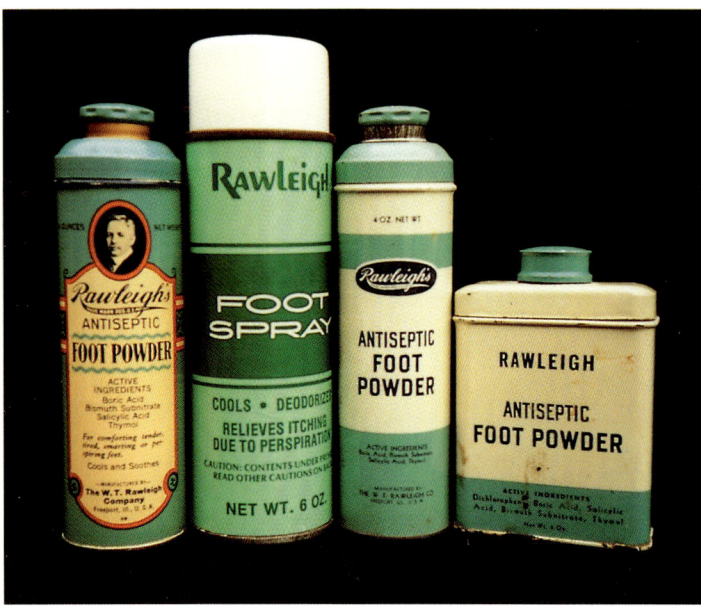

Foot Powder anyone? These three foot powders were manufactured by The W.T. Rawleigh Company Freeport, Ill. U.S.A. The spray was distributed by The W.T. Rawleigh Co. Freeport, Illinois 61032.

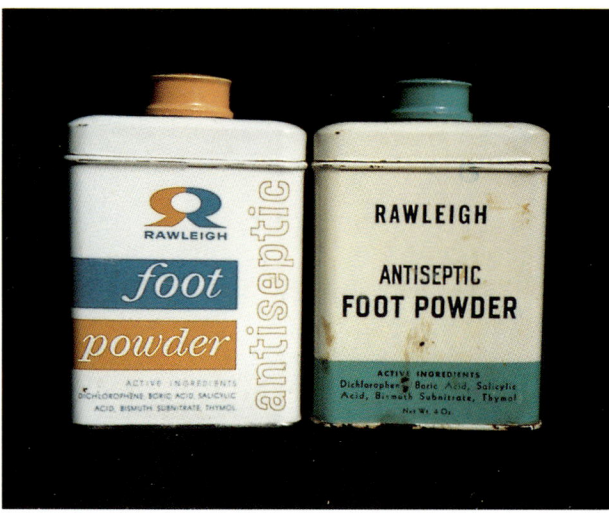

Two different Rawleigh Antiseptic Foot Powder containers. The blue container is marked "Manufactured by The W.T. Rawleigh Company Freeport, Illinois." The gold/blue container is marked "The W.T. Rawleigh Co. Freeport, Ill., U.S.A." Circa 1960s. *See* original advertisement in this chapter. $40-$50 ea.

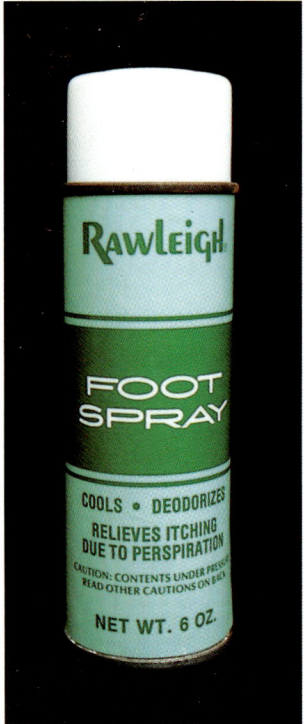

Rawleigh 6 ounce aerosol Foot Spray. Distributed by The W.T. Rawleigh Co. Freeport, Illinois 61032. $15-$20.

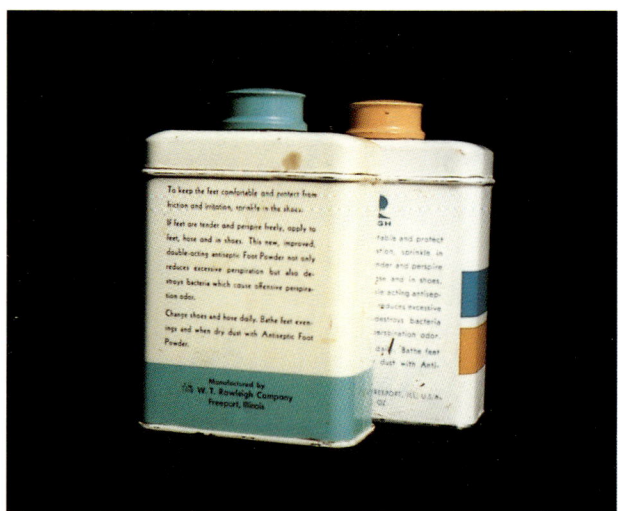

The reverse sides which provide directions for use. This was a new, improved, double-acting antiseptic foot powder. $40-$50 ea.

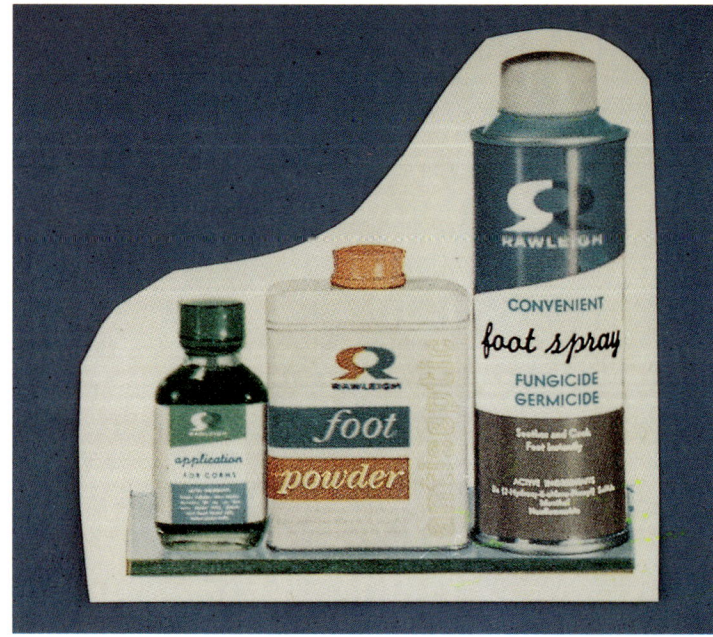

During the 1960s, Rawleigh promoted its application for corns or callus, 4 ounce foot powder, and its 8-1/2 ounce aerosol foot spray. $15-$20 ea.

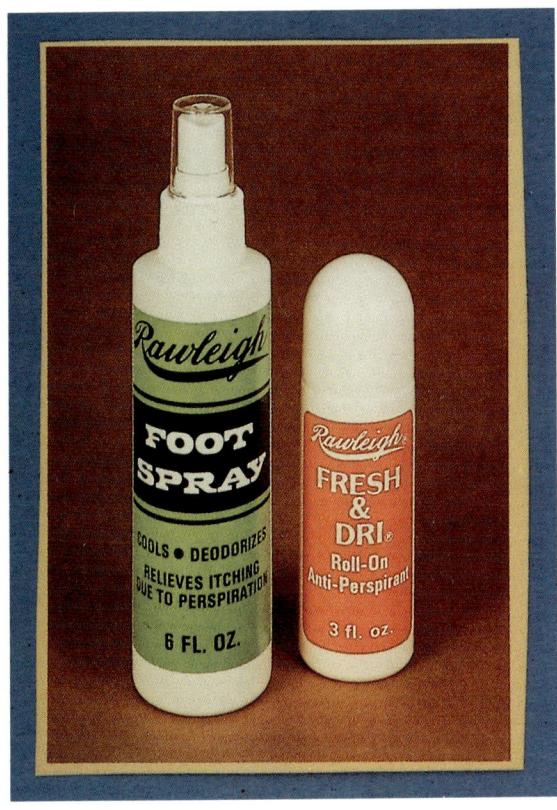

Rawleigh aerosol 6 ounce Foot Spray and Rawleigh "Fresh & Dri" 3 ounce Roll-On Anti-Perspirant. Circa 1986. $15-$20 ea.

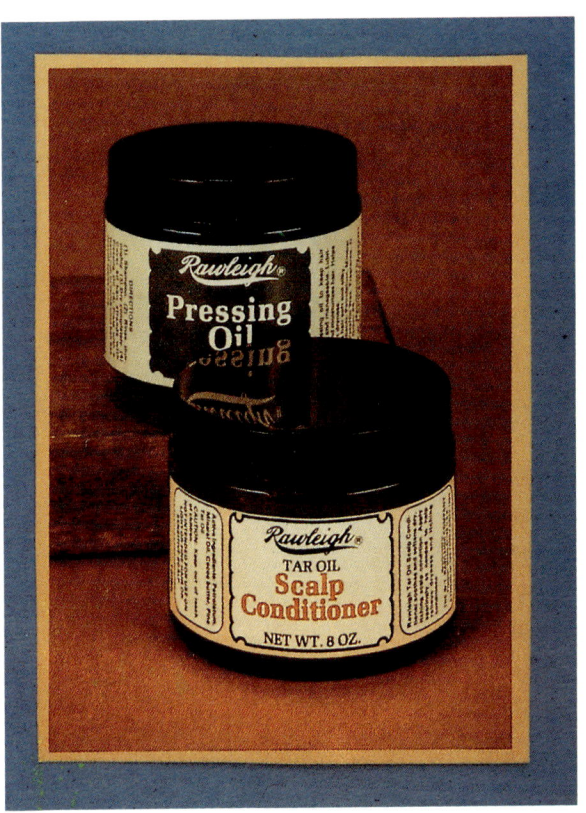

Rawleigh 8 ounce Pressing Oil and 8 ounce Tar Oil Scalp Conditioner. Circa 1986. $15-$20 ea.

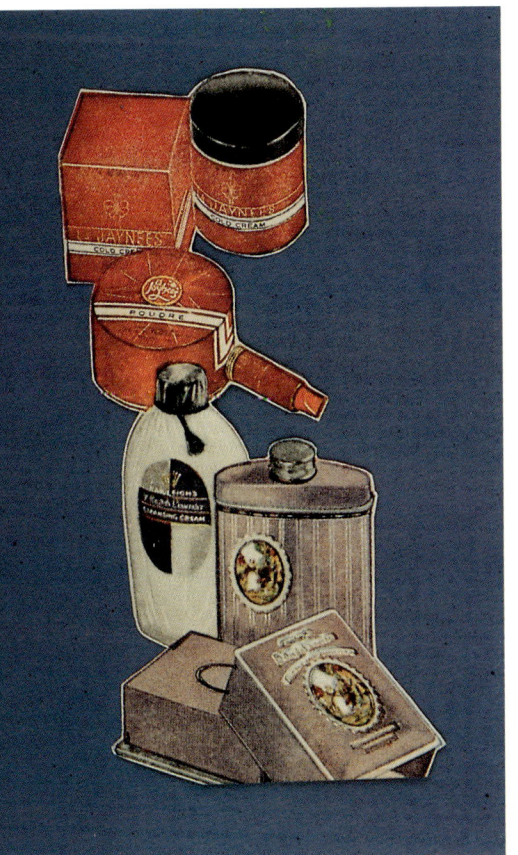

Rawleigh 8 ounce hair dressing, 8 ounce scalp conditioner, 8 ounce pressing oil, and 8 ounce marcel hair wax. Circa 1960s. $15-$20 ea.

Rawleigh's toilet preparations were familiar to hundreds of thousands of women throughout the United States, Canada, Australia, and New Zealand. In 1942 Rawleigh promoted grooming creams, powders, deodorants, rouge, and lipstick products.

Soaps, Shampoo and Shaving Cream

In 1917, Rawleigh indicated to their customers that over 500 establishments were engaged in the soap industry in the United States and that the total value of their annual products were over one hundred thirty-five million dollars.

In the Rawleigh industries the manufacture of toilet soaps had become an important part of their business. The purchase of crude materials in large quantities and the use of the best modern machinery, immense steam-jacketed heating kettles, iron cooling frames, quick action slabbers for cutting the soap into bars, and the automatic presses for shaping the bars and stamping the name of Rawleigh's, together with proper methods for wrapping and packing, enabled Rawleigh to produce soaps far above the average in quality, at prices that enabled them to give more real soap value for a specified price.

Rawleigh's toilet soaps were made by what is known as the cold process — the most expensive and the most exacting method of making soap, yet it was only by this cold process that soaps were good enough to bear the Rawleigh brand could be made.

"Only pure coconut oil and other fine materials were used. Nature's own ingredients were selected, tested, combined, and converted into soaps in a manner that every bar bearing the brand of Rawleigh added to the reputation which gained their first twenty-seven years of satisfactory service."

Users of Rawleigh's toilet soaps were assured that they were free from chalk, cheap talc, Fuller's Earth, Oatmeal, and other similar substances which were commonly used to lower costs, add bulk and increase profits.

Rawleigh's soaps came in generous sized cakes and produced a light and cleansing lather that was "soothing, healing, refreshing, pleasing, and which remained sweet and wholesome" indefinitely. They were pure and could be used on the most delicate skin. The perfumes used in Rawleigh's soaps were made in Rawleigh's laboratories from oils purchased first hand from leading European producers.

There was a Rawleigh soap for every purpose. Rawleigh's Vegetable Oil Soap (shown in an original advertisement in this chapter) was made from vegetable oils only and contained no animal fats, filler, or "coloring matter." Rawleigh's Alba Rose was made by a special French process while Rawleigh's Cocoa Castile Soap was prepared from East Indian coconut oil and the best soap stock. Rawleigh's Ideal Pine Tar Soap was produced from No. 1 tallow, vegetable oils, and first class refined, clean oil of tar. Rawleigh's Orange Glycerin Soap contained only the purest vegetable oils used for soap making. Rawleigh's Witch Hazel Soap was distinguished by its attractive green color and fragrant, refreshing perfume. Rawleigh's Derma-Tone Complexion Soap was highly medicated with balsams and antiseptic. Derma-Tone was recommended for infants and children. Rawleigh's Ideal Pumice Soap was made from a combination of oils and pumice. Rawleigh's Cream Shaving Soap softened the most obstinate beard and the round cakes were just right for the shaving mug. This Shaving Soap was offered in a trial size.

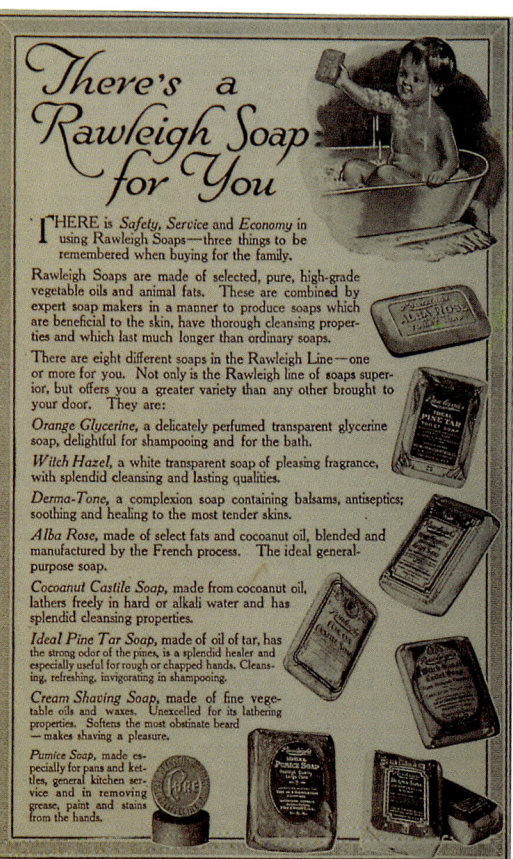

An original 1916 advertisement "There's a Rawleigh Soap for You." Original packaging may take some time to locate and can be expensive. $100-$125 complete.

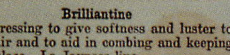

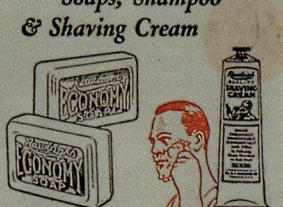

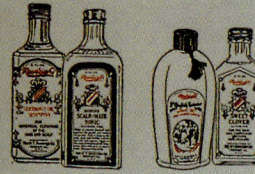

An original 1935 promotion for Rawleigh's Soaps, Shampoo & Shaving Cream providing a complete description of each product.

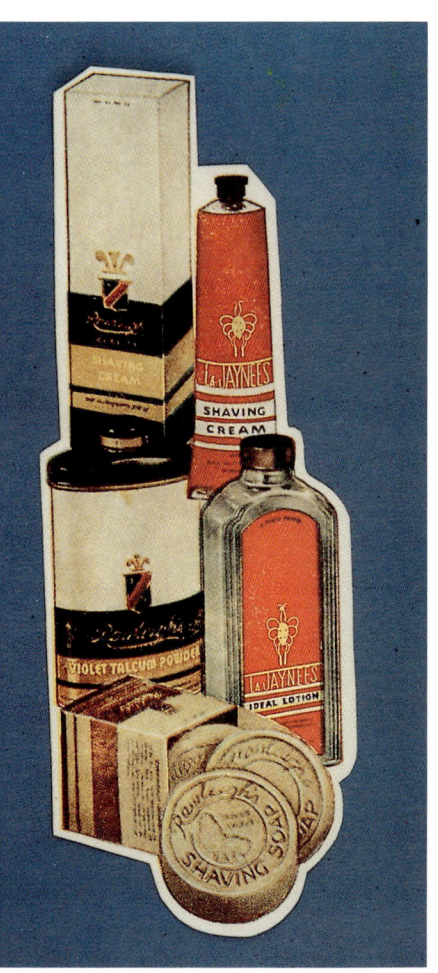

In 1941, men found it easy to keep their face clean-shaven and smooth with Rawleigh's Shaving Cream, Violet Talcum Powder, Shaving Soap, La Jaynees Shaving Cream, and La Jaynees Ideal Lotion. The Rawleigh Talcum Powder is shown elsewhere in this chapter.

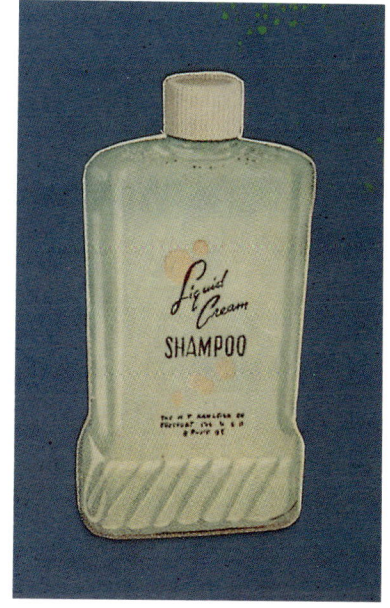

In 1954, Rawleigh's "Liquid Cream Shampoo" was a new shampoo with a refreshing perfume that cleaned hair and scalp perfectly, rinsed away, and left no film. $20-$25.

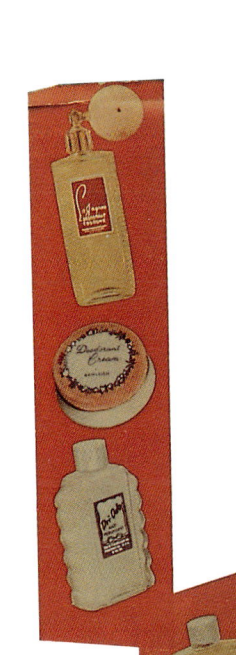

In 1957 these products were advertised as "Night or Day — Work or Play, fresh as a daisy the Rawleigh way." La Jaynees Deodorant Spray Cologne, Deodorant Cream, Dri-Odo Anti-Perspirant, After Bath Cologne, and Jasmine Bath Salts. $20-$25 ea.

In 1954, this was Rawleigh's new Antiseptic Hair Tonic. It had the ingredients hexachlorophene and dichlorophene. Rawleigh's hair tonic was easy to apply and gave the hair a well-kept appearance. $20-$25.

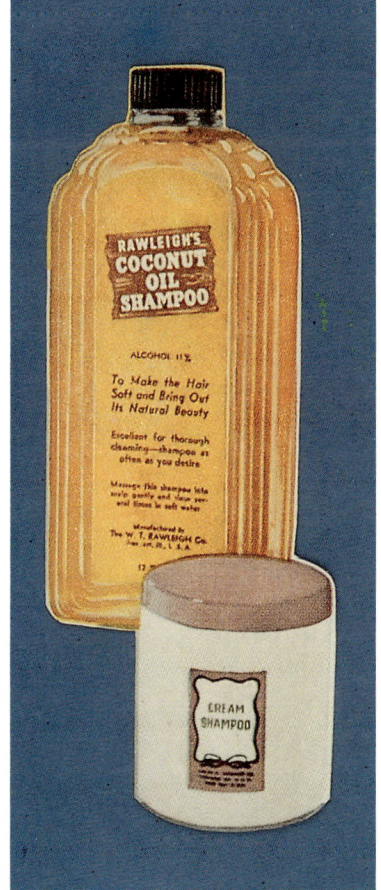

An original 1954 advertisement for Rawleigh's "Coconut Oil Shampoo" which was an old reliable that had given wonderful shampoos for years. Rawleigh's "Cream Shampoo" produced fragrant, rich, billowy suds that lifted dirt and dandruff out and contained natural oil that was good for the scalp and hair. $20-$25.

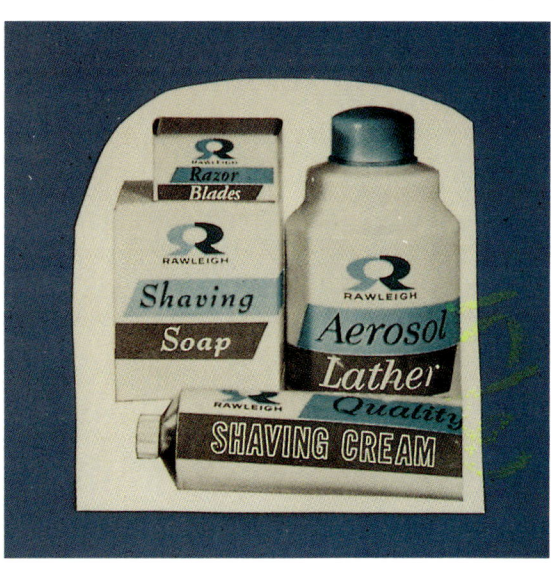

During the 1960s Rawleigh provided help for clean, fast shaves with Rawleigh quality Razor Blades, Aerosol 10 ounce Lather, Shaving Cream, and Shaving Soap in a handsome blue and white packaging. These were popular items for 60 years.

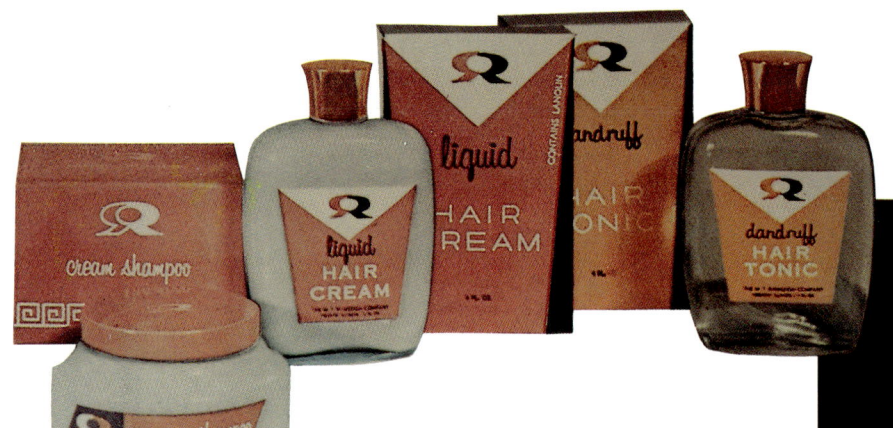

Promoted during the 1960s, these items appeared in a Rawleigh publication. They include a 5 ounce Cream Shampoo with carton, a 4 ounce Liquid Hair Cream with carton, and a 4 ounce Dandruff Hair Tonic with carton. $20-$25 ea.

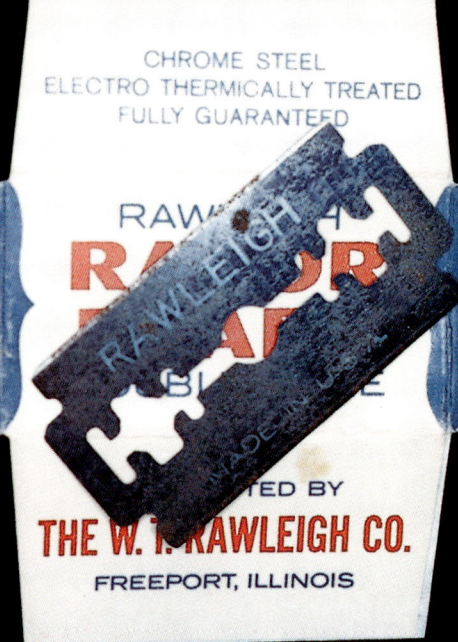

Rawleigh Double Edge Razor Blade and sleeve. This blade was of chrome steel, electro-thermically treated and fully guaranteed. *Courtesy Phillip L. Krumholz.* $5-$6.

Rawleigh Double Edge Razor Blade. *Courtesy Phillip L. Krumholz.* $5-$6.

The reverse side of the Rawleigh Double Edge Razor Blade. *Courtesy Phillip L. Krumholz.* $5-$6.

In 1915, Rawleigh promoted Shampoo Jelly. Manufactured By The W.T. Rawleigh Medical Co., Freeport, Ill., U.S.A. $95-$100.

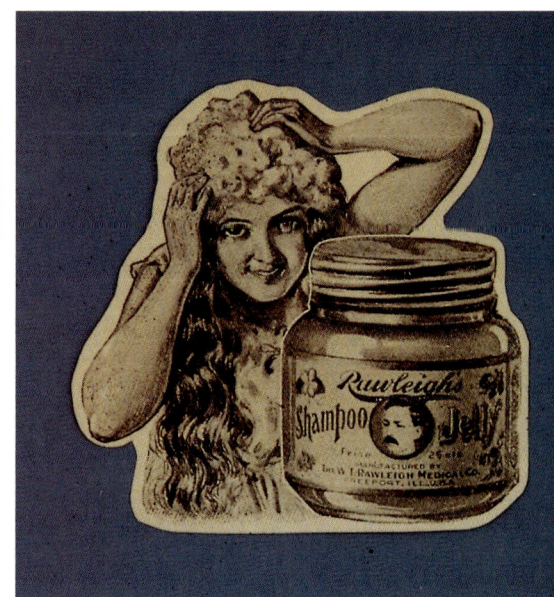

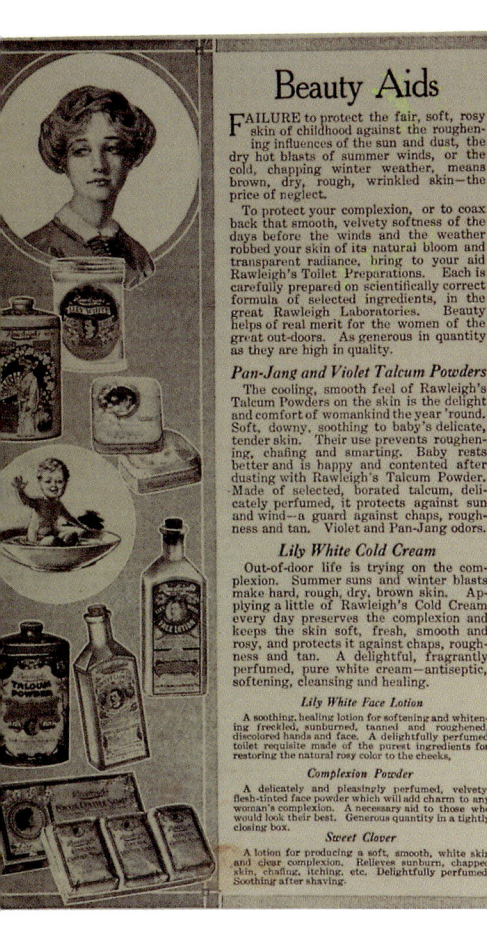

These original "Beauty Aids" appeared in Rawleigh's 1916 Almanac. $150-$200 ea.

An original "Pretty Hair Secrets" advertisement from Rawleigh's 1916 Almanac.

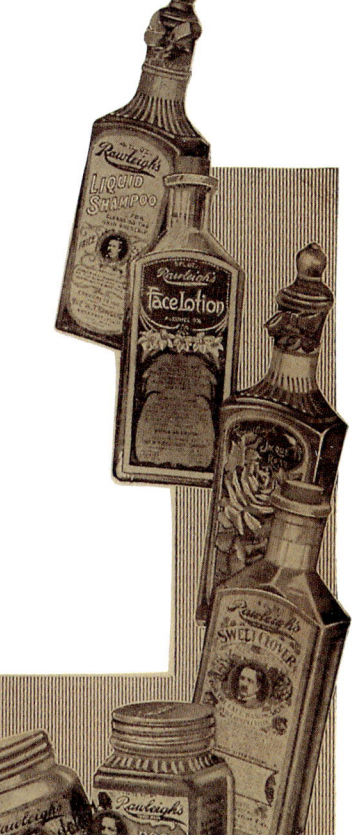

In 1917, Rawleigh promoted Rawleigh's Shampoo and Hair Tonic products.

All Rawleigh's Perfumes and Toilet Waters were made in Rawleigh's Perfume Making Laboratories under the supervision of Rawleigh's chief chemist who had years of experience in the manufacture of perfume. The chemist had studied the processes used by the most noted perfumeries both in the United States and abroad. Only the finest oils and other perfume-making materials were used in Rawleigh's scents. These oils were purchased direct from the countries where the flowers were grown and the odors were produced.

Rawleigh was fortunate in making a long term contract at prices prevailing before World War I, under which they purchased upwards of $100,000.00 worth of perfume making materials.

In 1917, Rawleigh's Perfumes and Toilet Waters were put up in larger and better looking bottles and packaging.

This miniature Perfume bottle is marked THE W.T. RAWLEIGH CO., FREEPORT, ILL. $75-$100.

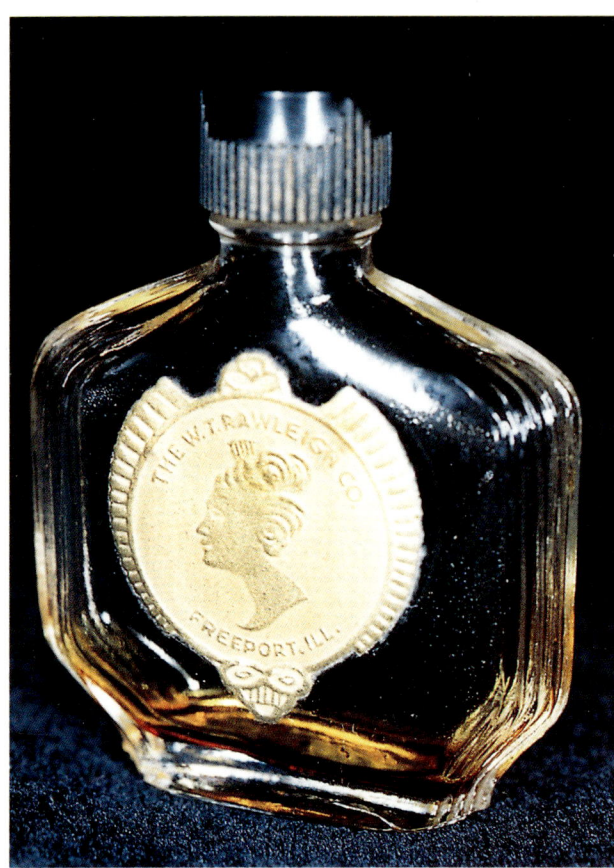

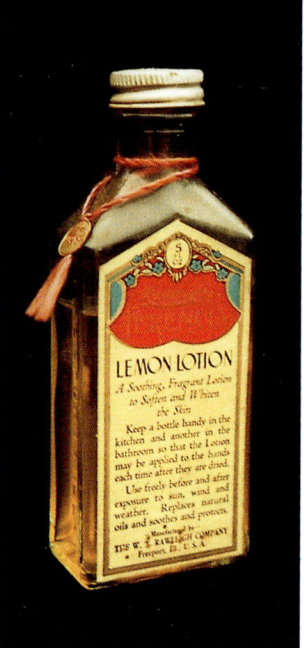

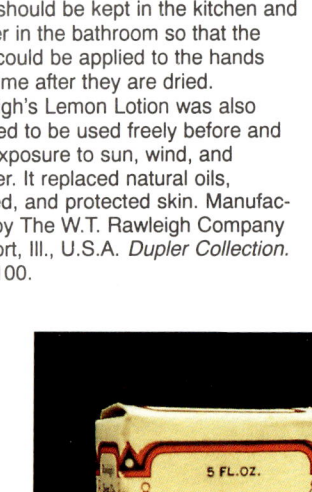

Rawleigh's Florencia Lemon Lotion, "A soothing, Fragrant Lotion to Soften and Whiten the Skin." This 5 fluid ounce bottle should be kept in the kitchen and another in the bathroom so that the lotion could be applied to the hands each time after they are dried. Rawleigh's Lemon Lotion was also intended to be used freely before and after exposure to sun, wind, and weather. It replaced natural oils, soothed, and protected skin. Manufactured by The W.T. Rawleigh Company Freeport, Ill., U.S.A. *Dupler Collection.* $75-$100.

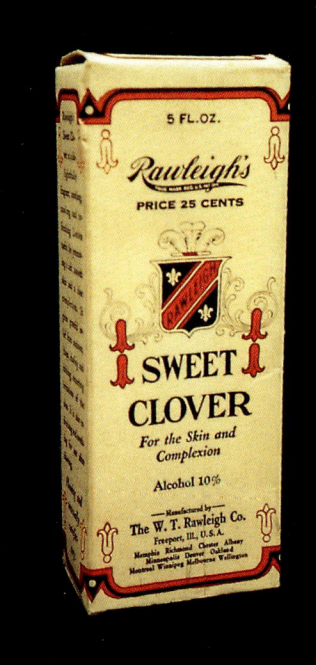

This miniature perfume bottle is only 2" high. A small amount of liquid inside the bottle has dried to a brown residue. A sweet fragrance is still present when the cap is removed. $75-$100.

This carton held 5 fluid ounces of Rawleigh's Sweet Clover. The original price was 25 cents. Sweet Clover was intended to be used for the Skin and Complexion. Manufactured by The W.T. Rawleigh Company Freeport, Ill., U.S.A. Rawleigh's Sweet Clover was a delightfully fragrant, soothing, cooling, and refreshing lotion useful for promoting a soft, smooth skin and a clear complexion. It provided relief from sunburn, chaps, chafing and itching, smarting irritations of the skin, and was refreshing and soothing for use after shaving. This carton is empty. *Dupler Collection.* $75-$100 complete.

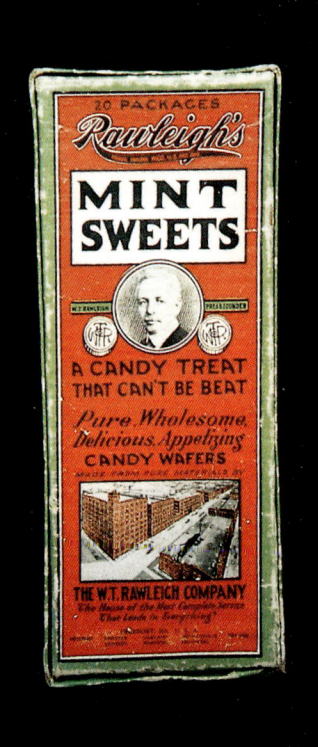

The carton held 20 packages of Rawleigh's Mint Sweets, a candy wafer. "A Candy Treat That Can't Be Beat." The W.T. Rawleigh Company, "The House of the Most Complete Service That Leads in Everything Freeport, Ill., U.S.A. Memphis - Chester - Oakland - Minneapolis - Denver - London - Winnipeg - Montreal." This carton is empty. *Dupler Collection.* $75-$100 complete.

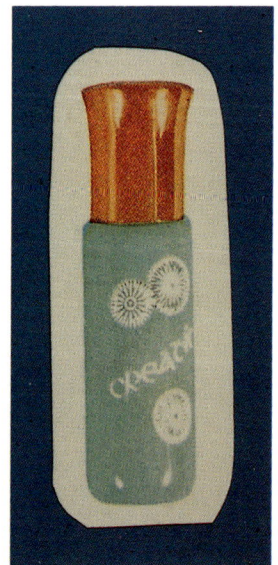

During the 1960s, "Creation perfume" was first in a line of NEW and lovely cosmetics. At the touch of a button, Creation released one of two hundred measured sprays of fragrance. $10-$15.

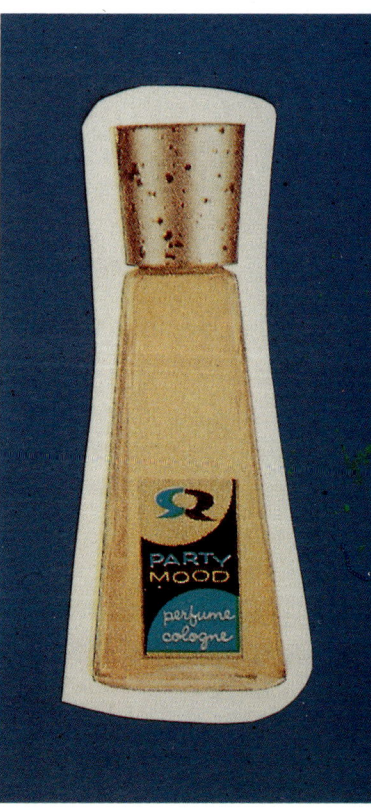

A 2 ounce container of Rawleigh's Party Mood, a perfume cologne with a blithe fragrance. $10-$15.

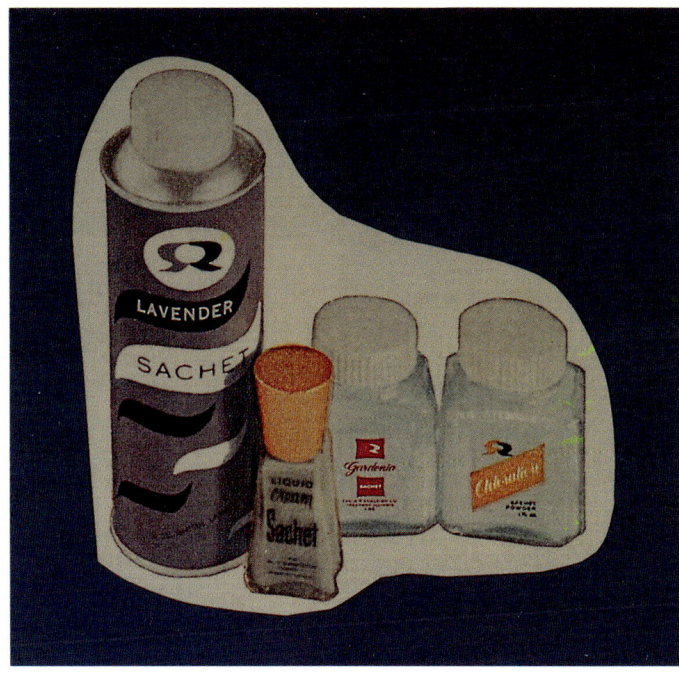

During the 1960s, Rawleigh promoted four sachets. Lavender Sachet in an 8 ounce can, liquid cream sachet in a 1/2 ounce jar, gardenia sachet in a 1-1/2 ounce powder and 1-1/2 ounce jar of Adoration sachet powder. $10-$15 ea.

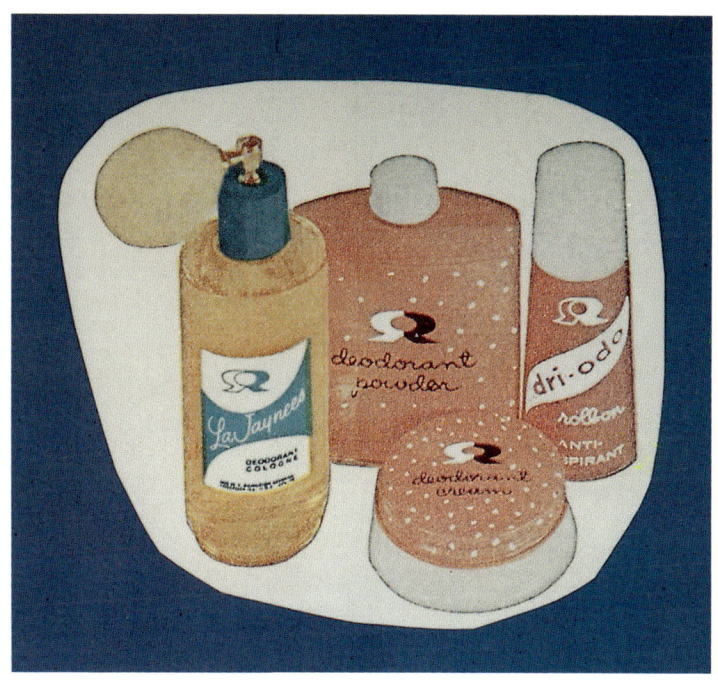

This selection of Rawleigh deodorants banished perspiration odor — La Jaynees deodorant 4 ounce cologne with atomizer, Deodorant 2 ounce powder, Deodorant 1 ounce cream, and Dri-Odo 2 ounce roll-on in an attractive pink containers. $10-$15 ea.

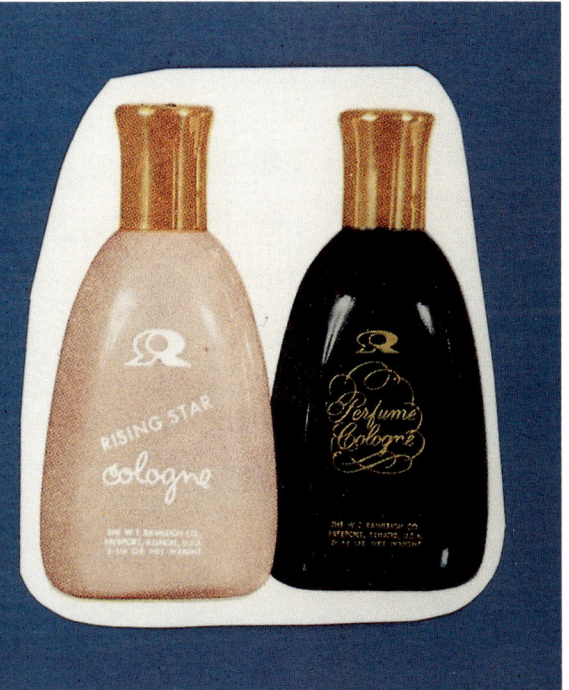

During the 1960s, Rawleigh provided a wide choice of fragrances to bring romance. A 2-1/4 ounce Rising Star Cologne in a pink aerosol bottle and — in a dramatic black and gold bottle — a Rawleigh's 2-1/4 ounce Perfume Cologne. $10-$15 ea.

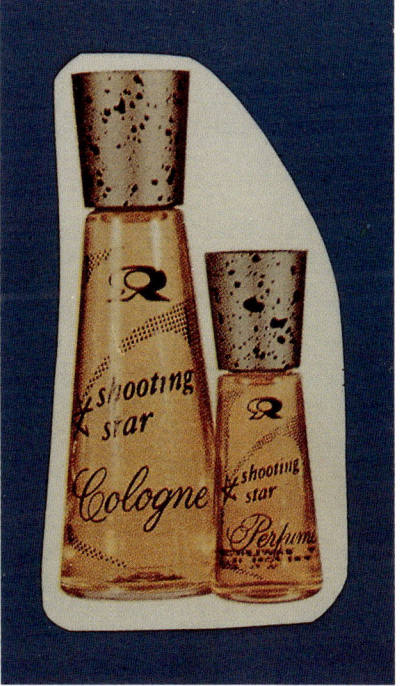

Rawleigh's Shooting Star Perfume is shown here in a 1/2 ounce container and Rawleigh's Shooting Star Cologne is displayed in a 2 ounce container. Both were rich and elegant French fragrances. $10-$15 ea.

Rawleigh's 1960 La Jaynees 1 ounce perfume and 1 ounce Gardenia Perfume. $10-$15 ea.

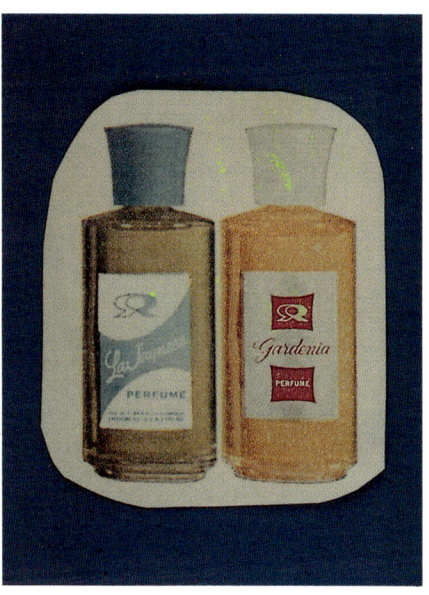

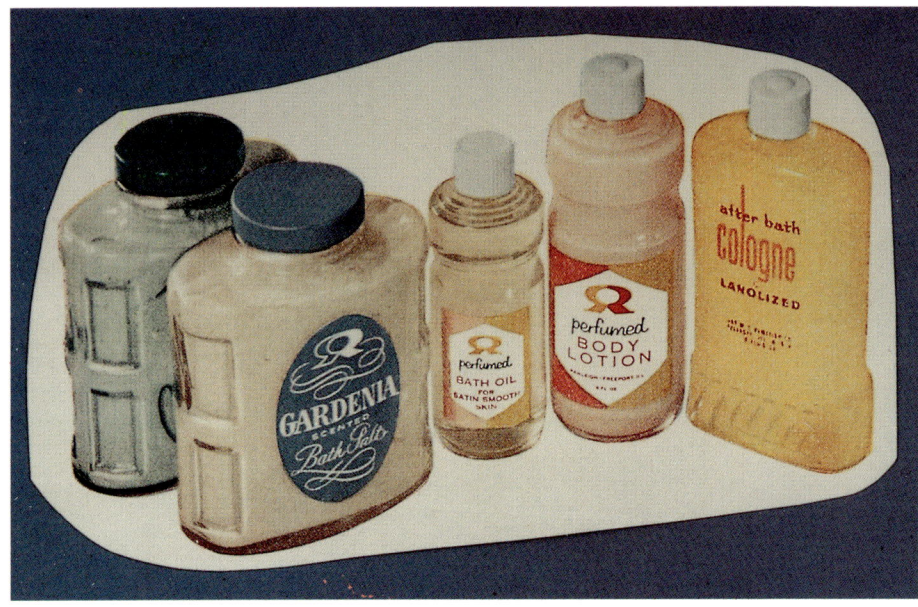

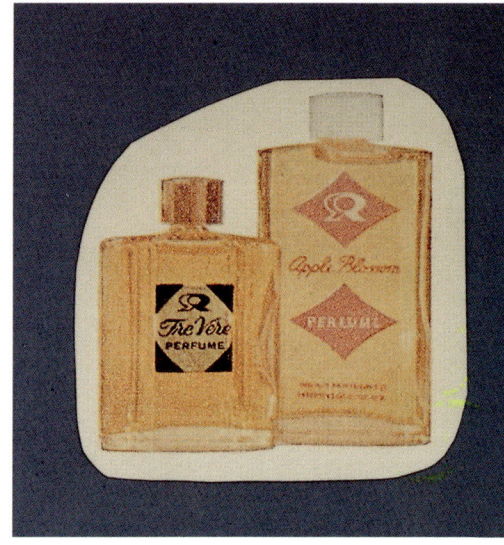

Rawleigh's 16 ounce bottle of Gardenia and Jasmine Bath Salts, perfume Bath Oil, perfume Body Lotion, and 8 ounce After Bath cologne. $10-$15 ea.

Rawleigh's 1/2 ounce TreVere Perfume and 1 ounce Apple Blossom Perfume. $10-$15 ea.

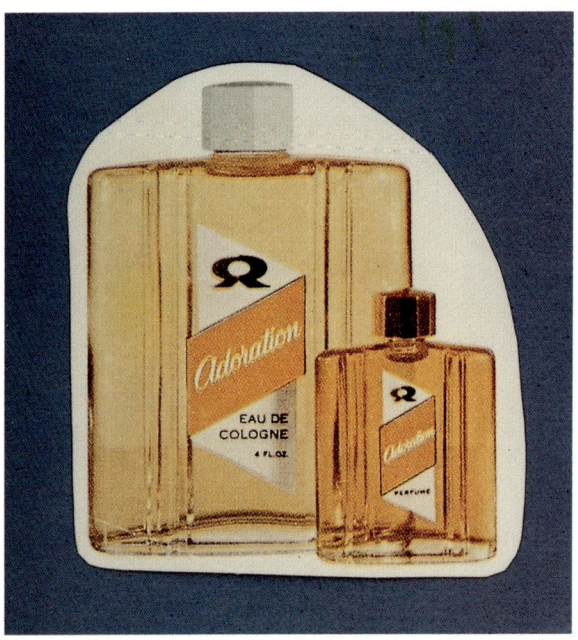

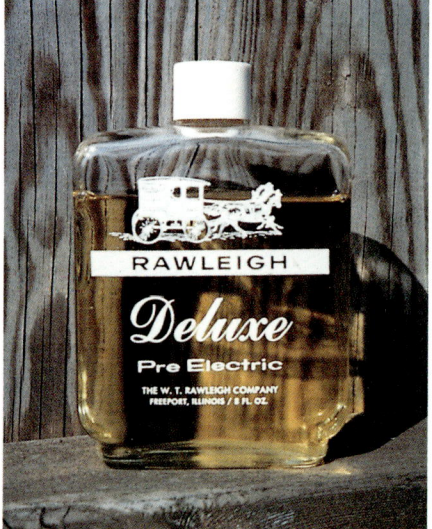

An 8 fluid ounce bottle of Rawleigh Deluxe Pre Electric. The W.T. Rawleigh Company Freeport, Illinois. *Dupler Collection.* $20-$30.

Rawleigh's Adoration 1/2 ounce perfume and 4 ounce Adoration cologne — both were promoted in the 1960s. $10-$15 ea.

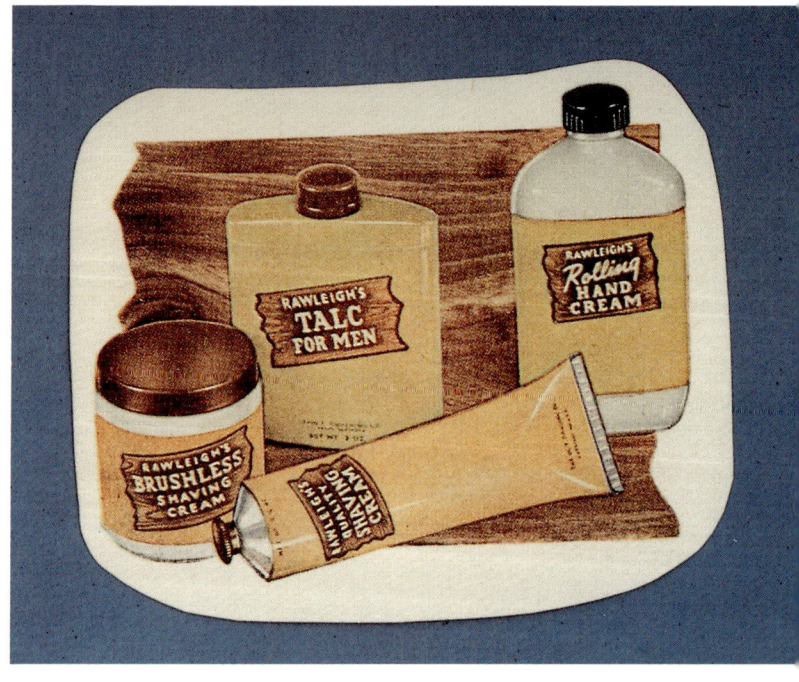

Rawleigh Brushless Shaving Cream, Talc for Men, Rolling Hand Cream and Shaving Cream. $20-$30 ea.

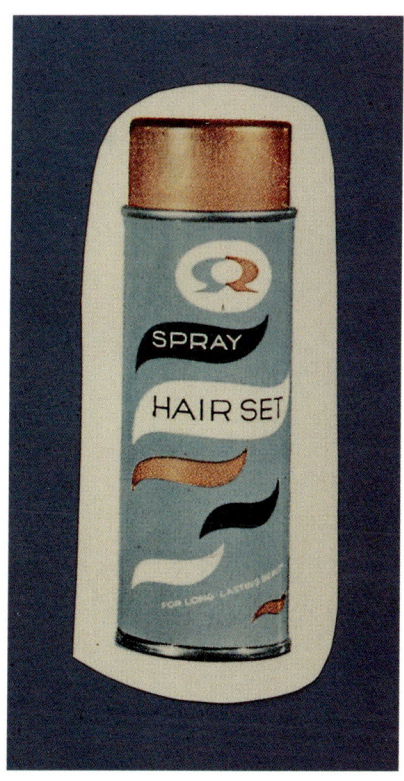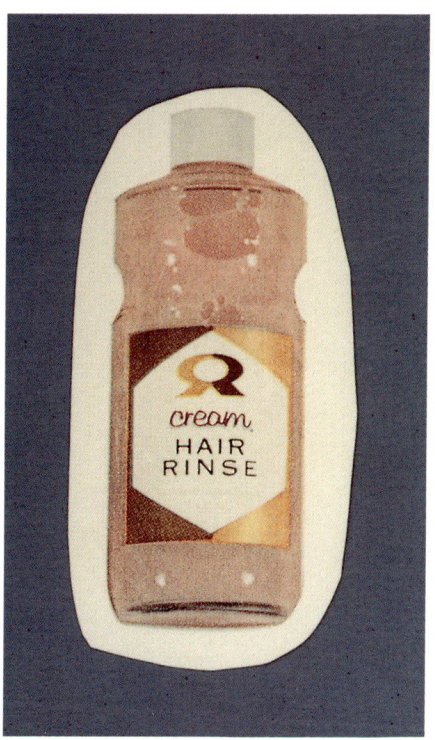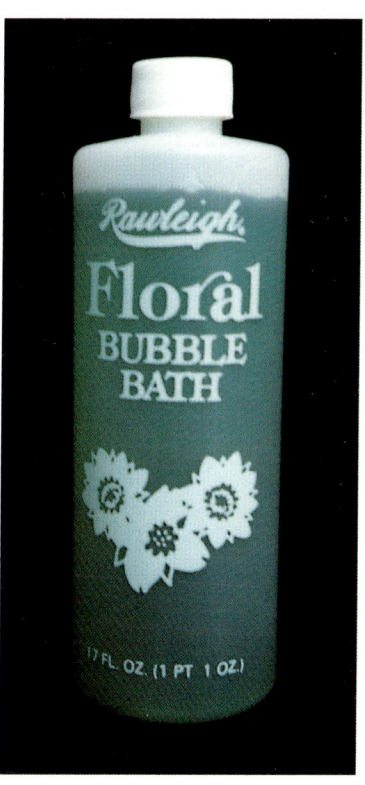

Rawleigh's "Hair Set" was a fragrant aerosol spray that kept hair in place all day. Circa 1960s. $10-$15.

The 8 ounce Rawleigh "Cream Hair Rinse" appeared in a 1960s publication. This special rinse for after shampoo helped to soften hair and provided a beautiful sheen. $10-$15.

Rawleigh's 17 fluid ounce Floral Bubble Bath. Manufactured by The W.T. Rawleigh Company Freeport, Illinois 61032 U.S.A. *Dupler Collection.* $10-$15.

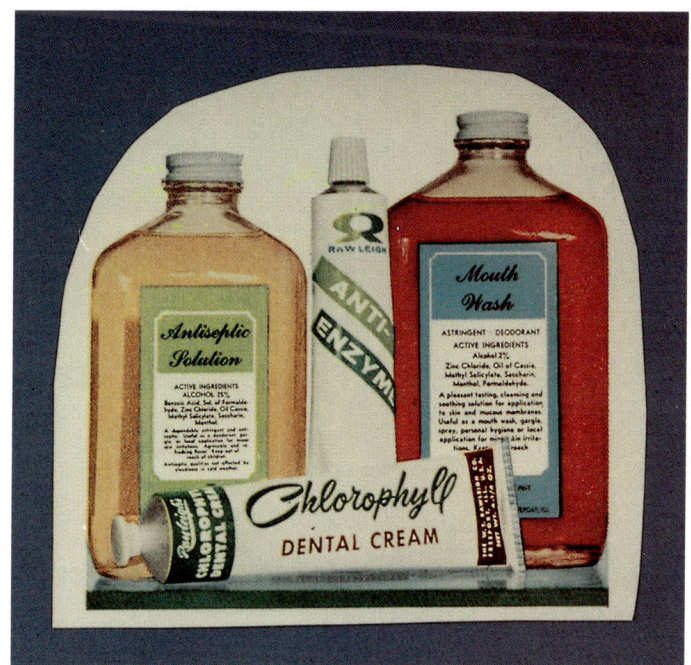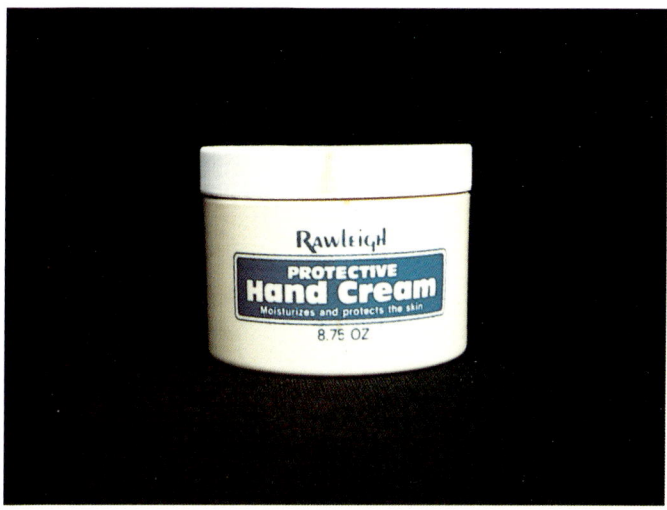

Rawleigh 8.75 ounce Protective Hand Cream. *Dupler Collection.* $10-$15.

An original 1960s advertisement for Rawleigh 4-1/4 ounce Chlorophyll Dental Cream, 10 ounce Antiseptic Solution, 1-pint Mouth Wash, and Anti-Enzyme Tooth Paste. Also offered but not illustrated were special adults and child's toothbrushes in boxes of three. $15-$25 ea.

In 1932, a specially prepared cleaner that quickly and easily removed dirt, grease, grime, ink stains, paint, oil, and left the hands clean, smooth and soft, was introduced. It was a hand soap that was economical and better than most cake soaps. Photograph not available.

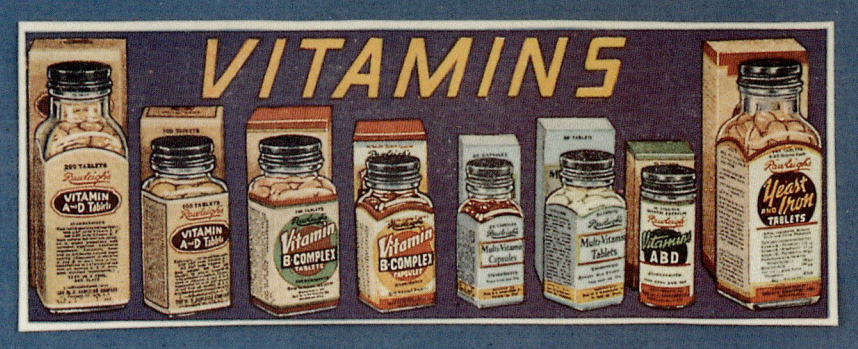

This selection of Rawleigh Vitamins appeared in a 1946 Rawleigh publication. $10-$15 ea.

Work Savers for Kitchen, Laundry and Bath

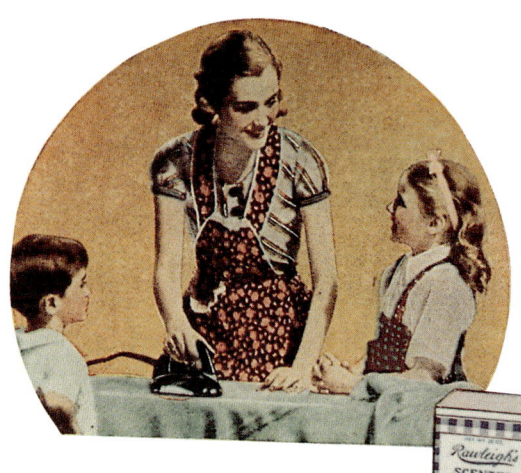

An original 1946 Rawleigh advertisement for Rawleigh's Scented Starch and Rawleigh's Starch-Aid. Remember your first lesson using an iron?

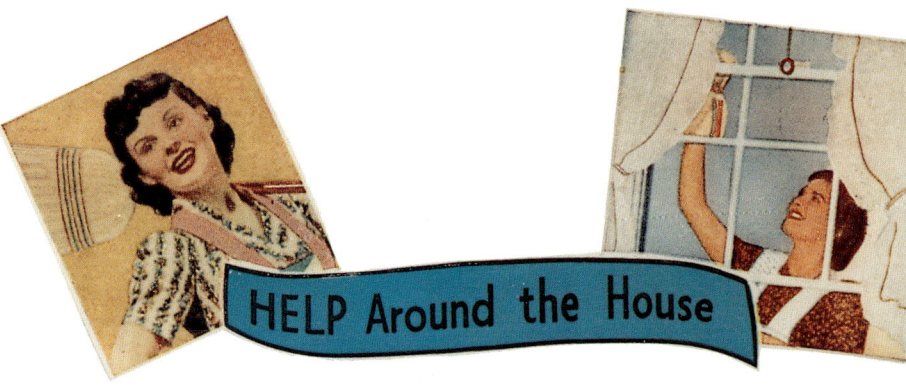

Help Around the House, advertisement, circa 1950.

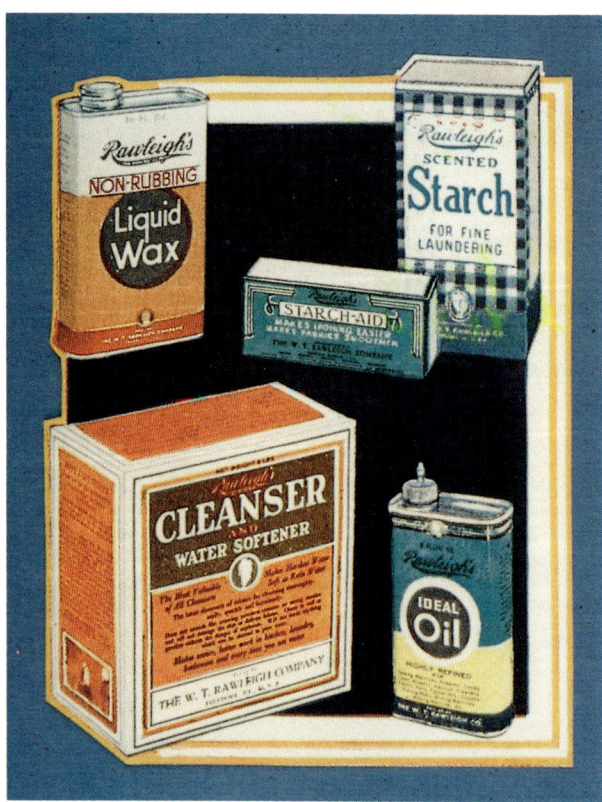

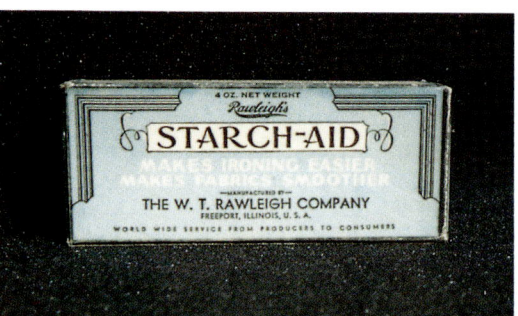

Rawleigh's Starch-Aid: a new, economical, laborsaving help that made ironing of starched fabrics and clothing easier and smoother. Gave a fine, firm, glossy finish and made clothing daintier and fresher. This full cardboard carton held 4 ounces. *Dupler Collection.* $75-$100 complete.

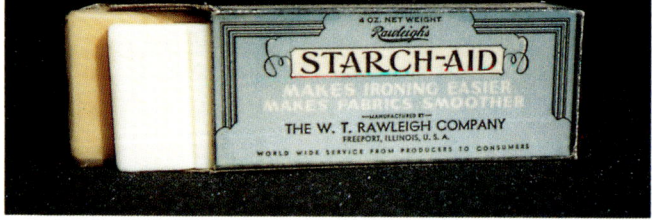

Sections of Rawleigh's Starch-Aid tablets. Manufactured by the W.T. Rawleigh Company Freeport, Illinois. U.S.A. Circa 1932. These tablets have never been used. *Dupler Collection.* $75-$100 complete.

These Rawleigh products were promoted as savers around the house in 1942. "Save Time and Trouble With Rawleigh Products" Rawleigh's liquid wax, scented starch, starch-aid, cleanser, and ideal oil.

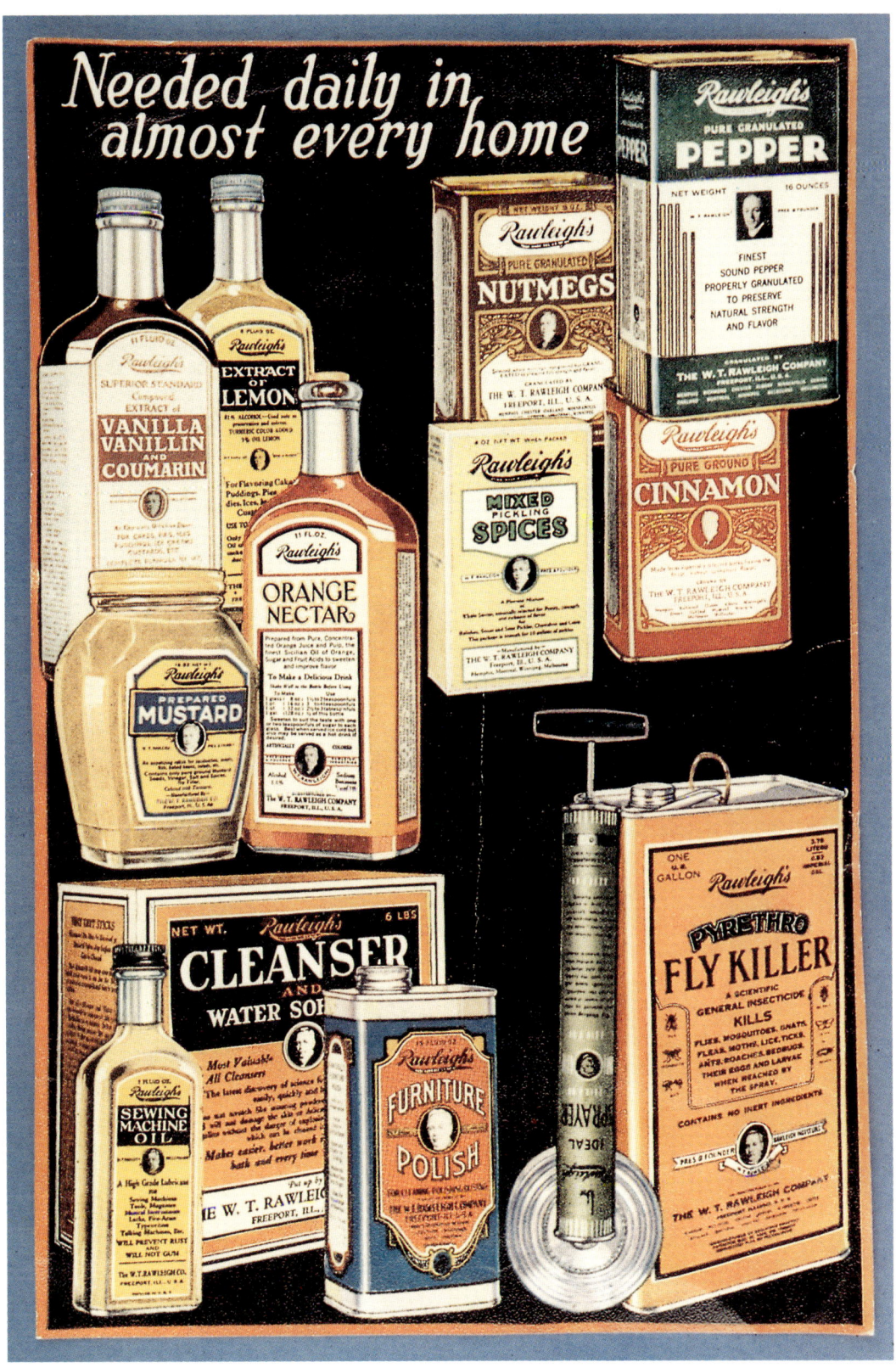

A promotional Rawleigh advertisement from 1935. Many of these "Needed daily in almost every home" products appear throughout this publication.

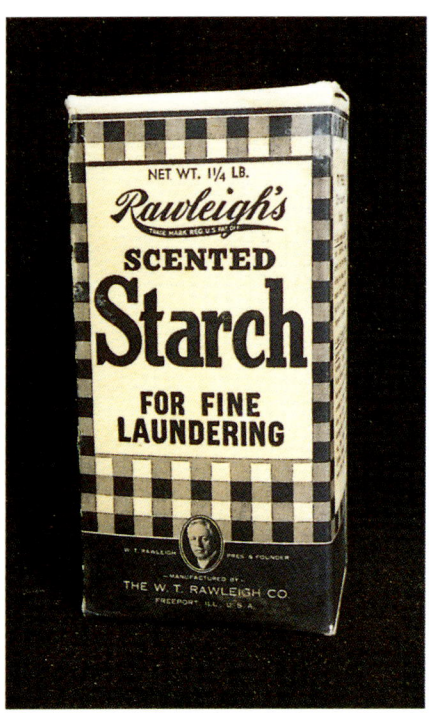

Rawleigh's 1-1/4 lb., Scented Starch "For Fine Laundering." Circa 1958. *Dupler Collection.* $50-$75.

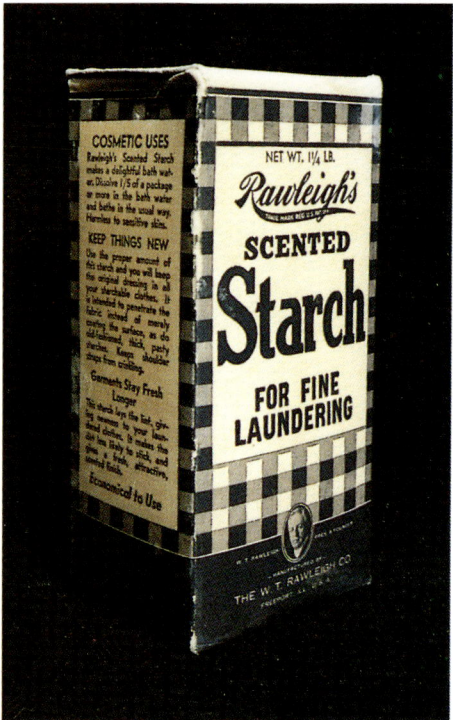

The side panel provided instruction for cosmetic uses and told the reader that it "kept Things New and Garments Stay Fresh Longer." Rawleigh's Scented Starch was economical to use. $50-$75.

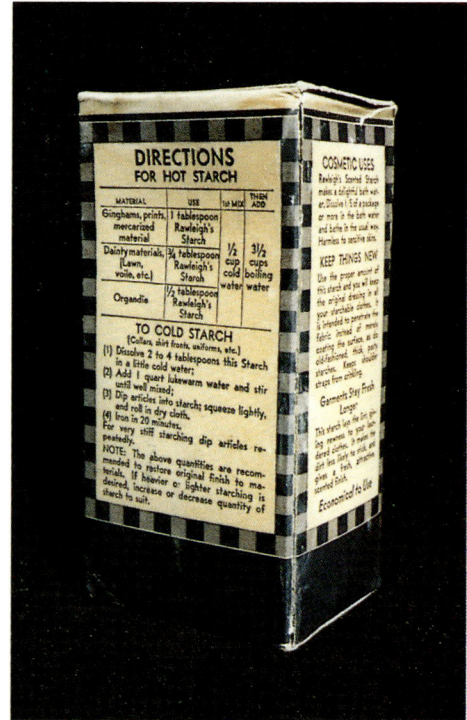

The back panel — DIRECTIONS for Hot Starch and To Cold Starch was provided. Manufactured By The W.T. Rawleigh Co., Freeport, Ill., U.S.A. *Dupler Collection.* $50-$75.

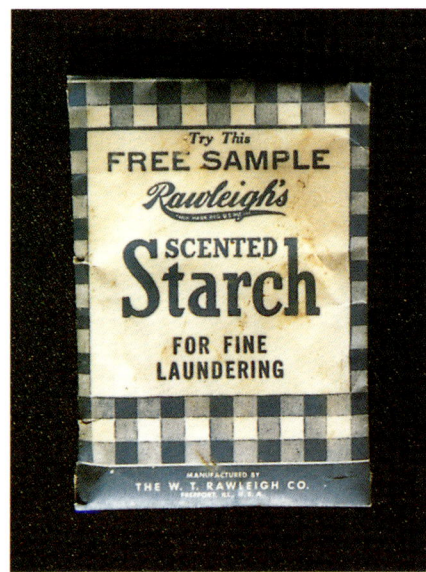

A FREE SAMPLE envelope of "Rawleigh's Scented Starch" for fine laundering. *Dupler Collection.* $40-$50.

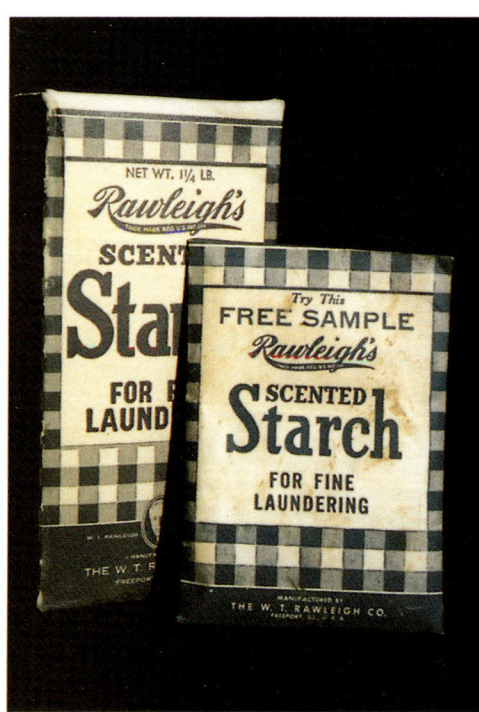

It was not uncommon for dealers to offer (when available) both the 1-1/4 lb., and the FREE SAMPLE of "Rawleigh's Scented Starch" as one unit and one price. *Dupler Collection.* 1-1/4 lb. $50-$75. SAMPLE $40-$50.

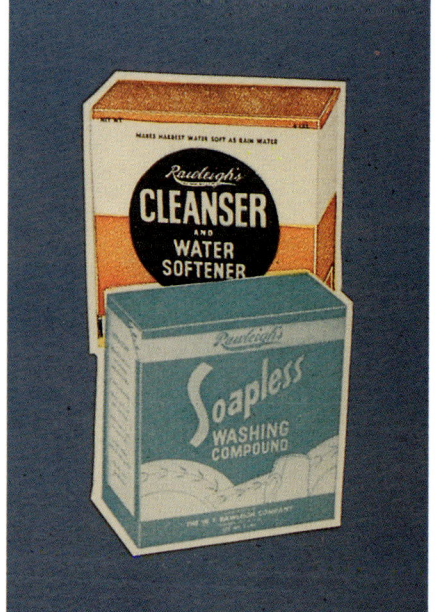

Rawleigh's Cleanser and Water Softener loosened dirt and grease and had over 50 daily uses. Rawleigh's new Soapless Washing Compound gently lifted dirt from the finest fabrics and lingerie. Circa 1950. $40-$50.

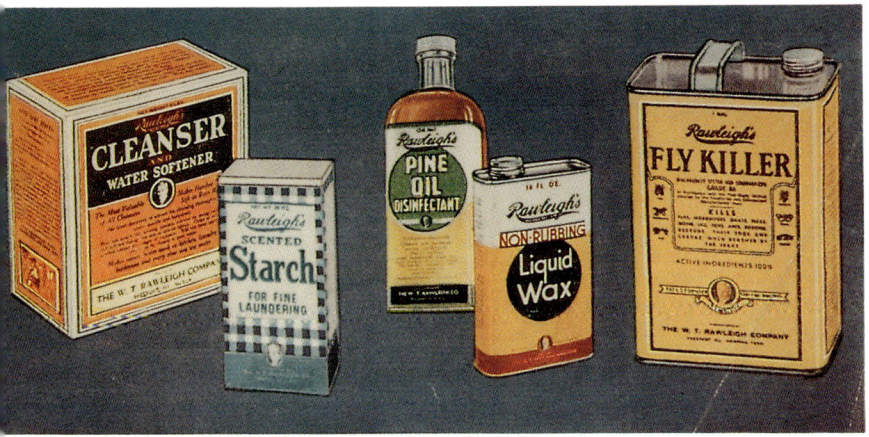

Rawleigh's Cleanser and Water Softener, Scented Starch, Pine Oil, Liquid Wax, and Fly Killer all appeared in this 1946 advertisement. Rawleigh's Fly Killer is shown elsewhere in this publication.

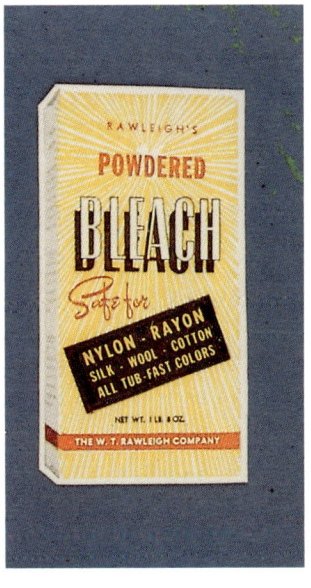

Rawleigh's Powdered Bleach was safe for nylon, rayon, silk, wool, cotton, and all tub fast colors. Circa 1958. $10-$15.

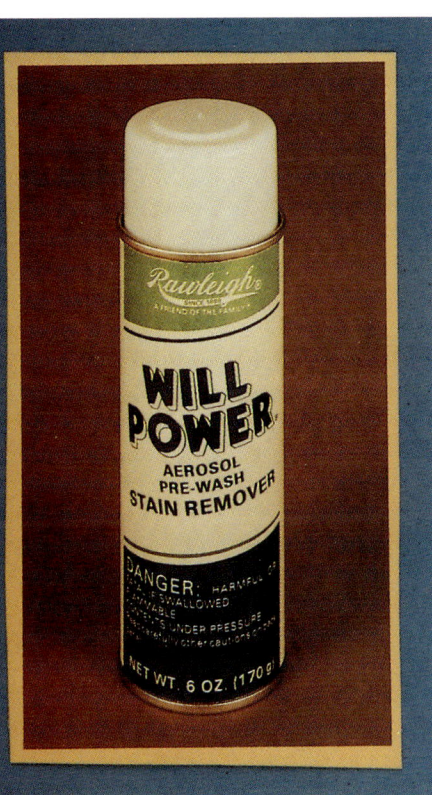

Rawleigh's "WILL POWER" was a 6 ounce aerosol prewash stain remover. A complete line of "WILL POWER" was offered in 1986 to make laundry day a breeze and included WILL POWER (Phosphate Free) Detergent, Laundry Detergent (With Phosphate), Liquid Laundry Detergent, Fabric Softener and Brightener, and WILL POWER Non-Chlorine All-Fabric Bleach. $10-$15 ea.

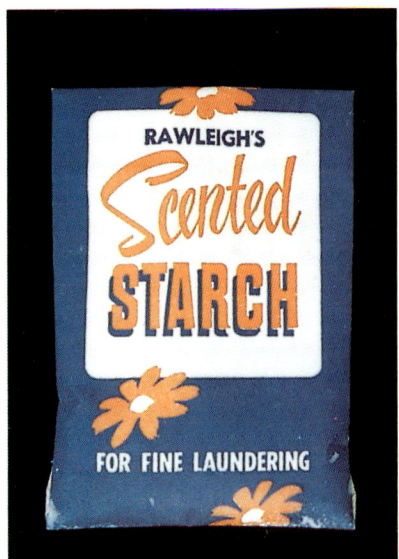

"Rawleigh's Scented Starch" for fine laundering. This is a FREE SAMPLE. *Dupler Collection.* $40-$50.

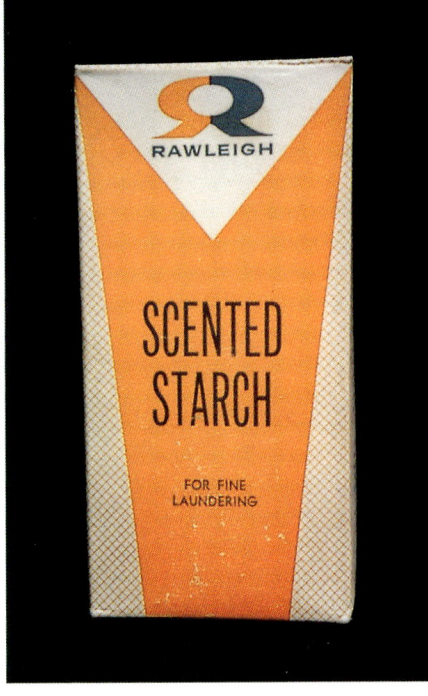

The Rawleigh Scented Starch was used for fine laundering. Manufactured by The W.T. Rawleigh Company Freeport, Ill. 1-1/4 pounds. *Dupler Collection.* $50-$75.

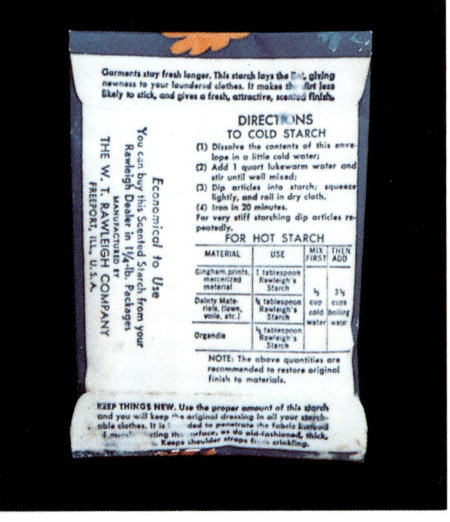

The reverse panel provided DIRECTIONS for "Rawleigh's Scented Starch." This SAMPLE was Manufactured by The W.T. Rawleigh Company Freeport, Ill. "You can buy this Scented Starch from your Rawleigh Dealer in 1-1/4-lb. packages." *Dupler Collection.* $40-$50.

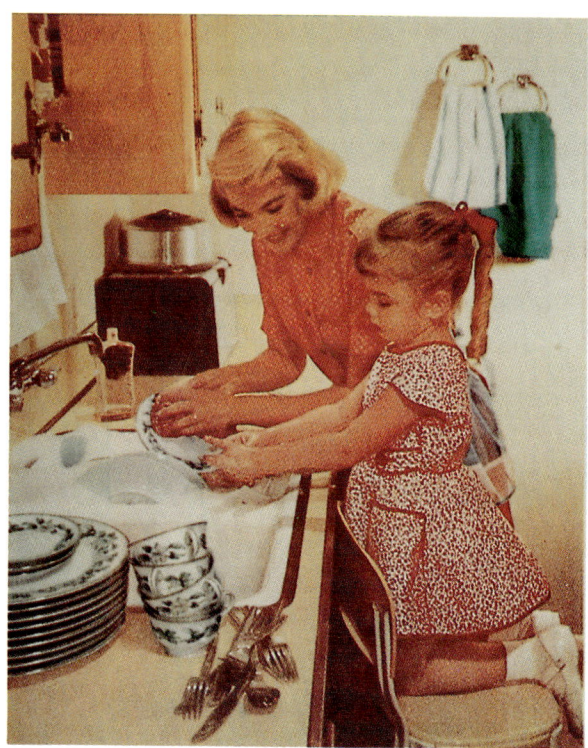

Mild suds made dishes sparkle and were kind to hands and fine dishes. The original illustration of a mother and daughter appeared in a 1960s Rawleigh publication.

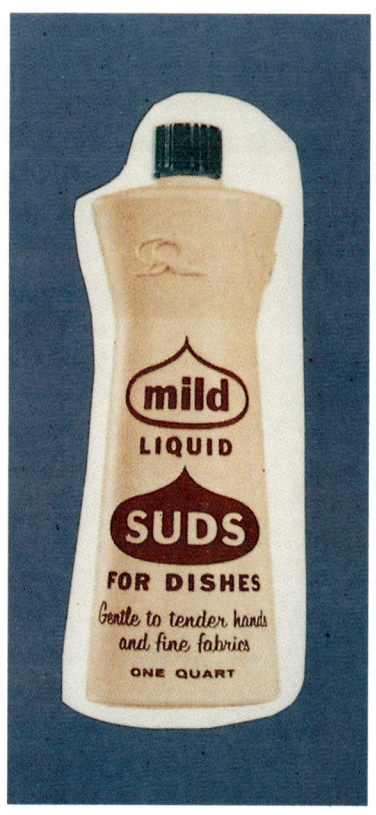

Rawleigh's One Quart Mild Liquid Suds for dishes was gentle to tender hands and fine fabrics. Circa 1960s. $10-$15.

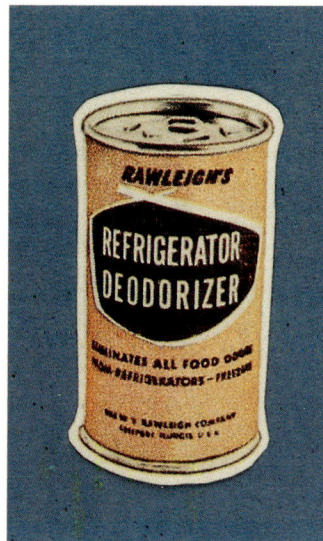

Rawleigh's Refrigerator Deodorizer. Circa 1957. No work was involved; just set the can on the refrigerator shelf and it did the rest. One can lasted one year. $15-$20.

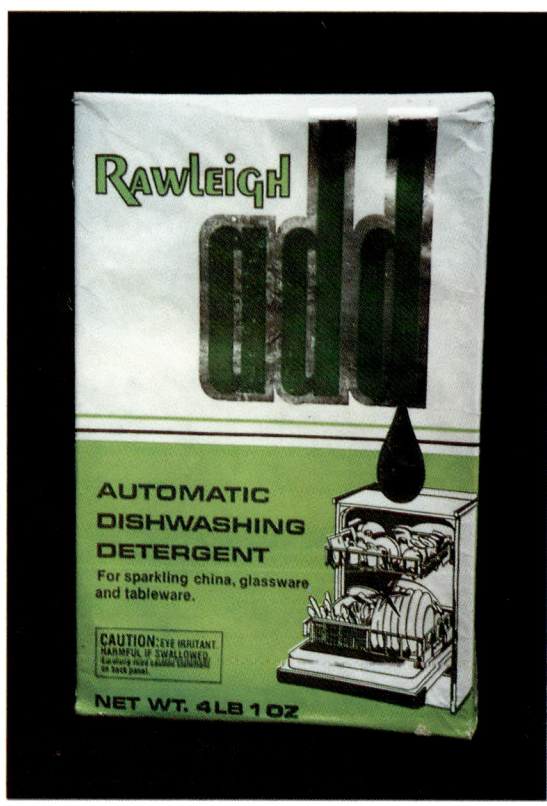

A 4 pound, 1 ounce box of Rawleigh add (Automatic Dishwashing Detergent) for china, glassware, and tableware. $10-$15.

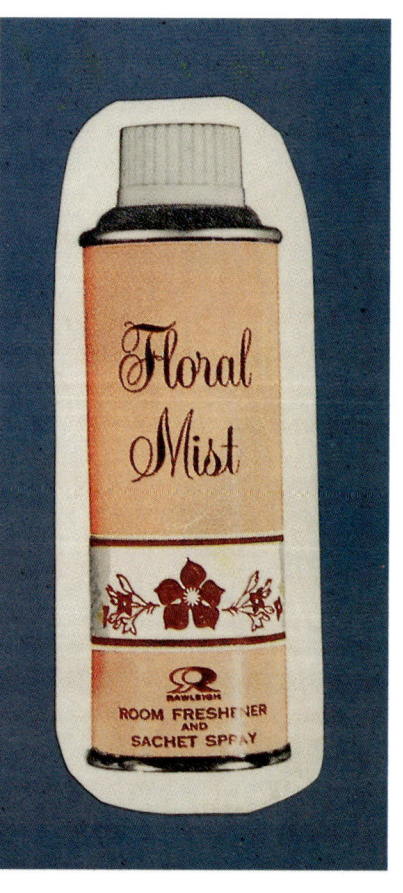

During the 1960s, Rawleigh's Floral Mist Room Freshener and Sachet Spray was a NEW sachet spray and room freshener. The 8 ounce container was a blend of flowers and spices. $10-$15 ea.

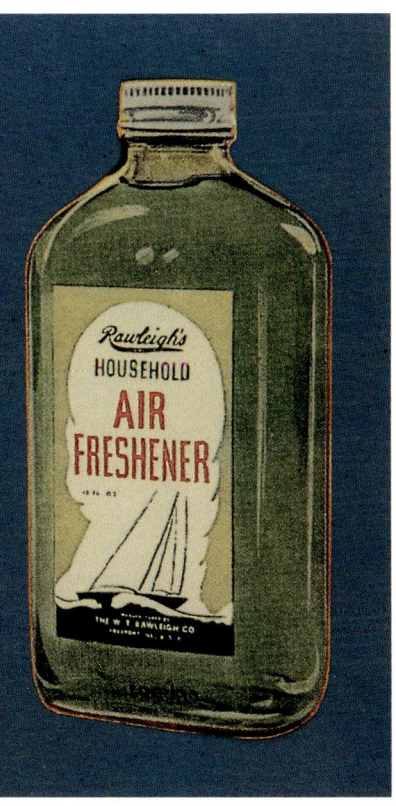

Promoted in 1958 as "Easy Ways To Keep a Home Fresh." Touch a button on Rawleigh's Aerosol Air Freshener and unpleasant odors were replaced with the fresh fragrance of clover fields, also available in a wick type. Just raise the wick to banish the smell. Rawleigh's Perfumed Deodorant Blocks kept the bathroom and closets fresh. There were five fragrance blocks, Mint in green (shown), Lilac in blue, Rose in red, Pine in clear and New-Mown Hay in amber. Rawleigh's Pine Oil Disinfectant was a safe disinfectant that smelled good and wouldn't harm the skin. $10-$15 ea.

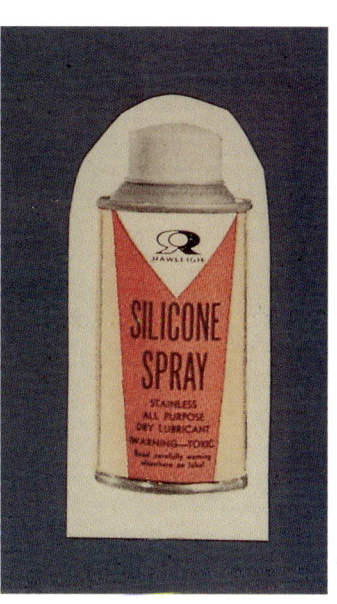

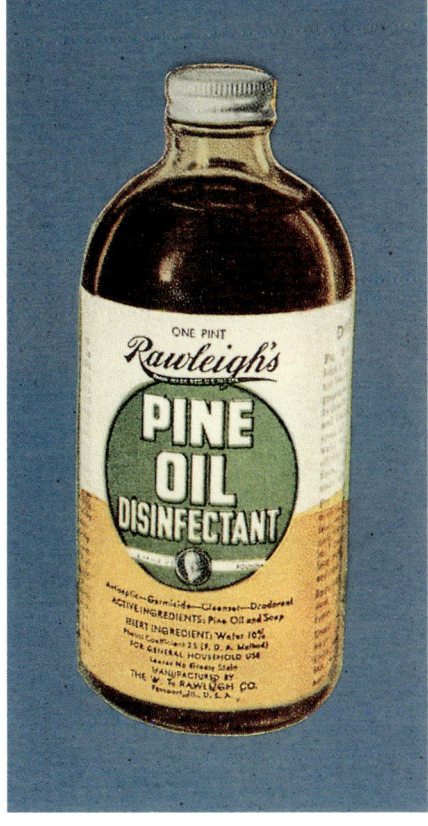

Rawleigh's NEW 7 ounce Silicone Spray (without oil or grease). This NEW Spray lubricated hinges, locks, springs, zippers, garden tools and skates in the 1960s. $10-$15.

Rawleigh's Pine Oil Disinfectant was manufactured by The W.T. Rawleigh Co., Freeport, Ill., U.S.A. Circa 1954. $20-$30.

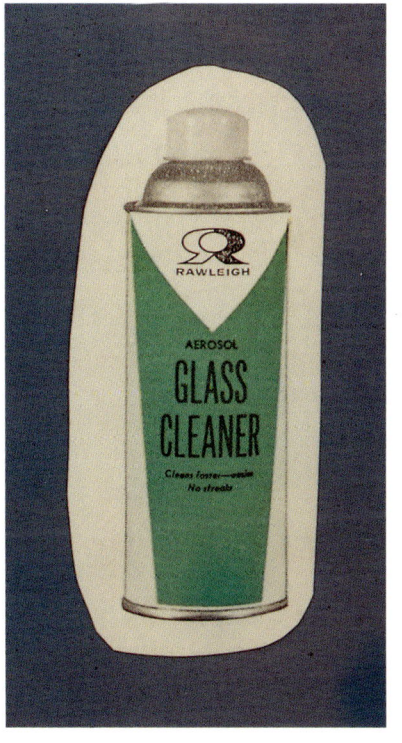

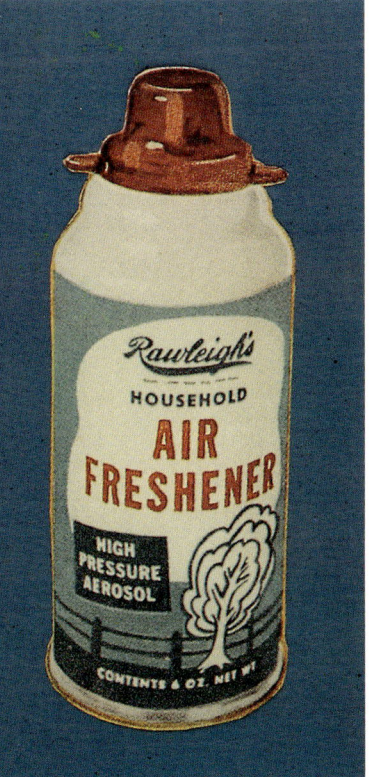

Rawleigh's 6 ounce Household High Pressure Aerosol Air Freshener. Circa 1954. $20-$30.

Rawleigh's 16 ounce Aerosol Glass Cleaner. Circa 1960s. $10-$15.

Rawleigh's Aerosol 12 ounce Oriental Spice Air Freshener, Rawleigh's Aerosol 12 ounce Clover Blossom Air Freshener, 10 ounce Bottle with wick, and Rawleigh's Floral Air Freshener in a 5-1/2 ounce apothecary jar. Rawleigh's 10 ounce refill Floral Freshener for use in jar or with wick. Circa 1960s. $10-$15 ea.

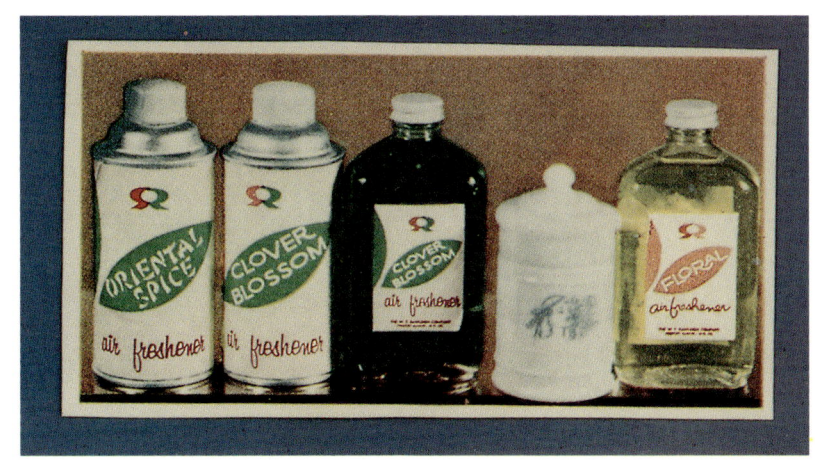

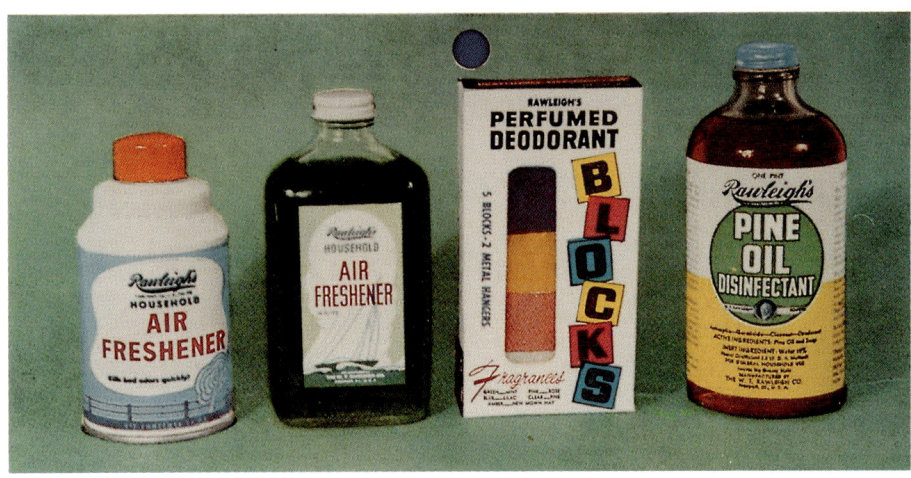

Four easy ways to keep a home fresh. Rawleigh's Aerosol Air Freshener also came in a wick type; raise the wick to banish the smell. Rawleigh's Perfumed Block Deodorant and Rawleigh's Pine Oil Disinfectant. Circa 1958. $10-$15 ea.

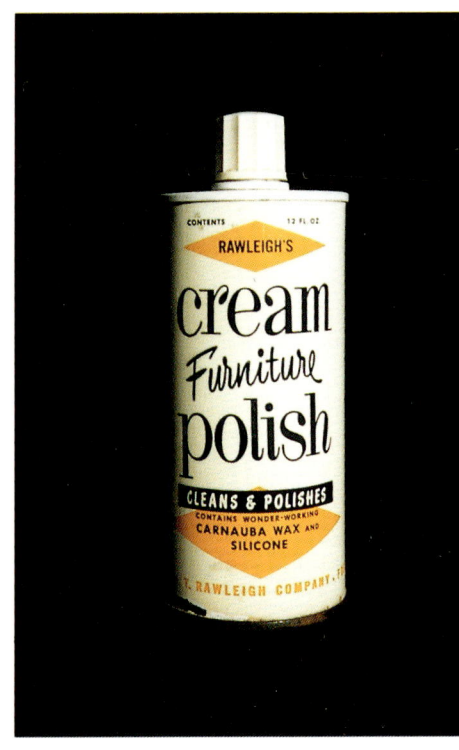

Rawleigh's Cream Furniture Polish "Cleans & Polishes." Manufactured By The W.T. Rawleigh Company, Freeport, Illinois, U.S.A. Circa 1960s. *Dupler Collection.* $15-$20.

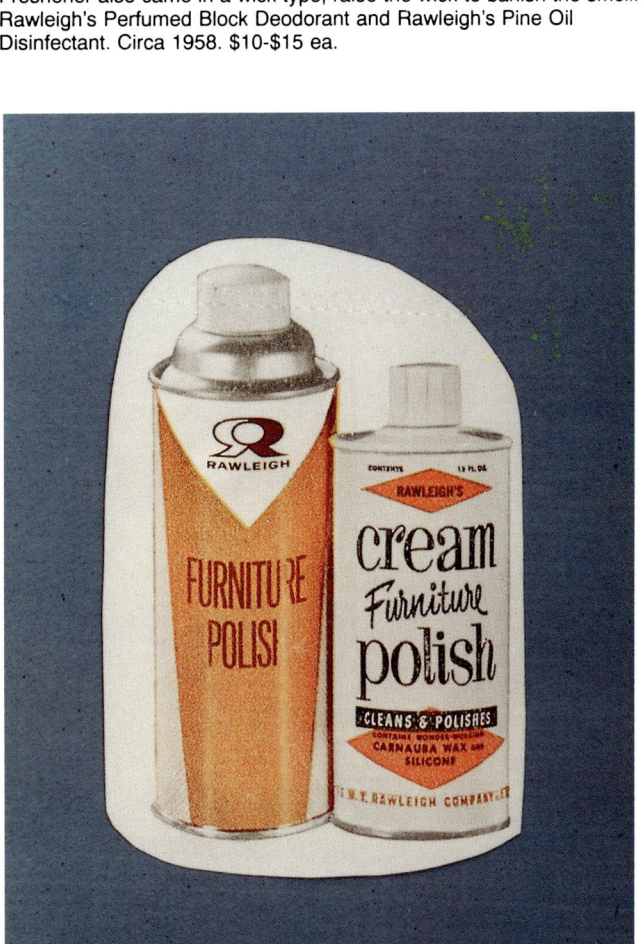

Rawleigh's 14 ounce Aerosol Furniture Polish and Rawleigh's 12 ounce Cream Furniture Polish. Circa 1960s. $10-$15 ea.

Rawleigh's Floor Shine. Available in either one qt. or two qt. containers. Floor Shine made an invisible shield that would not scuff. Rawleigh's Self-polishing Floor Wax dried to a hard wax finish. Available in 1/2 gal. or one qt. containers. Circa 1960s. $15-$20.

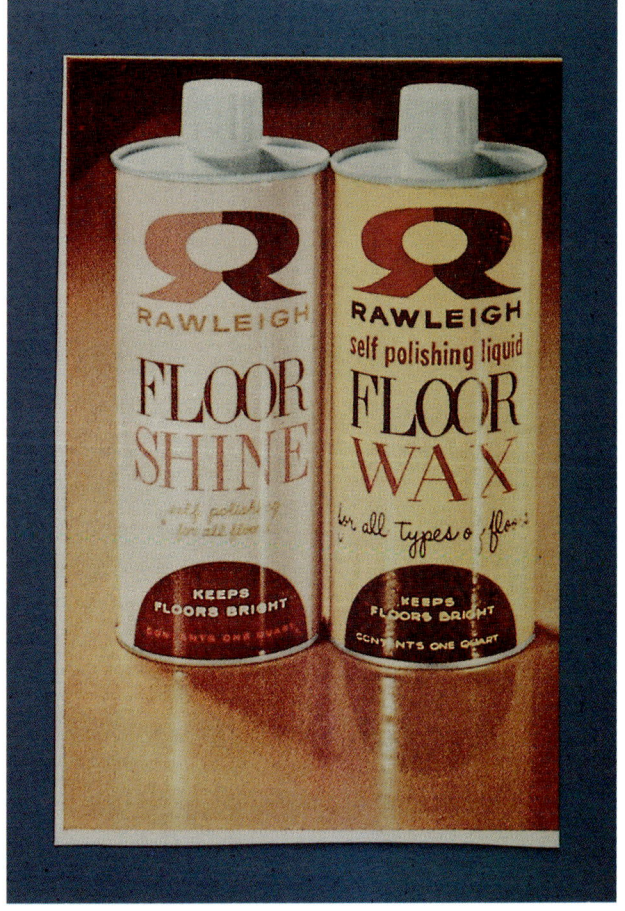

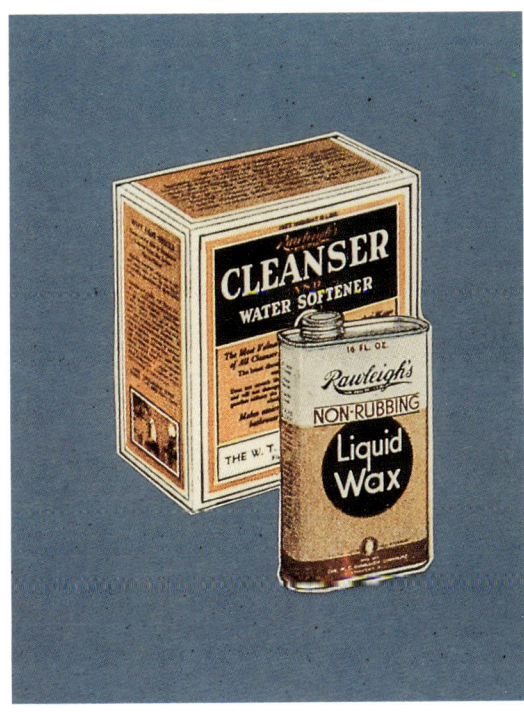

An original 1946 Rawleigh advertisement for Rawleigh's Cleanser and Water Softener and Rawleigh's Non-Rubbing Liquid Wax. $20-$25 ea.

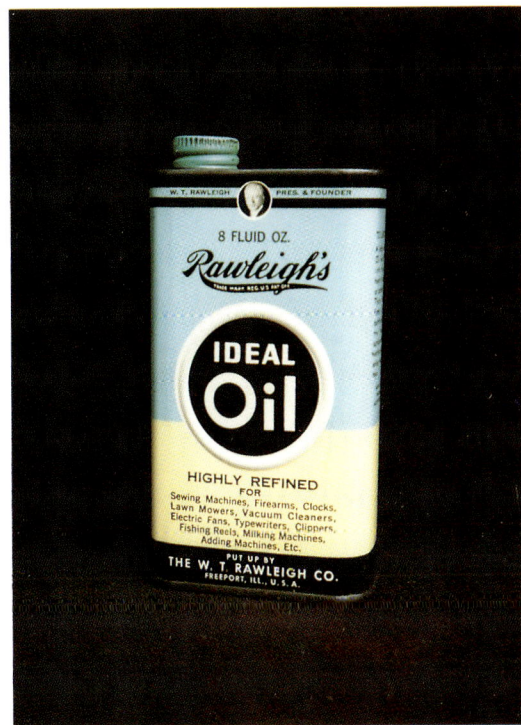

Rawleigh's 8 ounce Ideal Oil. Highly refined for sewing machines, firearms, clocks, lawn mowers, vacuum cleaners, fans, typewriters, clippers, fishing reels, milking machines, and adding machines. Put Up By The W.T. Rawleigh Co., Freeport, Ill., U.S.A. $50-$75.

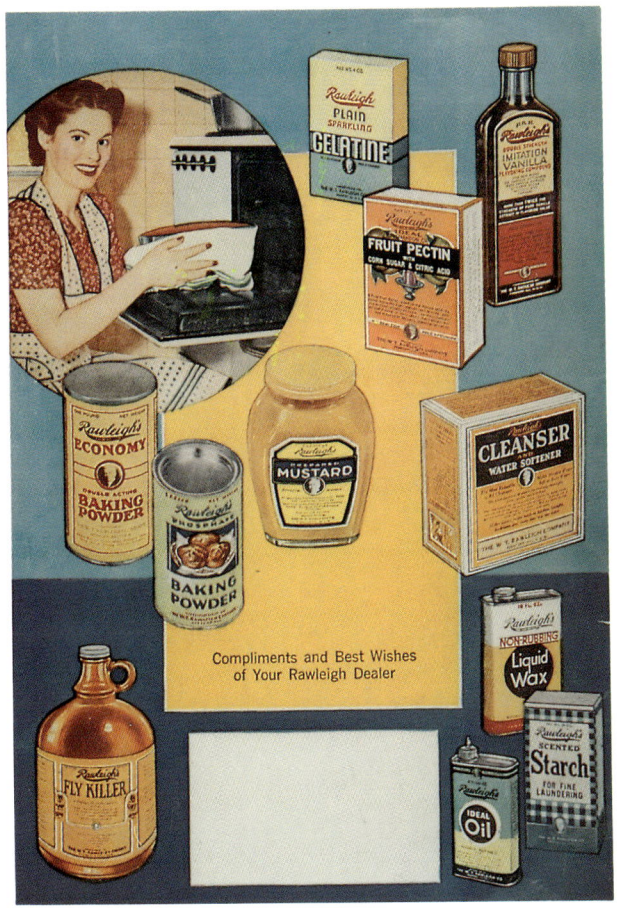

An original 1944 Rawleigh advertisement. Many of these products appear throughout this publication. It is wise to use original advertisements as references. Remember Rawleigh products very seldom changed in packaging and the product always remained the same.

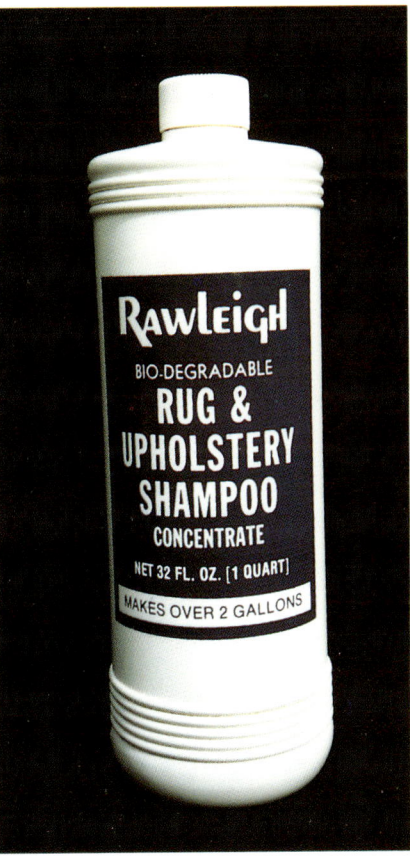

Rawleigh Bio-Degradable Rug & Upholstery Shampoo made over 2 gallons. Manufactured by The W.T. Rawleigh Company Freeport, Illinois 61032. $10-$15.

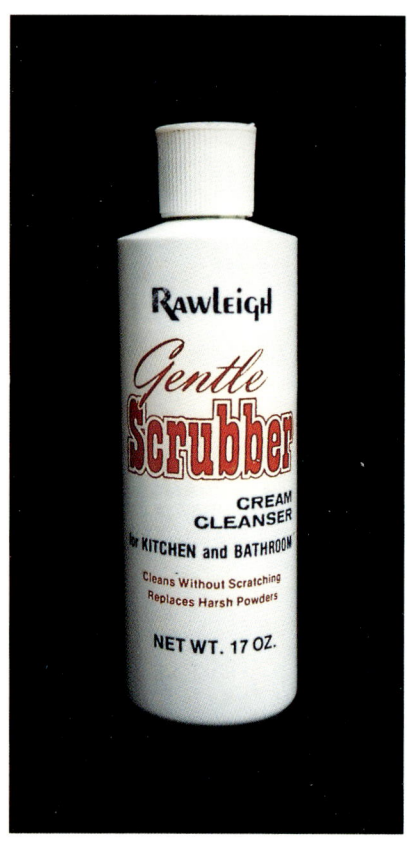

Rawleigh Gentle Scrubber Cream Cleanser for Kitchen and Bathroom. This was a new cream cleanser that scrubs away dirt and grime without scratching. Manufactured by The W.T. Rawleigh Company Freeport, Illinois 61032. $10-$15.

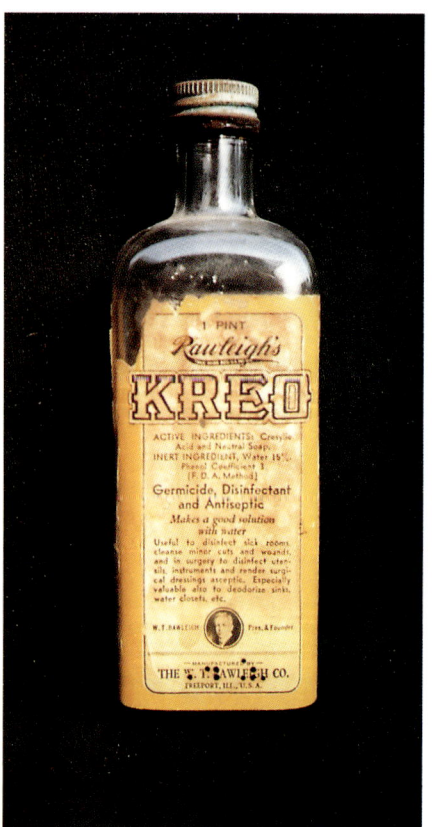

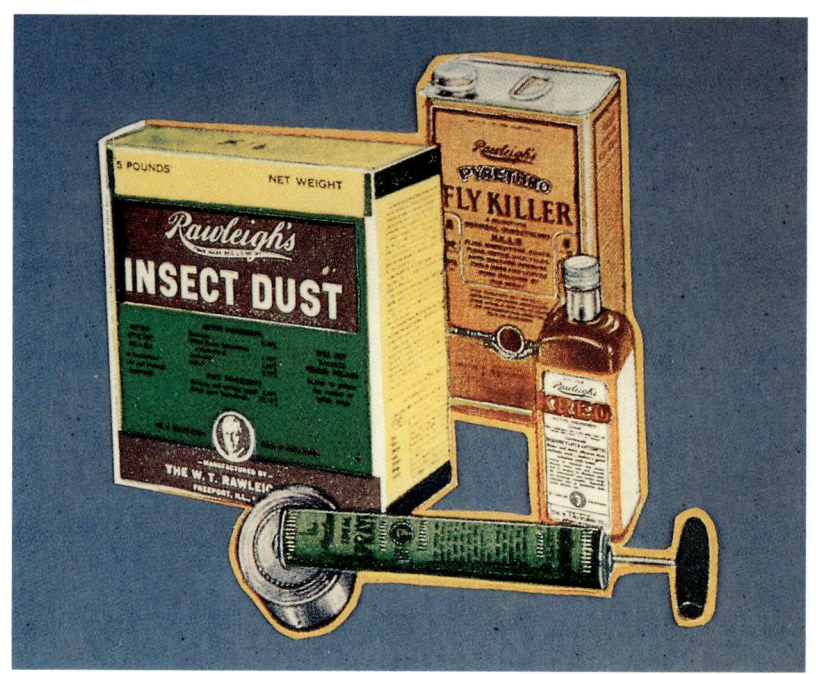

An original 1942 Rawleigh advertisement promoting insect dust, flyer killer, sprayer, and KREO.

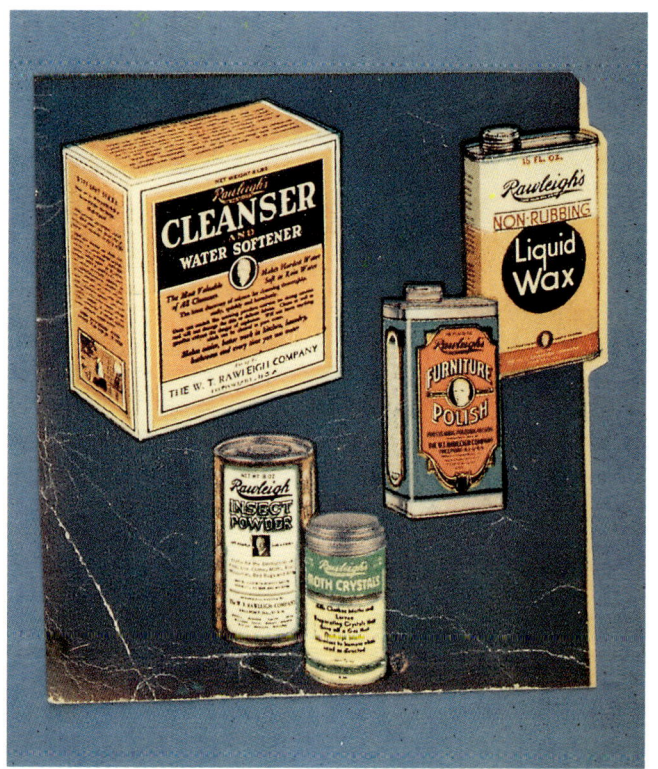

An original 1941 Rawleigh advertisement promoting moth crystals, furniture polish, liquid wax, water softener, and insect powder.

Rawleigh's KREO. Germicide, Disinfectant, and Antiseptic. Useful to disinfect sick rooms, cleanse minor cuts and wounds, and in surgery to disinfect utensils, instruments, and render surgical dressing antiseptic. Especially valuable to deodorize sinks and water closets. Manufactured by The W.T. Rawleigh Company Freeport, Illinois. $40-$50.

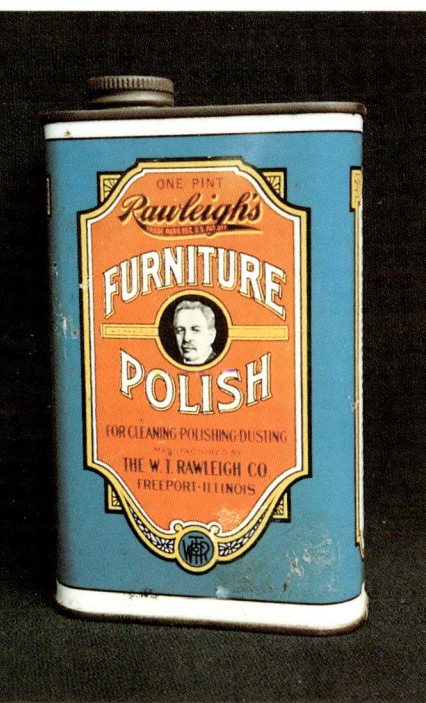

Rawleigh's Furniture Polish. Manufactured by The W.T. Rawleigh Company Freeport, Illinois. $10-$15.

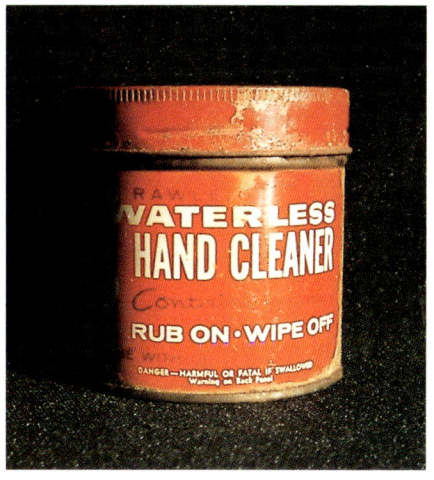

Rawleigh Waterless Hand Cleaner. *Dupler Collection.* $10-$15.

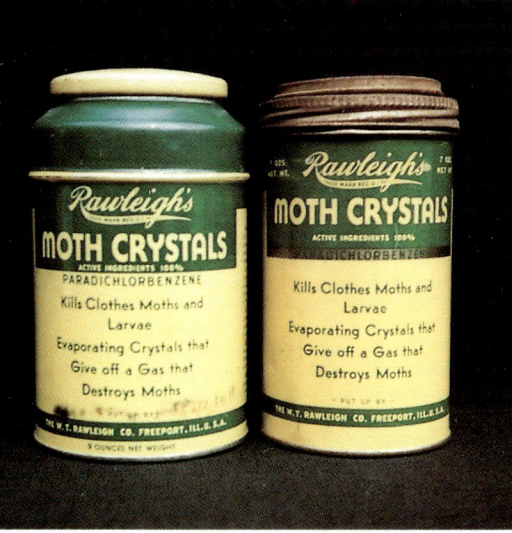

Two variations of Rawleigh's Moth Crystals. "Put Up By The W.T. Rawleigh Company Freeport, Ill., U.S.A." $25-$30 ea.

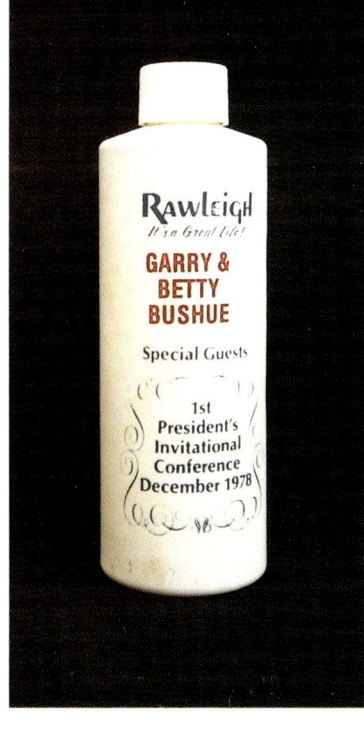

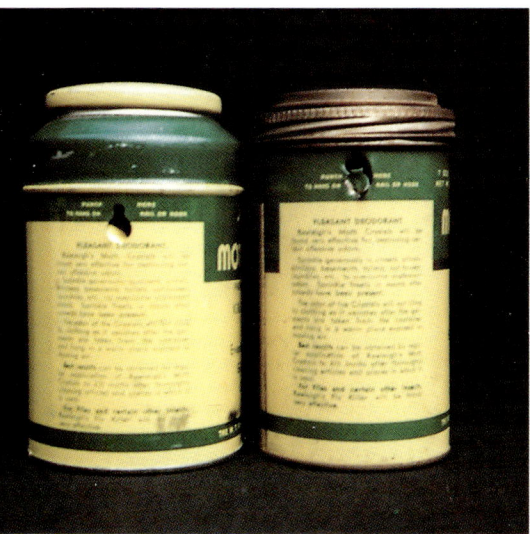

Rawleigh Cream Hair Rinse. *Dupler Collection.* $10-$15.

A give-away at the "1st President's Invitational Conference December 1978. Rawleigh It's a Great Life! Garry & Betty Bushue Special Guests." *Bushue Collection.* $75-$100.

The reverse side of Rawleigh's Moth Crystals. On this section a hole was provide for customers to "Punch Here To Hang on Nail Or Hook." Rawleigh's Moth Crystals were found to be very effective for destroying certain offensive odors and killing clothes moths and larvae. $25-$30 ea.

Chapter 7. Rawleigh Brushes, Mops, Dusters, and Toothbrushes

The Rawleigh Brush Factories were equipped with modern machinery that produced brushes, mops, and dusters rapidly, accurately, and uniform in size, shape, and design at the lowest production costs which gave the customer better and more attractive brushes for less money.

Rawleigh claimed, "With the careful selection of materials, manufactured on the best of equipment, and inspected by experienced operators, there was no question that Rawleigh brushes, mops and dusters were of the highest quality and better values at lower prices than could be obtained elsewhere."

Upon request from customers, the Rawleigh Dealer would show and explain their unusual values, usefulness and lower prices.

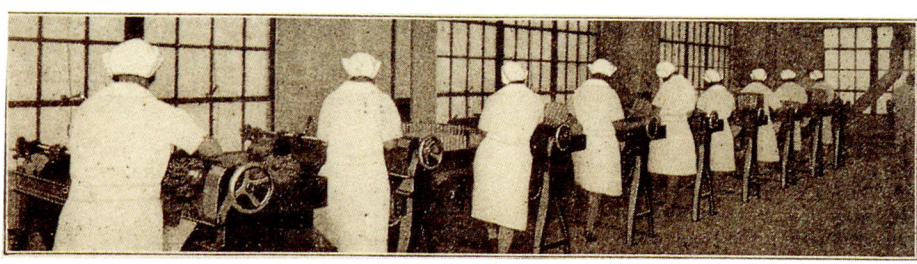

"In 1932, Rawleigh understood that the brush twisting machinery was formerly crude in construction, difficult and tiresome to operate which resulted in slow production." Improvements were developed slowly and it was not until Rawleigh Industries decided to manufacture brushes, mops, and dusters that the machines featured in this photo were developed and built according to Rawleigh's specifications and under their supervision. The Rawleigh Modern Brush Factory was the first to be equipped with these new special improved brush twisting machines.

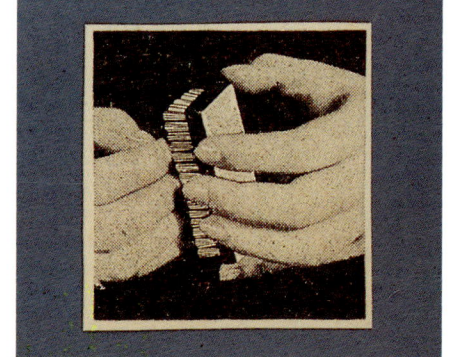

Rawleigh's Nail Brush was available in six assorted colors, had pearl on amber handles, and was made of the best imported Chinese bristles of the right stiffness to thoroughly clean the hands and nails without injury to the skin. $50-$75.

Customers were delighted with the ease with which they could keep their home clean and tidy, having extra hours for social activities by using Rawleigh brushes, mops, and dusters in their home. Only the best materials — Chinese bristle, Siberian and Australian hair, Mexican and India fibers, and Delta yarn were used in the production of Rawleigh's brushes, mops and dusters. Each was made of the best material obtained for the purposes of which the brush was recommended.

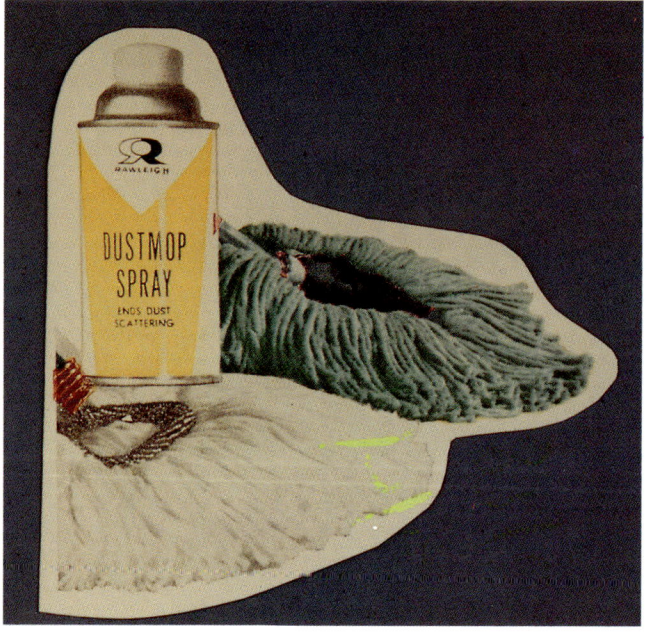

An original advertisement promoting Rawleigh's 12 ounce Dust Mop Spray, a Turquoise Dustmaster Mop, and a White Nylon Wet Mop. Circa 1960s. $15-$25 ea.

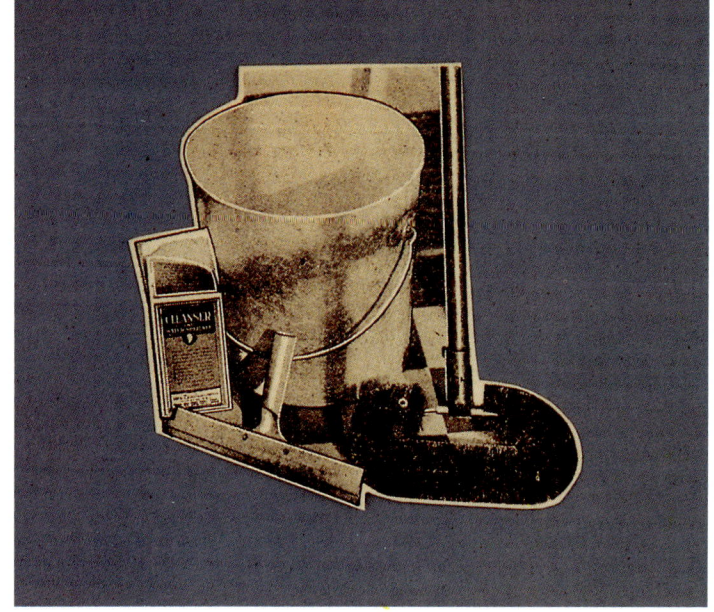

An original 1932 advertisement for Rawleigh Brushes, Mops, Dusters, and Cleanser. $6-$8 advertisement; $10-$15 brushes, mops, & dusters; $20-$25 cleanser.

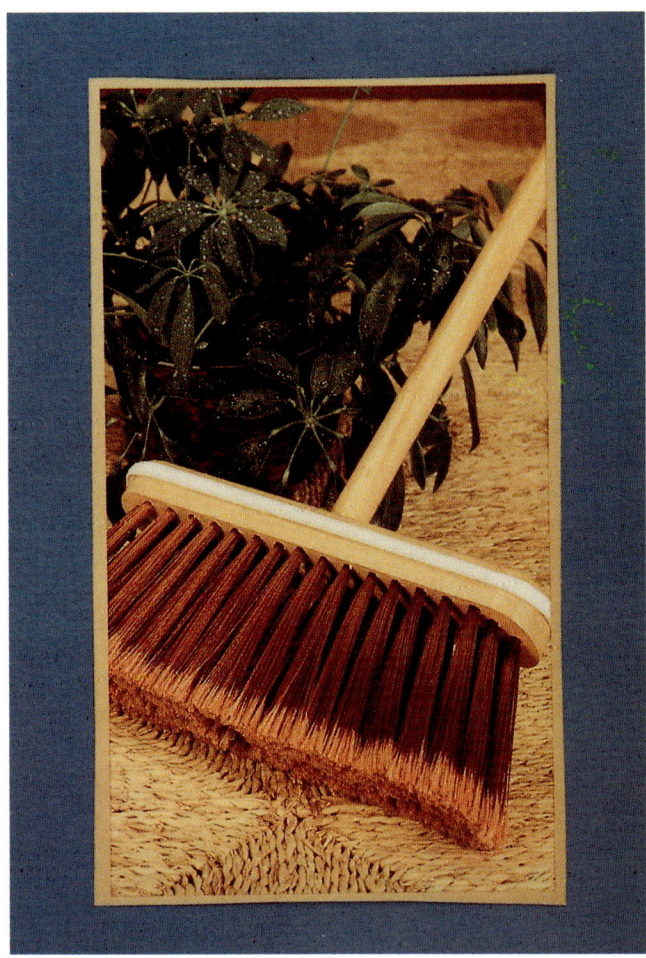

An original advertisement for the Rawleigh Magnetic Broom that appeared in Rawleigh's 1986 Family Shopping Guide. The Magnetic Broom attracted dust like a magnet, while the rubber bumper protected walls and furniture from scratches. Listed as Item #28130 and sold for $8.85. $10-$15.

Rawleigh's new line of toothbrushes included four different models: 1) Rawleigh Special (Adult), 2) Rawleigh Special (Child's), 3) Rawleigh Ideal and, 4) Rawleigh Good Health. These artistic brushes were made of beautiful transparent, translucent, and pearl on amber handles in six colors — rose, orange, light and dark green, lemon, and purple.

For years toothbrushes were handmade, a slow and expensive procedure. Rawleigh's toothbrushes were made on a rapid, automatic machine which drilled the holes, filled them with the correct number of bristles, and then fastened them securely in the handles at the rate of four brushes or 148 tufts per minute. This reduced production costs and created a better brush for less money.

Rawleigh's toothbrushes were made of imported white sterilized bristle which were carefully selected and were of the right stiffness and elasticity to properly clean the teeth. The handles were made of celluloid. Company literature explained, "Celluloid is a colloid of complex chemical composition — the greater portion of which is soluble nitro-cellulose and camphor to which pigment colors were added as desired. These handles were the best quality, most attractive colors, and best values obtainable."

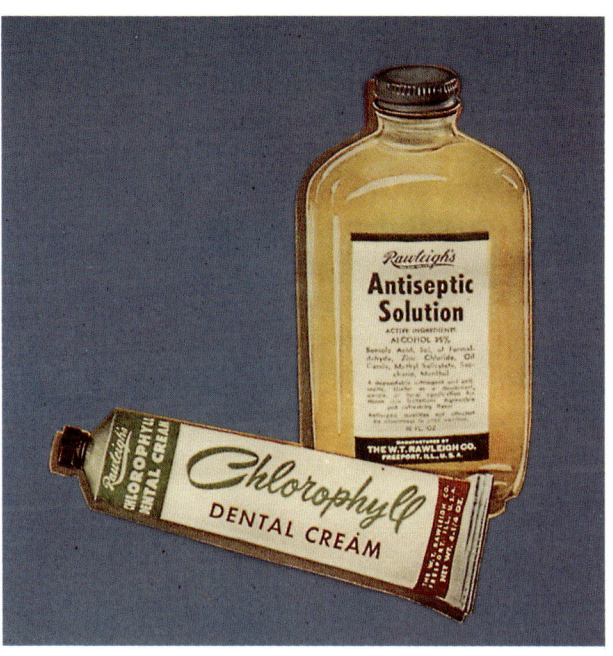

Rawleigh's "ANTISEPTIC SOLUTION" was a dependable antiseptic with an agreeable refreshing flavor. Rawleigh's "CHLOROPHYLL DENTAL CREAM" was especially popular with children and adults. Circa 1954. Antiseptic and dental cream are shown elsewhere in this publication. $25-$35.

In 1932, a new line of Rawleigh toothbrushes was being manufactured in the Freeport factories on modern automatic machines at the rate of several thousand a day. These brushes were the latest ideas and newest designs in toothbrushes. $25-$35 ea.

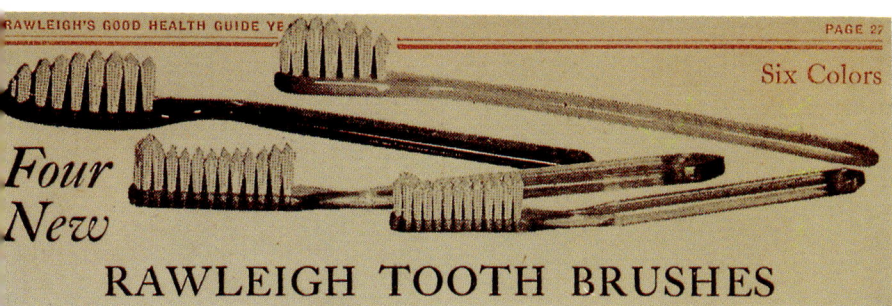

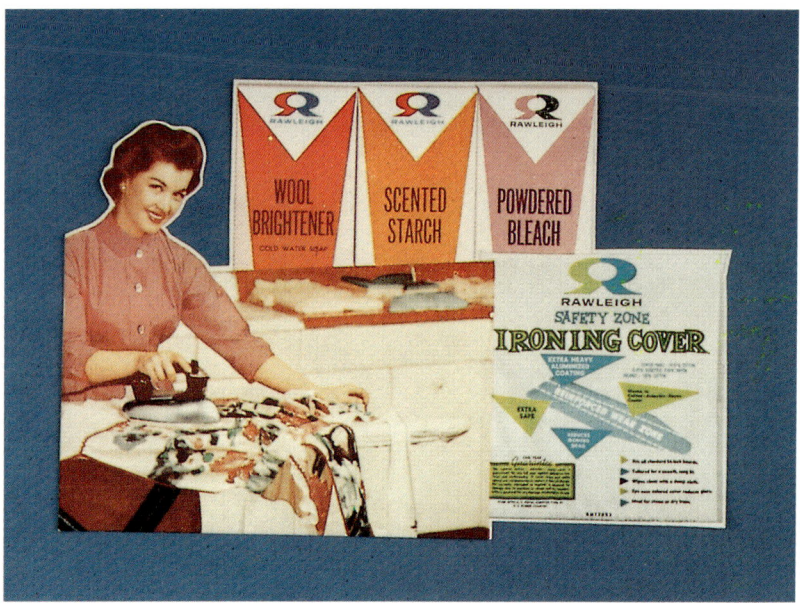

Rawleigh Safety Zone Ironing Cover was promoted with Rawleigh Wool Brightener, Scented Starch and Powdered Bleach. Circa 1960s. Rawleigh Scented Starch is also shown elsewhere in this publication. $75-$100 complete.

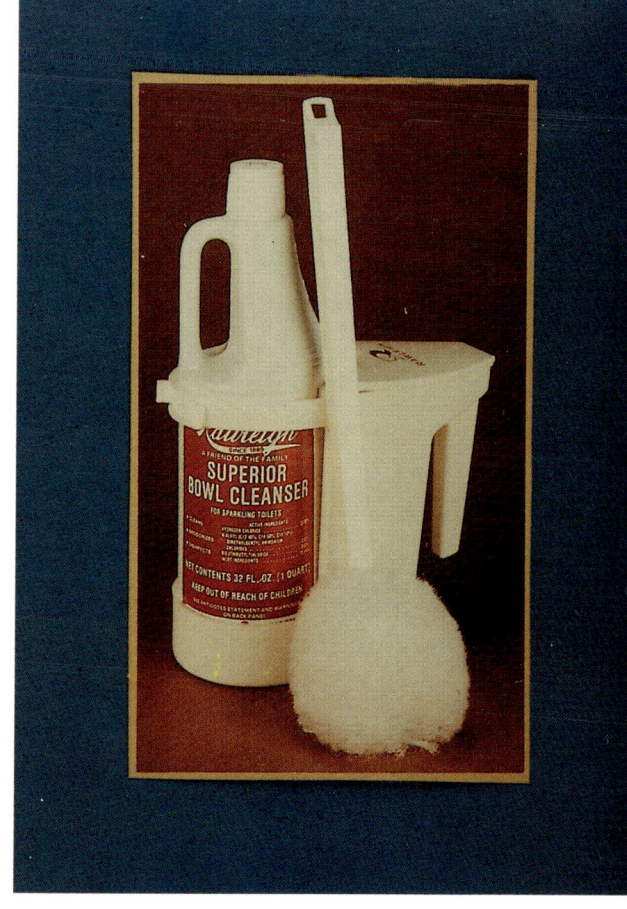

Rawleigh's Superior Bowl Cleaner, Caddie, and Applicator. These super products cleaned, deodorized, and disinfected, leaving toilets sparkling. Circa 1986. $10-$15 ea.

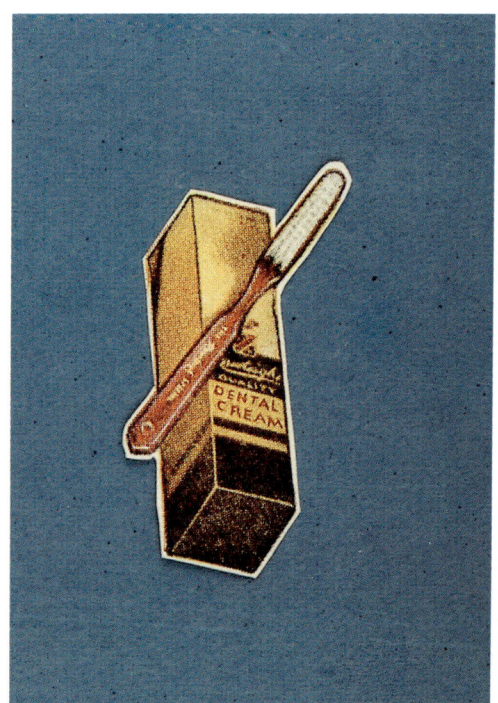

In 1942, Rawleigh promoted their toothbrushes, powder, dental creams, and mouth wash. Rawleigh toothbrushes were made of durable, natural, sterilized bristles anchored with nickeled silver wire which locked them securely into the socket, making for longer use.

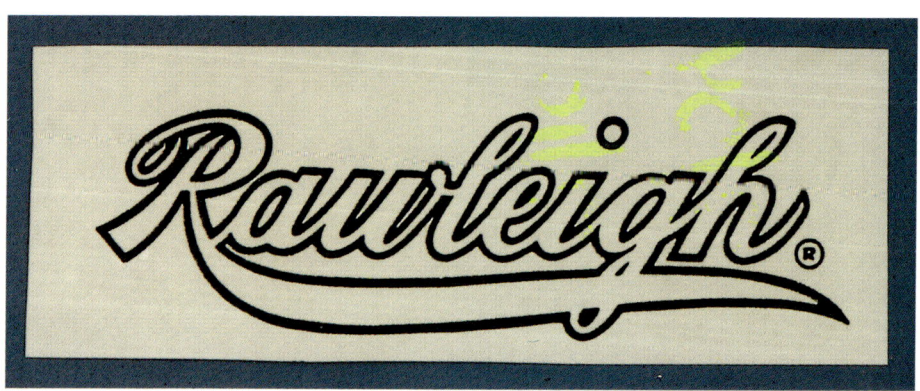

This trademark appeared on all genuine Rawleigh Quality Products.

Chapter 8. Rawleigh's Experimental Farm

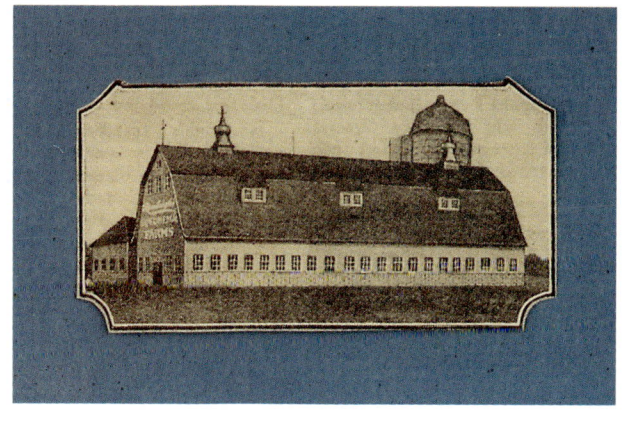

A dairy barn at Rawleigh's Experimental Farms, circa 1922.

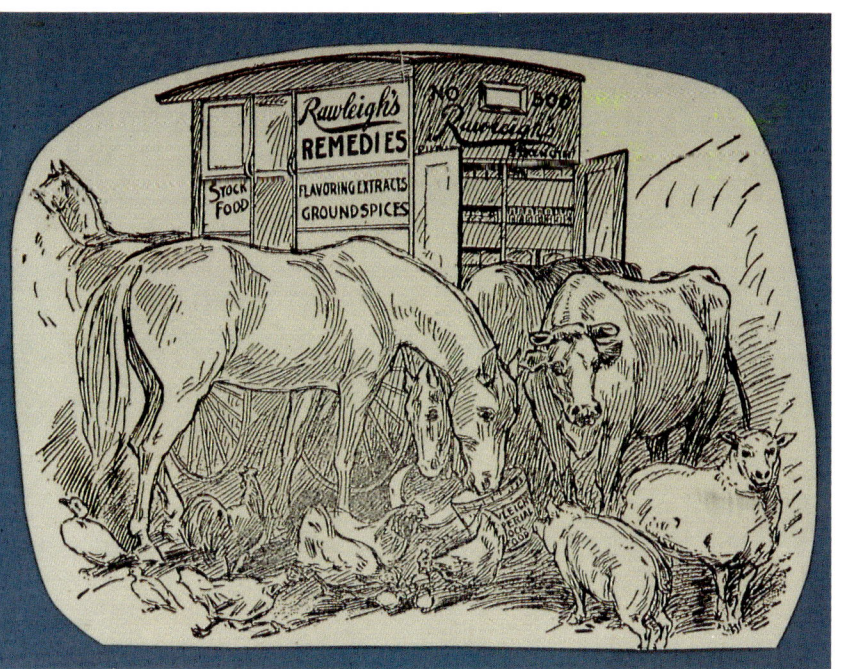

This illustration appeared in Rawleigh's 1905 Almanac Cook Book & Medical Guide. "THE MORE THEY EAT OF IT THE GREATER WILL BE YOUR PROFITS." Rawleigh was promoting "Rawleigh's Imperial Stock Food," a medicinal food containing highly concentrated food elements which improved digestion, created appetite, and caused proper assimilation. A GREAT STOCK TONIC.

A portion of Rawleigh's Experimental Farms, 1922.

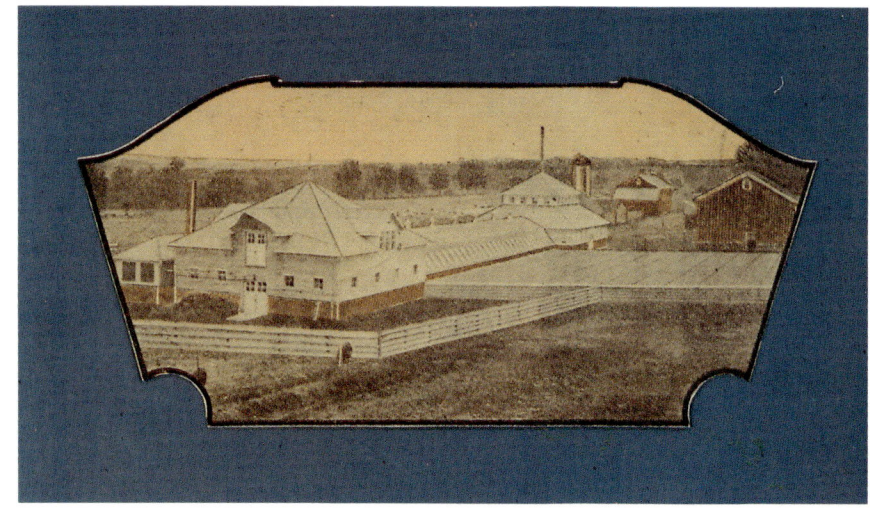

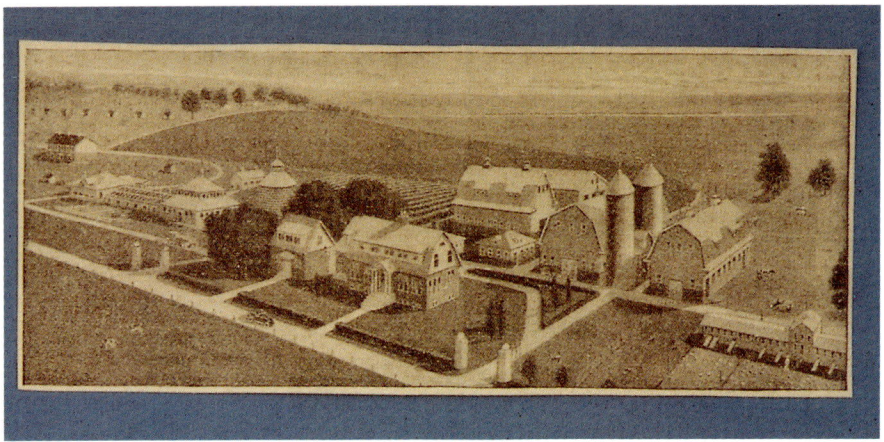

This illustration of Rawleigh's Ideal Farms appeared in 1927. Among the fundamental purposes of Ideal Farms was to improve the usefulness of Rawleigh's Veterinary Products and to develop ways of using them that provided the most valuable service. Another purpose was to develop (by constructive breeding, feeding, and care) the highest type of pure bred stock and to provide farmers and breeders the benefit of the methods followed and the information and experience gained.

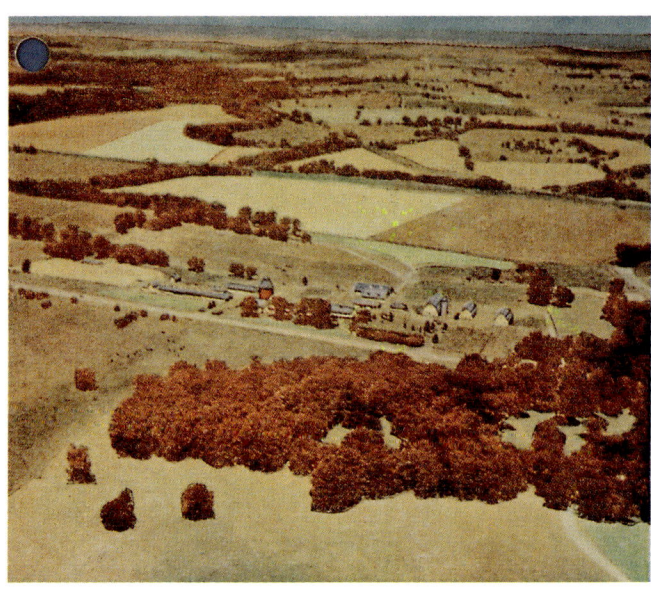

Autumn arrives at the Rawleigh Farms. In October 1951, this aerial view of Rawleigh Farms was taken. Only part of the nearly thousand acres can be seen. Fields and wooded pastures stretch almost to the horizon. The main farm buildings are in the immediate foreground and many other buildings are not in view. Rawleigh products were extensively used for the famous purebred cattle, hogs, and poultry at the farm.

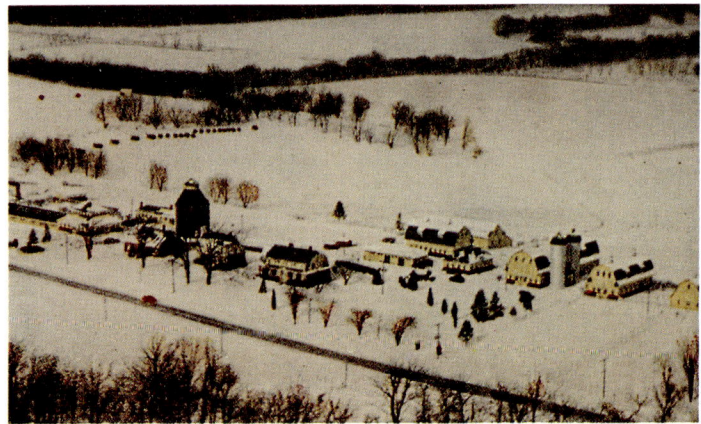

This winter aerial view of Rawleigh Farms was taken in 1950. To the extreme right is the bull barn; next on the left is the cow-testing barn. The main milking barn is next, featuring double silos. Other buildings include a garage and work shop, cattle barn, residences for the manager and herdsman, a dormitory for men, 12,000-bushel granary, a sausage factory, and a hog building. Additional housing facilities for several families, livestock barns, and other buildings were located on other parts of the 954-acre farm.

In the early 1920s, W.T. Rawleigh established a 240 acre experimental stock farm called Ideal Farms a mile west of Freeport, Illinois on the scenic Grant Highway. Additional land would be purchased over the next few years. By 1926-27, nearly 1000 acres of prime farmland had been acquired and incorporated into the farm.

The prime object of the farm was to increase the food supply by creating better herds and flocks. Through practical and scientific work in cooperation with the Rawleigh Laboratories, one of the fundamental purposes of Ideal Farms was to test and improve the veterinary products and to find improved ways of using them to give the most valuable service.

Ideal Farms also helped farmers to solve their problems and improve their stock by developing — through constructive breeding, feeding, and care — the highest type of purebred stock. The Ideal Farms staff gave farmers and breeders the benefit of the methods followed and the information and experience gained. They also made the best breeding stock available at reasonable prices for herd improvement.

In 1925, thirty-two head of pure bred Holstein cows at Rawleigh's Ideal Farms averaged 10-1/4 months in milk with 1,120 pounds of milk per month for each cow. Five averaged better than 19,000 pounds. Four produced over 30 pounds of butter in seven days and one produced 41.14 pounds. The herd held one world's record and eight state records.

In 1925, 150 farmers from Mississippi traveled by train to study the methods of livestock raising and to see first hand the modern agricultural procedures in use at the Rawleigh Ideal Farms.

W.T. Rawleigh himself developed an interested in the improvement of hogs through his connection with research into the stock medicines and feeds his company manufactured. His interest centered on Poland China hogs.

Rawleigh's Ideal Farms held the world's record ton liters of 15 and 16 pigs weighing 4511-1/2 and 4789 in 1925. In 1926 a liter of 17 that weighed 5117 when 180 days old established the leadership of Ideal Farms Poland Chinas. A representative from the Mexican government spent two days studying the farm's modern hog raising methods.

Ideal Farms' White Rocks chickens provide hatching eggs, thousands of broilers, and stock birds to improved farm poultry.

A sub-division now occupies most of the former Rawleigh Ideal Farms and land. All that is left of this once popular farm is a renovated horse barn, one of the former dairy barns, and an old stone quarry.

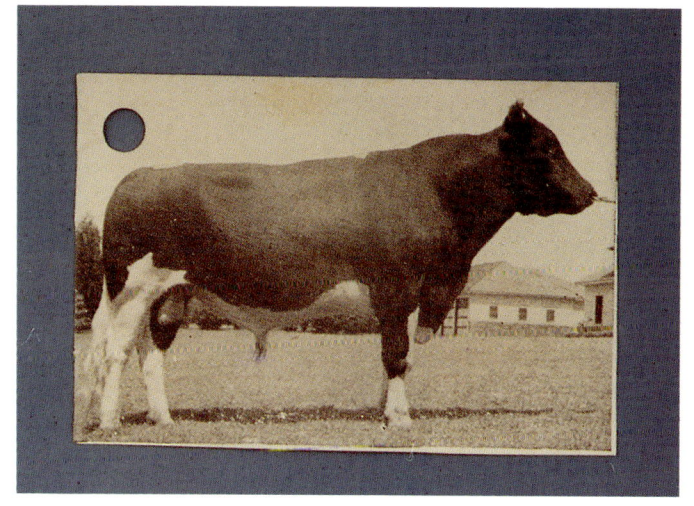

Sir Ormsby Fobes Dictator 39th, Senior Herd Sire at Rawleigh's Ideal Farms, Freeport, Illinois. Circa 1946.

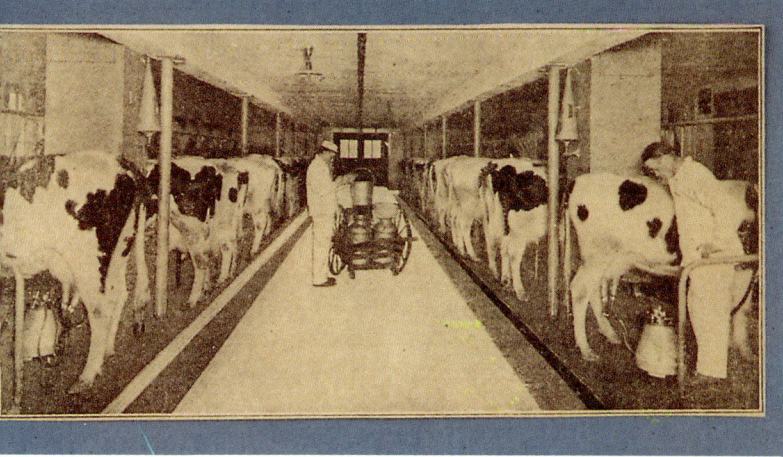

Milking time in the dairy barn of Rawleigh's Ideal Farms. Circa 1927.

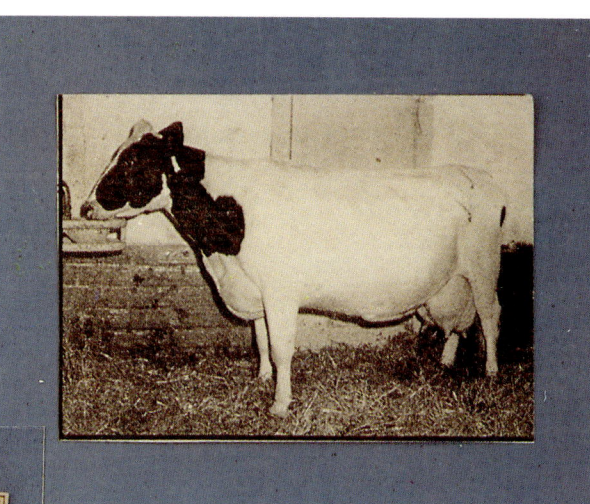

Della Buttercup pure-bred Holstein-Friesian owned by Rawleigh Farms. This cow was born and raised at Rawleigh Farms. Circa 1950.

Nearly five tons of geese were presented each Christmas to Rawleigh employees. Circa 1927.

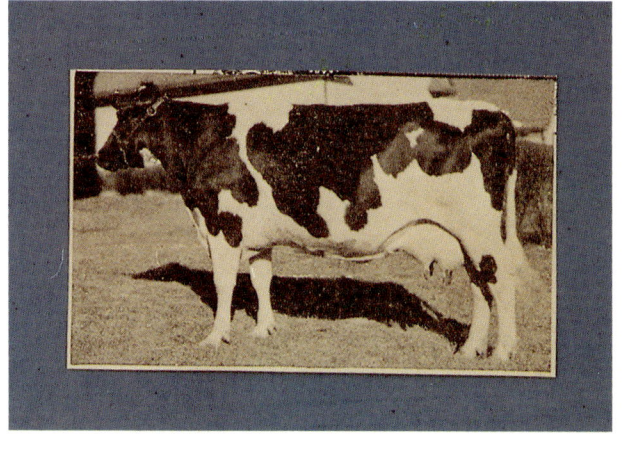

Rawleigh's prized cow Mapleon Colantha Segis Aaltje. Circa 1939.

Originators of the All-Medicine Mixtures

In 1908, the Rawleigh Company, through its staff of chemists, assisted by a veterinarian of professional standing and experience, originated Rawleigh's All-Medicine Mixtures. One mixture was for horses, cattle, and sheep while the other for hogs only.

Company literature claims that Rawleigh was first to recognize the inferiority of cheap stock tonics that contained little medicine and were mixed with fillers used as diluents that made up a large bulk of the ingredients. The W.T. Rawleigh Company created pure, full-strength compounds, mixtures of medicines adapted to the physiological requirements of the animal system, without diluents or fillers of any kind.

Rawleigh knew that while all stock tonics had some value, the reason most had failed to provided general satisfaction was because they did not contain sufficient medicines to produce the desired results. Rawleigh also knew farmers were buying these lesser products at medicine prices, largely for the medicines they were supposed to contain but did not. He recognized that the farmers wanted medicines and were willing to pay a fair price, provided they could get exactly what they wanted.

Rawleigh was the first to supply that need, and by 1916 Rawleigh's Medicinal Mixtures had gradually taken the place of the inferior stock tonics used and were endorsed by breeders of prize horses, dairy cattle, and swine all over the country.

Rawleigh's Medicinal Mixtures cost more, but they were cheaper and worth from two to five times as much as the average stock tonic regulator.

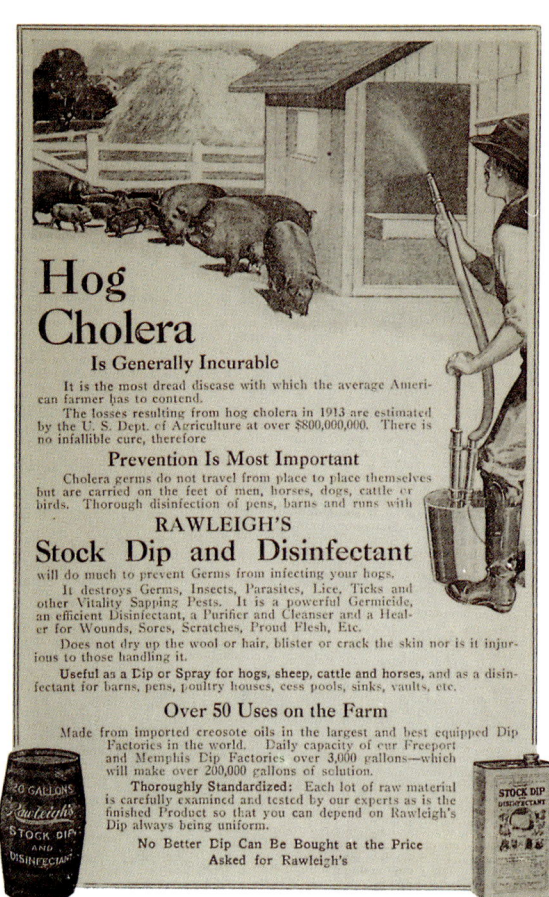

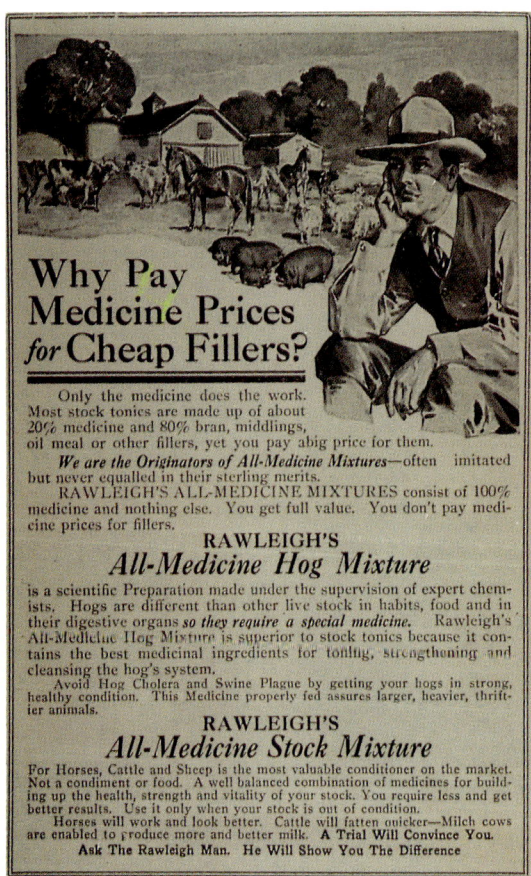

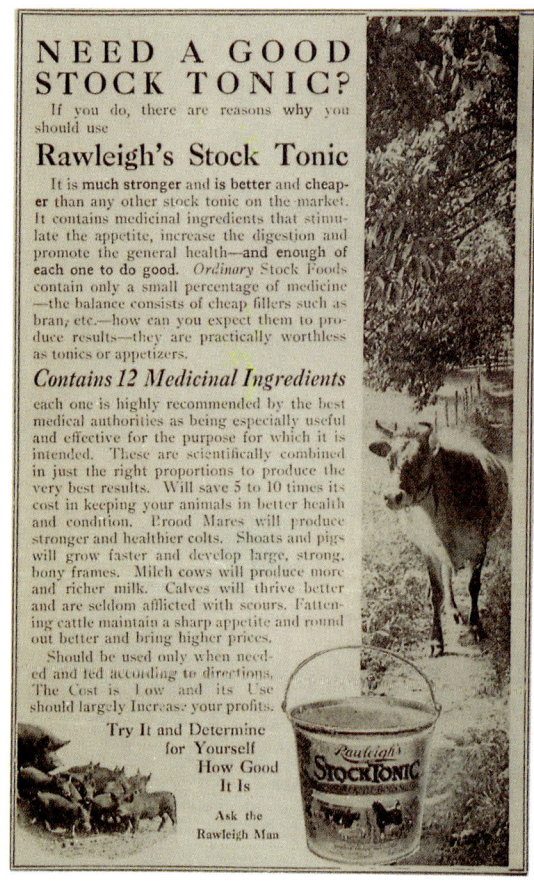

"Why Pay Medicine Prices for Cheap Fillers?" appeared in Rawleigh's 1915 Almanac.

These original advertisement's — "Hog Cholera" and "Need A Good Stock Tonic?" — appeared in Rawleigh's 1915 Almanac.

Livestock and Poultry Losses

During 1926-27, Rawleigh's supplied a line of medicines, applications, specific, disinfectants, insecticides, and veterinary products and poultry supplies that sold throughout the United States and Canada. The company pointed to increased sales and general use as proof that their service was valuable to owners of stock and poultry in preventing diseases and losses and in promoting profitable production.

Rawleigh's Veterinary Preparations included: Dip and Disinfectant, All-Medicine Hog Mixture, Iodized Stock Tonic, Fly Chaser, Colic and Bloat Compound, Fly Fluid and Sprayers, Veterinary Ointment, Application, Healing Powder, Healing Salve, Liniment, Camphor Balm, and Louse Killer.

Rawleigh's Poultry Supplies include: Poultry Powder, Louse Powder, Roup Powder, Poultry Worm Capsules, Cholera Tablets, and Louse & Roach Powder.

Care of Livestock the Rawleigh Way

As Rawleigh provided instruction for the general upkeep of human health, they also had suggestions for keeping livestock fit. Insufficient or improper foods, bad quarters, and neglect put animals in a bad rundown condition, causing weight loss, indigestion, serious ailments, and diseases.

By 1922, Rawleigh fully understood that in order to be profitable animals must be kept healthy, thrifty, and strong so that they could resist disease, do more work, produce more milk, and maximize profits to their owners. To avoid losses caused by disease, horses, cattle, sheep, and hogs needed proper feed. They also needed to be kept in clean sanitary quarters and exercised with an abundance of water, fresh air, and sunshine.

In 1898, The W.T. Rawleigh Company created their pure "All Medicine Mixtures." These pure medicinal preparations met with favor right from the beginning. Intelligent feeders quickly recognized their purity, strength, and real merits. Sales increased from year to year and the real value and superior merit of these pure preparations practically revolutionized the sale of stock preparations throughout the country.

Rawleigh made two different kinds of mixtures, both pure and made entirely of medicines; one made for horses, cattle and sheep whose anatomy and needs are similar. Another was made for hogs only, because hogs peculiar nature required an entirely different preparation. Both mixtures were the strongest, best, cheapest, and most efficient on the market and both were five times stronger than the average stock tonic sold.

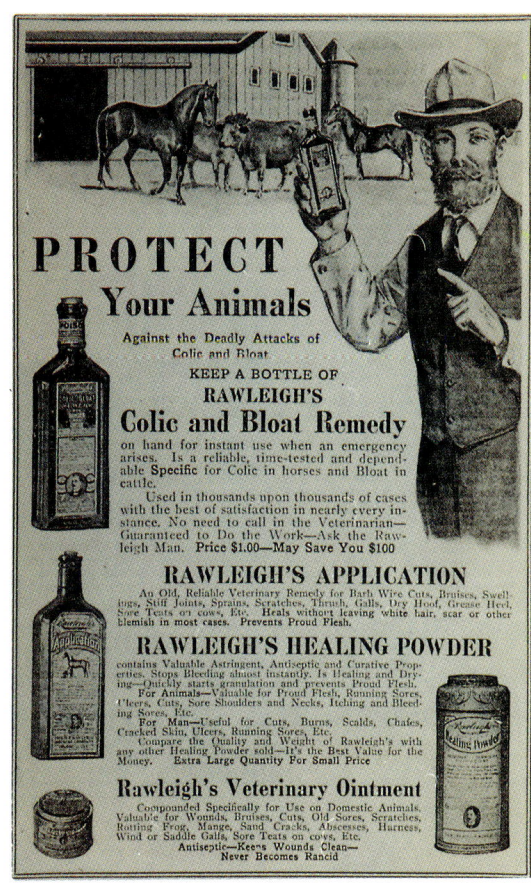

Rawleigh's Colic and Bloat Remedy, Rawleigh's Application, Healing Powder, and Rawleigh's Veterinary Ointment were promoted in "Protect Your Animals" 1915.

Rawleigh's Antiseptic Veterinary Ointment manufactured by The W.T. Rawleigh Company Freeport, Ill., U.S.A. This ointment appears in the original 1915 advertisement shown previously. $40-$50.

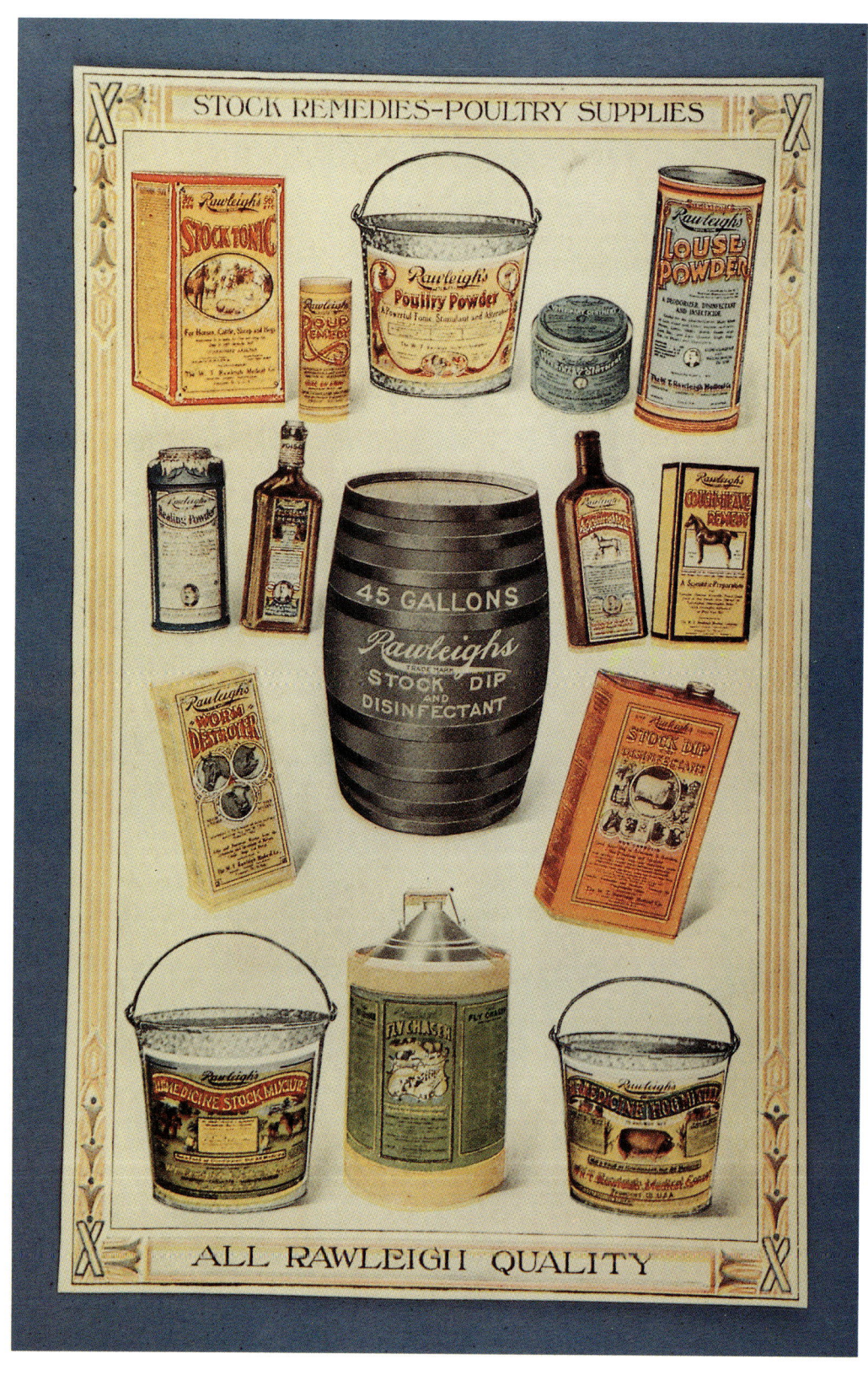

An original 1915 "Stock Remedies — Poultry Supplies" advertisement.

Farm and Gardening Products

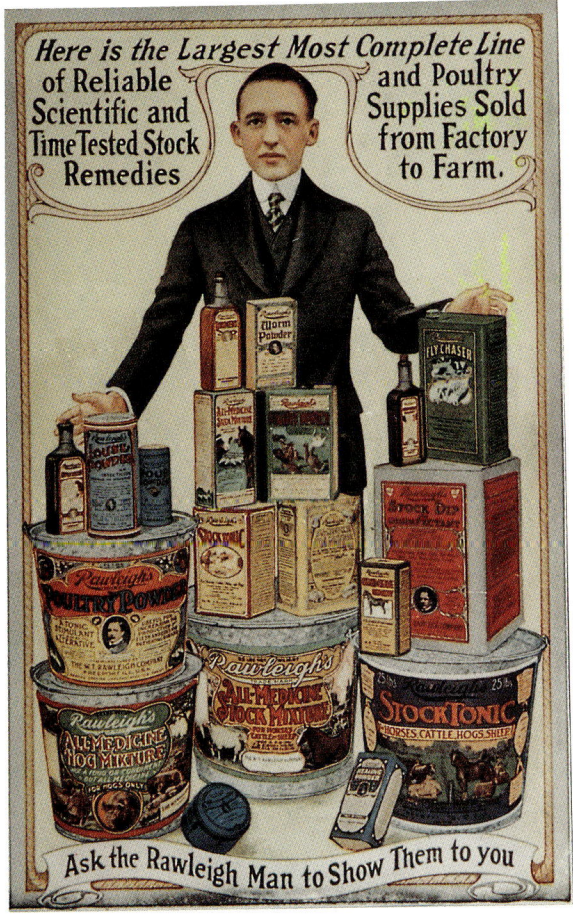

An original 1917 advertisement for Rawleigh's largest and most complete line of stock remedies and poultry supplies. These products will demand a higher price than later products.

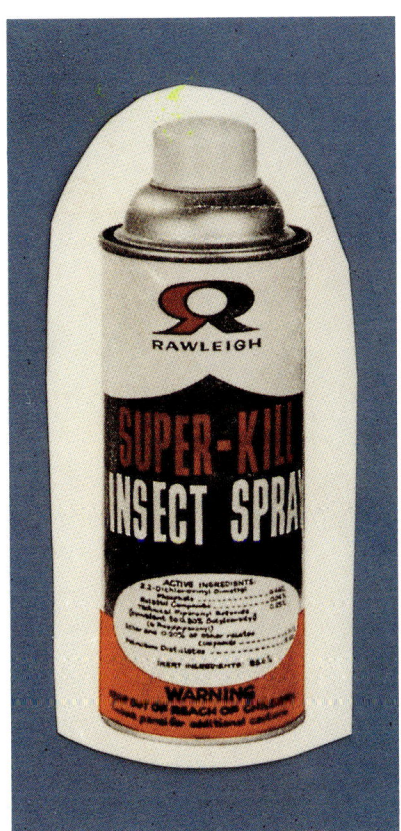

Rawleigh's 14 ounce "SUPER-KILL INSECT SPRAY." This aerosol product controlled 15 different insects in barns, homes, and outdoor areas. Contained Vapona and pyrethrins for fast knockdown and kill. Non-flammable. Pleasant odor. Circa 1960s. $10-$15.

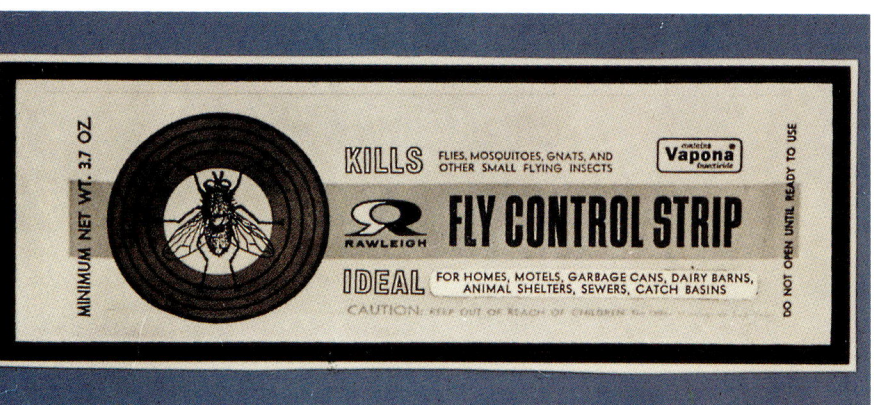

Rawleigh's 3.7 ounce "FLY CONTROL STRIP" hung on a nail. It volatilizes — no spraying necessary. Effective for three months when used according to directions. Circa 1960s. $15-$20.

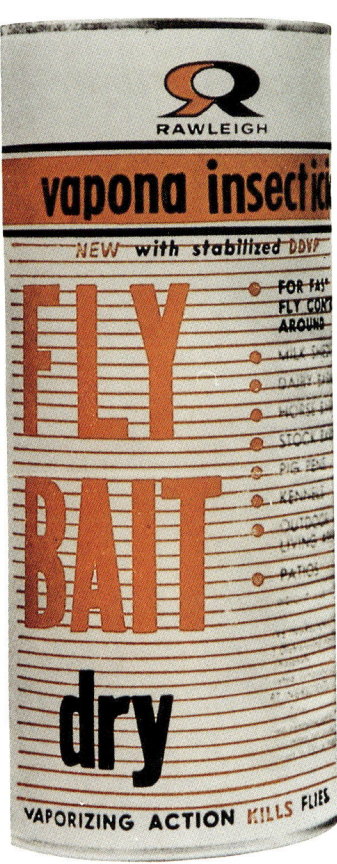

Rawleigh's 1 pound 10 ounce "FLY BAIT" killed flies in 2 ways: (1) by contact with the bait, (2) by volatilizing action. Circa 1960s. $10-$15.

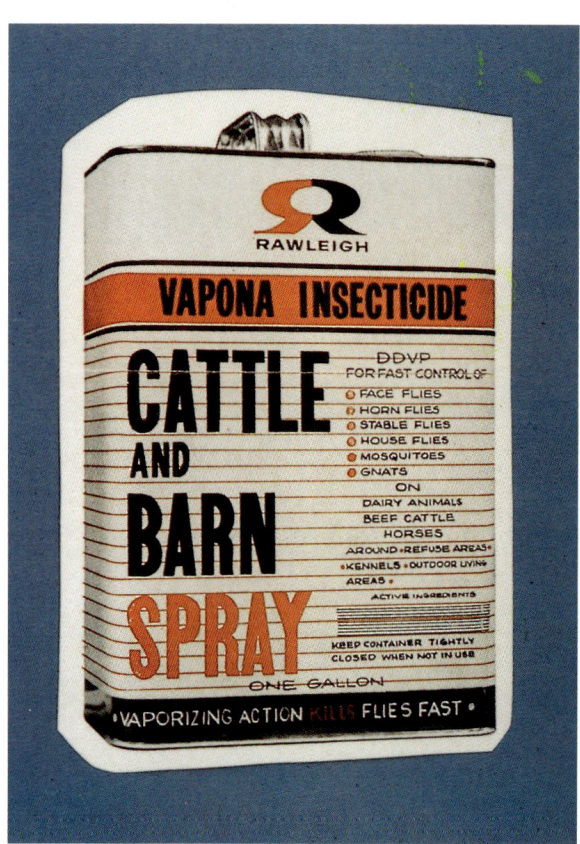

Rawleigh's "CATTLE AND BARN SPRAY" was available in 1, 5, 30, and 50 gallon containers. This spray was safe, powerful, effective, and odorless. It controlled roaches, ants, fleas, sow bugs, fly maggots, and brown dog ticks. Circa 1960s. $20-$25.

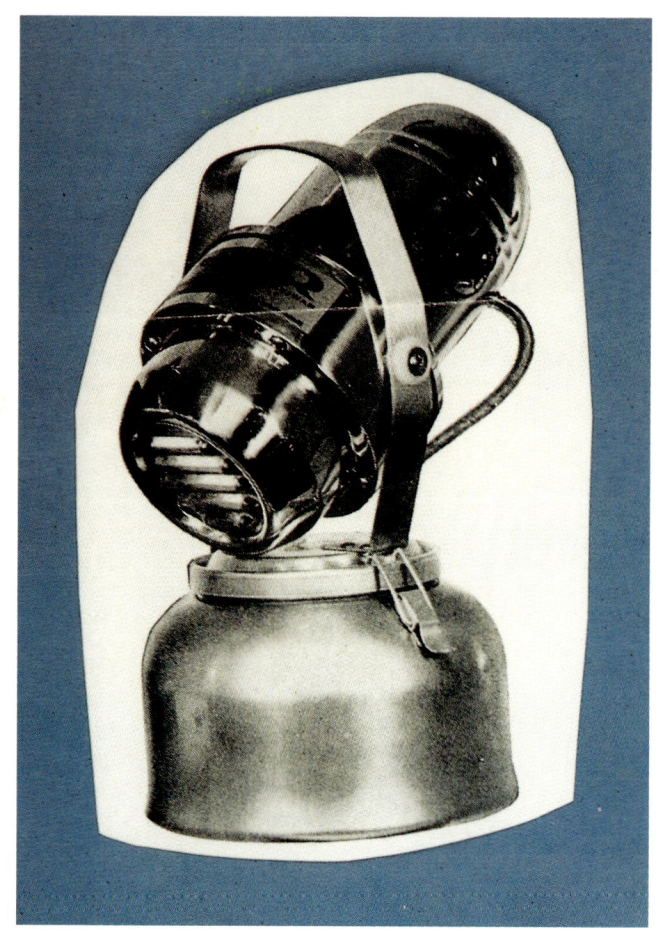

Rawleigh's "FOGMASTER SPRAYER" sprayed 1 to 5 gallons of insecticide an hour. Circa 1960s. $40-$50 complete.

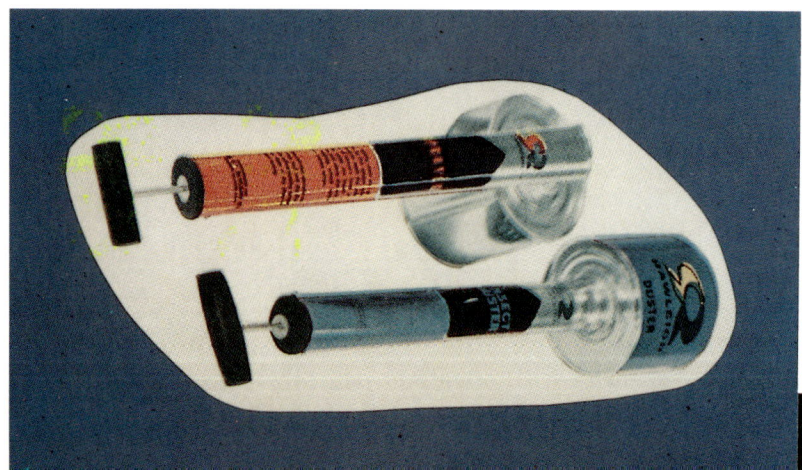

Rawleigh Sprayer, "The floating vapor mist produced by this sprayer makes it easier to reach the underside of an animal's head and body, under the leaves of plants, and along the seams of clothing where insects usually escape sprays." $20-$25.

Rawleigh's "SPRAYER" (orange) had a removable plunger and a leather washer. Rawleigh's "DUSTER" (blue) was sturdy, well made metal with a removable plunger and leather washer. Both were easy to use. Circa 1960s. $20-$25 ea.

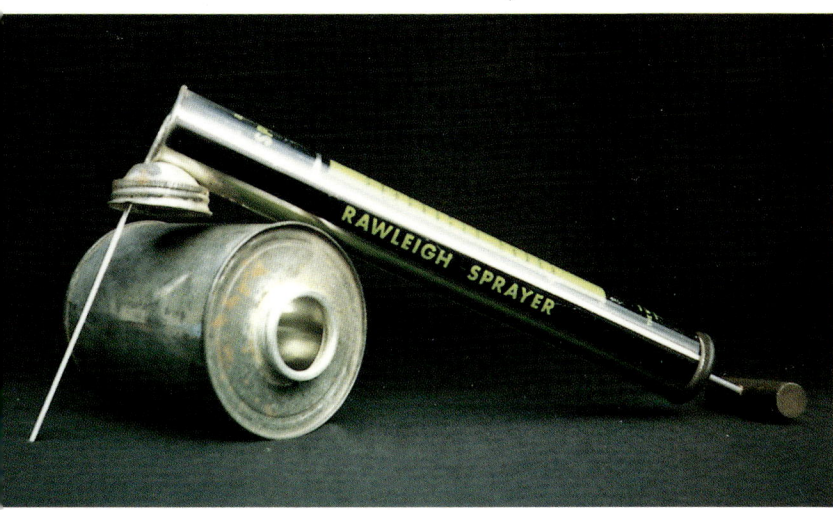

This Rawleigh Sprayer was manufactured for The W.T. Rawleigh Co., Freeport, Ill., U.S.A. The canister could be removed to add solution. $20-$25.

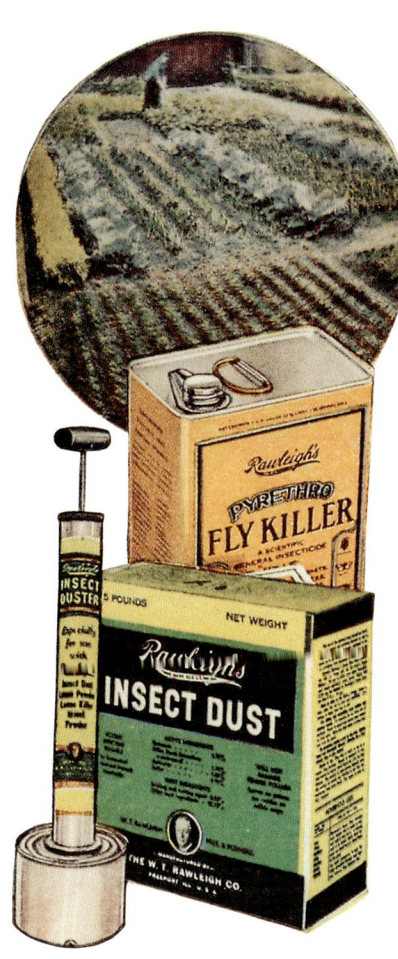

In 1942, Rawleigh promoted the improved compressed Pyrethro Fly Killer spray duster which was convenient and effective. Rawleigh's NEW Insect Dust was a wetting agent that adhered to a surface, keeping it in contact with insects or vegetation on which they feed. $20-$25.

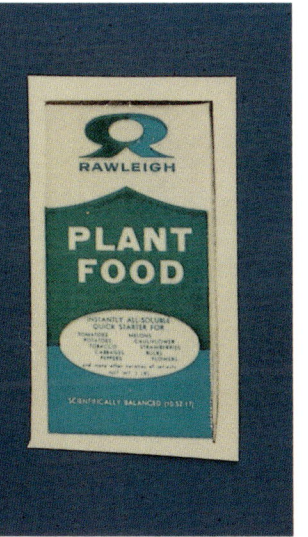

Rawleigh's "PLANT FOOD" was for transplants and general garden use. This product provided faster growth and better produce. It was odorless and fine for house plants. Available in 2 lb. and 5-5/6 ounces. Circa 1960s. $10-$15.

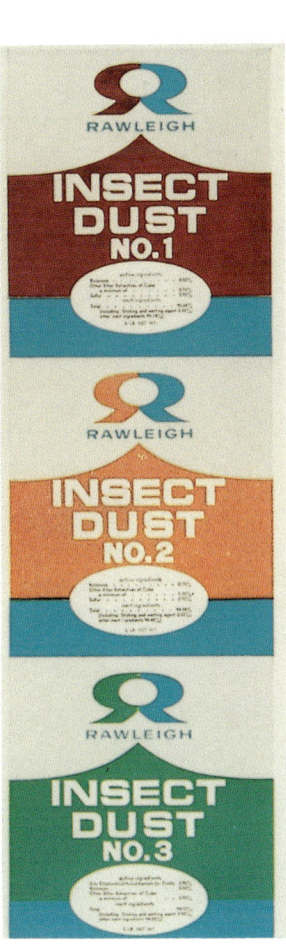

Three Rawleigh "INSECT DUST" packages. Insect Dust No. 1 was for general control and was available in 1-1/4, 5, and 25 pound amounts. Insect Dust No. 2, 1-1/2 times stronger than No. 1, was available in 1-1/4, 5, and 25 pound packages. Insect Dust No. 3 was the same as No. 1 but also controlled many plant diseases. No. 3. was available in 1-1/4 and 5 pound packages. Circa 1960s. $10-$15 ea.

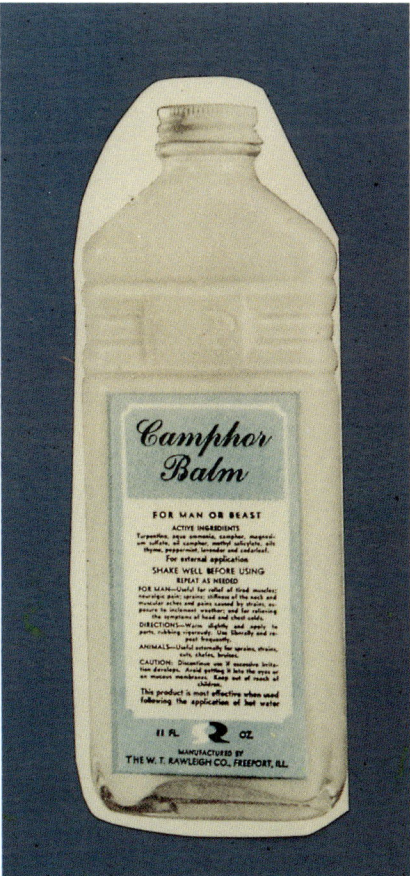

Rawleigh's 11 ounce "CAMPHOR BALM" was manufactured by The W.T. Rawleigh Co., Freeport, IL. The famous Rawleigh white liniment Camphor Balm was good "For man or beast." Circa 1960s. It is also shown elsewhere in this publication. $15-$20.

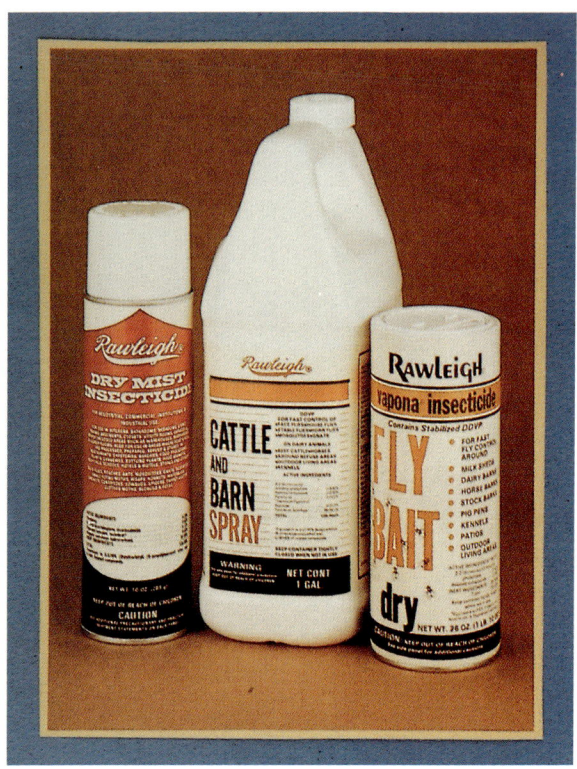

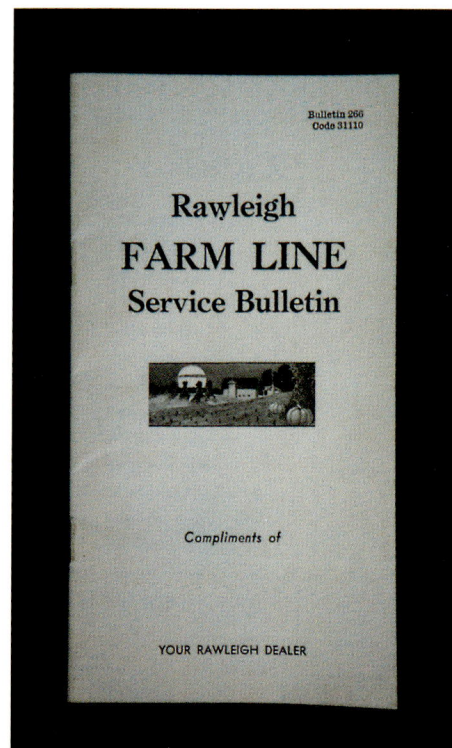

A 3-3/4" x 7" 21 page bulletin No. 266 "Rawleigh Farm Line Service Bulletin." This bulletin provided information and directions for use of Rawleigh's Antiseptic Salve, Calf Scour Tablets, Colic and Bloat Ease, Daily Water Requirements Chart, Fortified Vita-Biotic, Hydro-Cort Mastitis Ointment, Liniment Internal, Normal Body Temperatures Chart, Oral-Iron for Suckling Pigs, Poultry/Swine Wormer, Rat and Mouse Killer (Dry Bait), Rumen-etts, Udder Balm, and Veterinary Application and Ointment. Circa 1966. $15-$20.

These products appeared in the 1986 Rawleigh Family Shopping Guide. Left to right: Dry-Mist 10 ounce Aerosol Insecticide, Cattle and Barn Spray available in either 1-gallon or 5 gallons, and 1 lb. 10 ounce Dry Fly Bait.

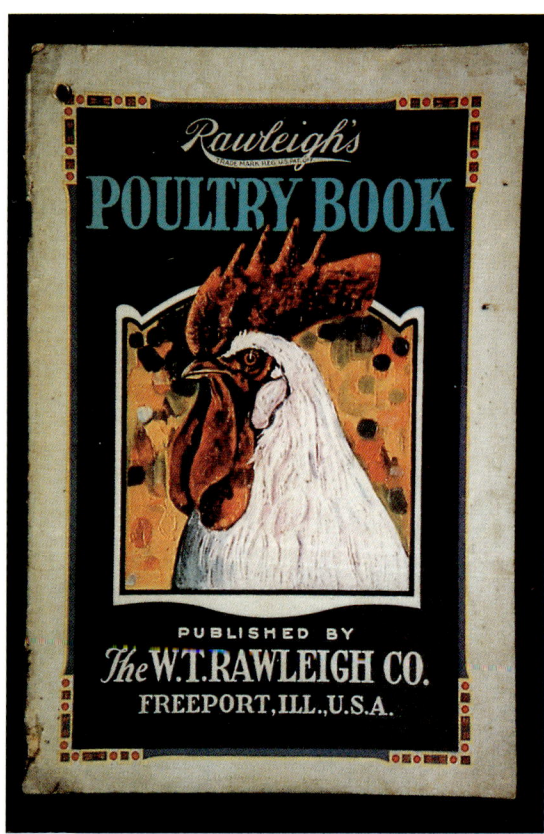

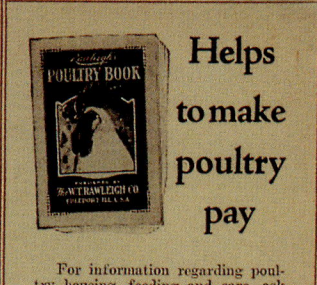

Rawleigh's 32 page Poultry Book. 6-1/2" x 0-1/2" © 1929 The W.T. Rawleigh Co. Freeport, Ill., U.S.A. Compiled by The Rawleigh Veterinarian. $20-$25 ea.

Rawleigh's 32 page Poultry Book. 6-1/2" x 0-1/2" © 1929 The W.T. Rawleigh Co. Freeport, Ill., U.S.A. Compiled by The Rawleigh Veterinarian. $20-$25 ea.

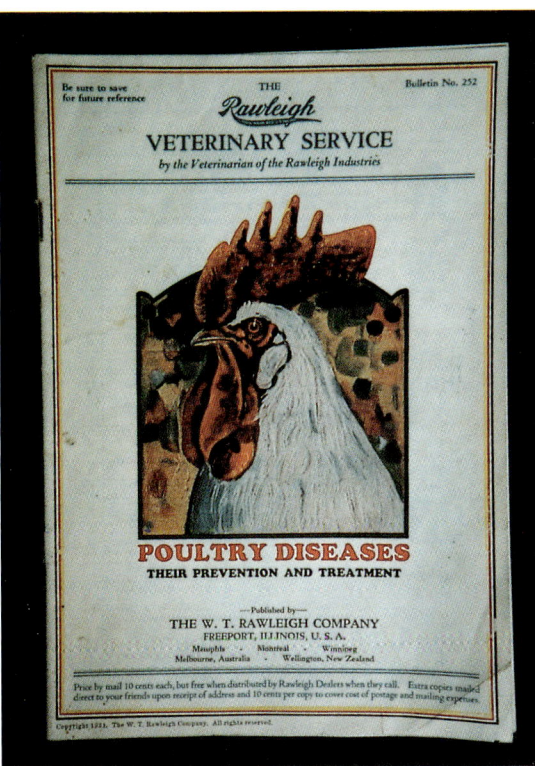

Rawleigh's 22 page "Poultry Diseases Their Prevention and Treatment." © 1931 The W.T. Rawleigh Company by the Veterinarian of the Rawleigh Industries. $20-$25.

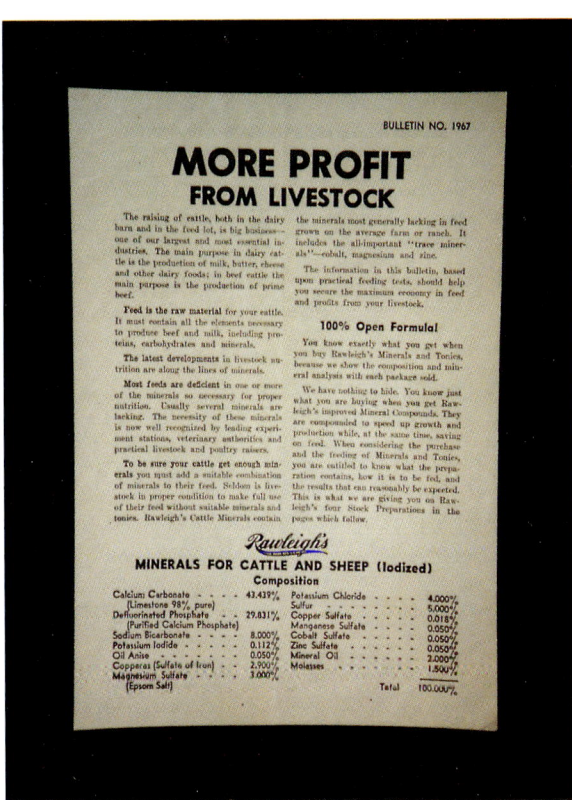

Rawleigh's Bulletin No. 1967 "More Profit From Livestock." $10-$15.

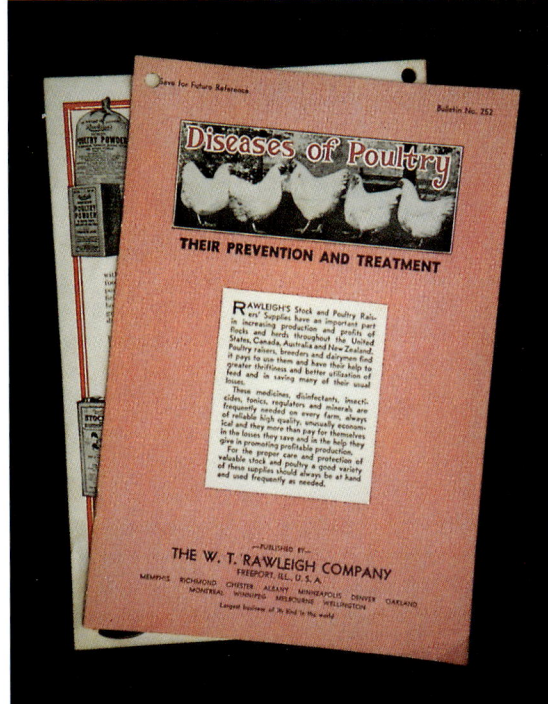

Two copies of Rawleigh's 11 page "Diseases of Poultry Their Prevention and Treatment." Published by The W.T. Rawleigh Company Freeport, Ill., U.S.A. Circa 1940. $20-$25 ea.

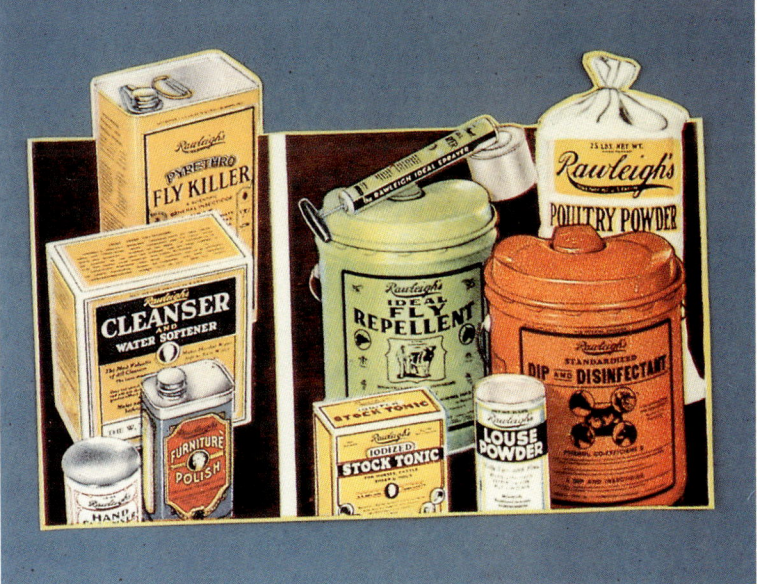

An original advertisement "For Home and Farm." Circa 1937.

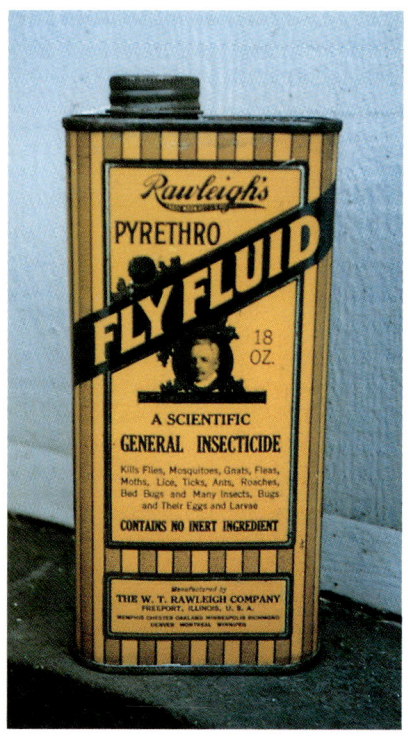 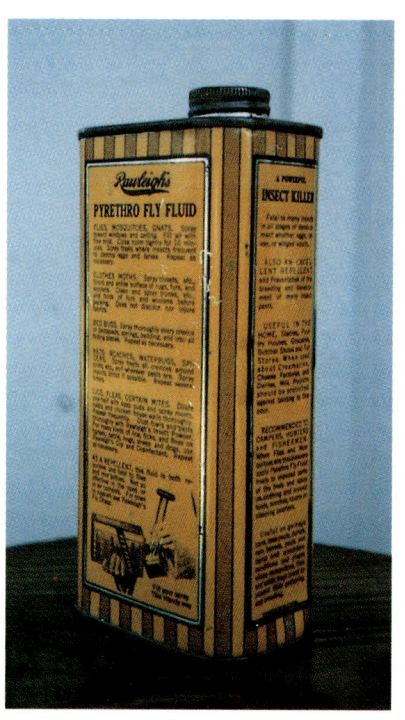 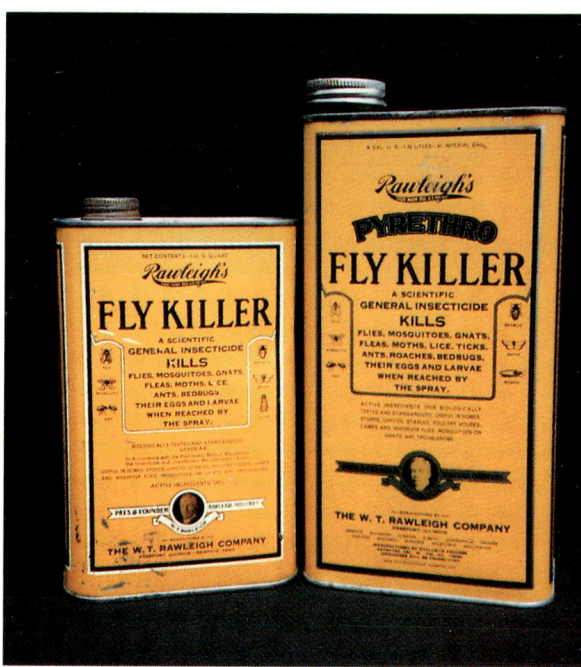

Rawleigh's Pyrethro Fly Fluid, an 18 ounce "Scientific general insecticide. Manufactured by The W.T. Rawleigh Company Freeport, Illinois U.S.A." *Heritage on High Antique Mall Foster/Miller.* $40-$50.

The back and side panels of "Rawleigh's Pyrethro Fly Fluid" provided instructions and directions for the use of this insecticide. *Heritage on High Antique Mall Foster/Miller.* $40-$50.

Two different sizes of Rawleigh's Fly Killer. Left: 1 quart; right: 1/2 gallon. *Dupler Collection.* $40-$50 ea.

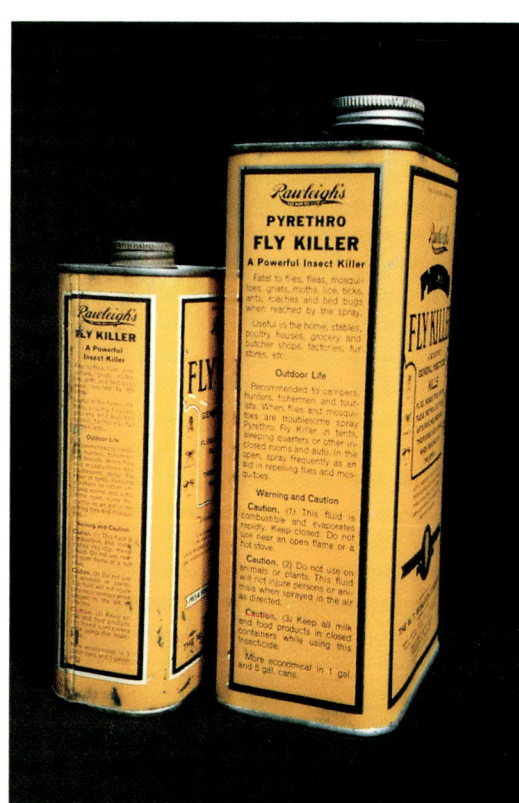 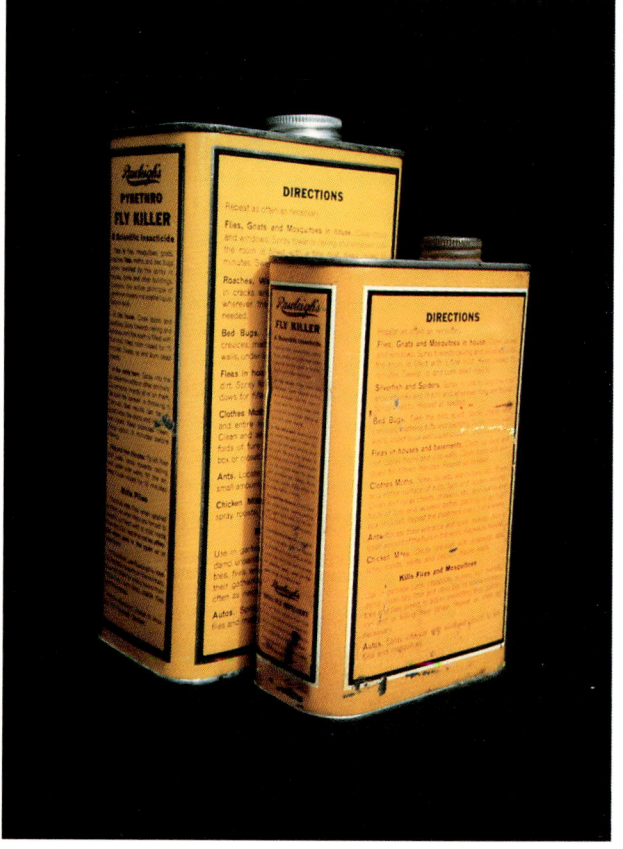

Rawleigh's Fly Killer was a powerful insect killer. The side panels listed directions for use inside the home and outside. Warnings and cautions were also provided. *Dupler Collection.* $40-$50 ea.

The back panels with complete directions. Rawleigh's Fly Killer could be used as often as necessary and could be sprayed into a car with windows closed to kill flies and mosquitoes. *Dupler Collection.* $40-$50 ea.

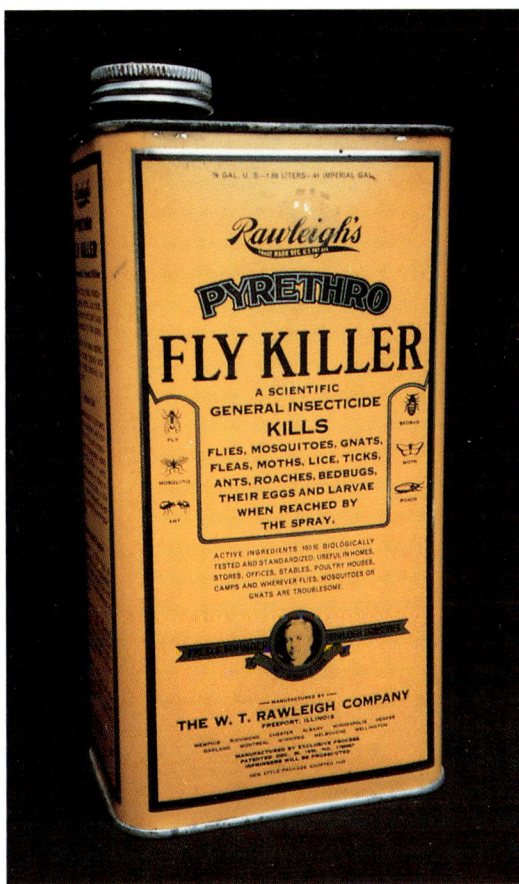

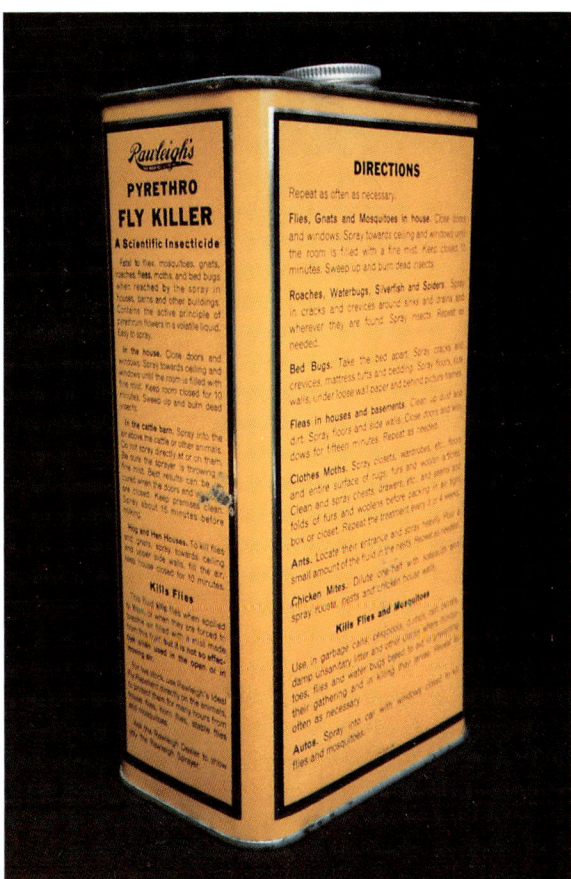

This container of Rawleigh's Pyrethro Fly Killer has never been used. It was labeled as a scientific general insecticide and was manufactured by The W.T. Rawleigh Company Freeport, Illinois - Memphis - Richmond - Chester - Albany - Minneapolis - Denver - Oakland - Montreal - Winnipeg - Melbourne - Wellington. *Dupler Collection.* $40-$50.

Rawleigh's Fly Killer 1 quart was biologically tested and standardized Grade AA. Manufactured by The W.T. Rawleigh Company, Freeport, Illinois - Memphis, Tenn. *Dupler Collection.* $40-$50.

Rawleigh's Pyrethro Fly Killer was fatal to flies, mosquitoes, gnats, flys, moths, and bed bugs when reached by the spray in houses, barns and other farm buildings. The container is marked "Manufactured By Exclusive Process Patented Dec. 30, 1930. No. 1786967 Infringers will be Prosecuted New Style Package Adopted 1935." *Dupler Collection.* $40-$50.

Rawleigh's Fly Killer, back panels, was not effective when used in the open air or in moving air. *Dupler Collection.* $40-$50.

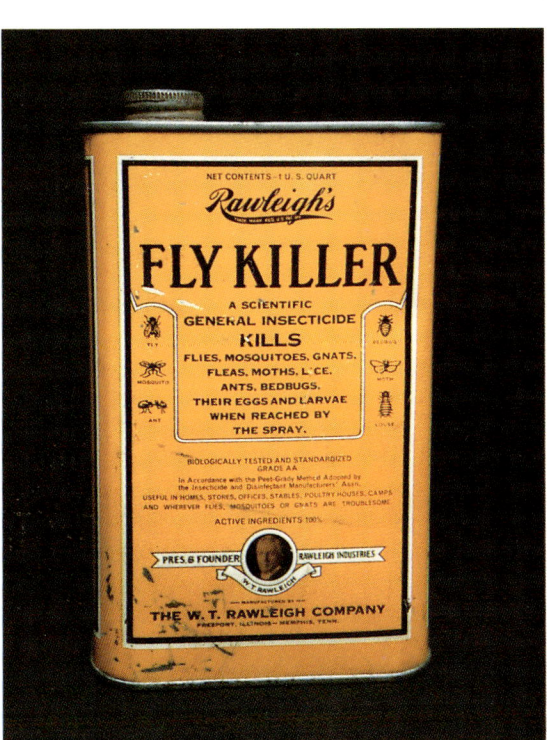

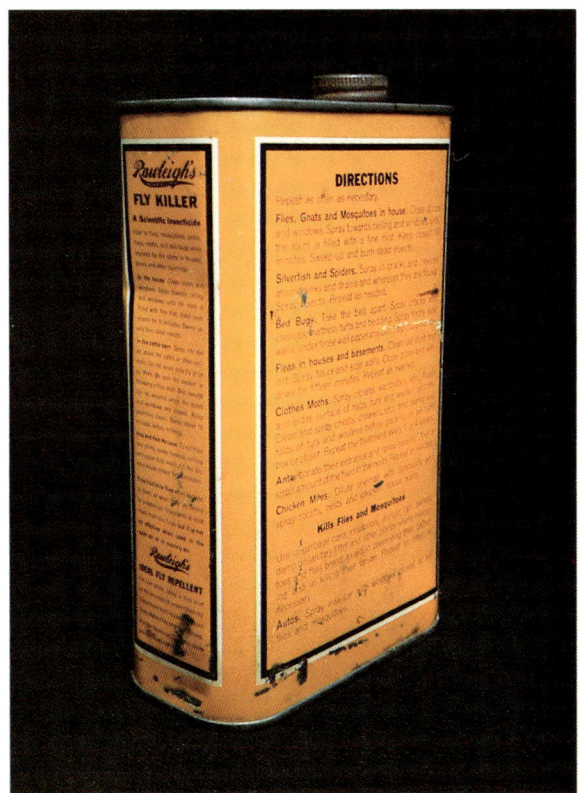

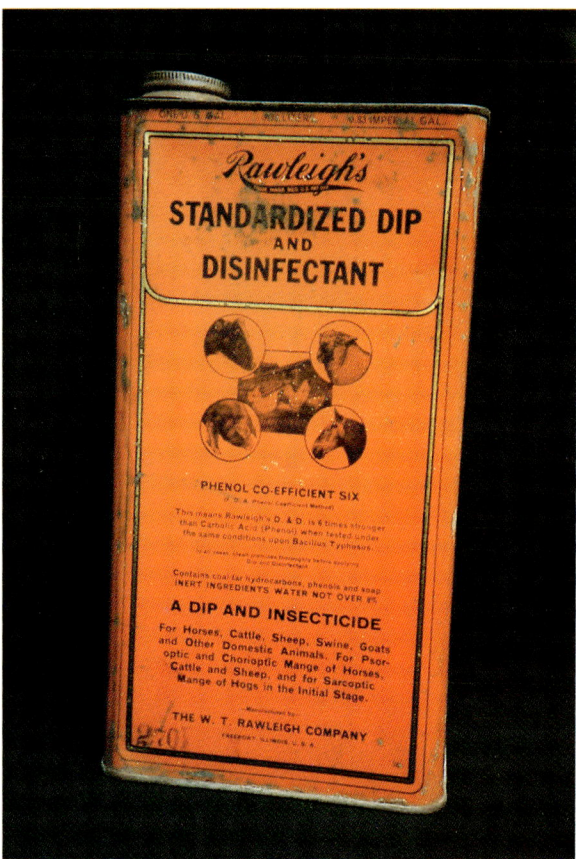

A 1 gallon container of Rawleigh's Standardized Dip and Disinfectant. A dip and insecticide for horses, cattle, sheep, swine, goats, and other domestic animals. Manufactured by The W.T. Rawleigh Company Freeport, Illinois U.S.A. *Dupler Collection.* $45-$55.

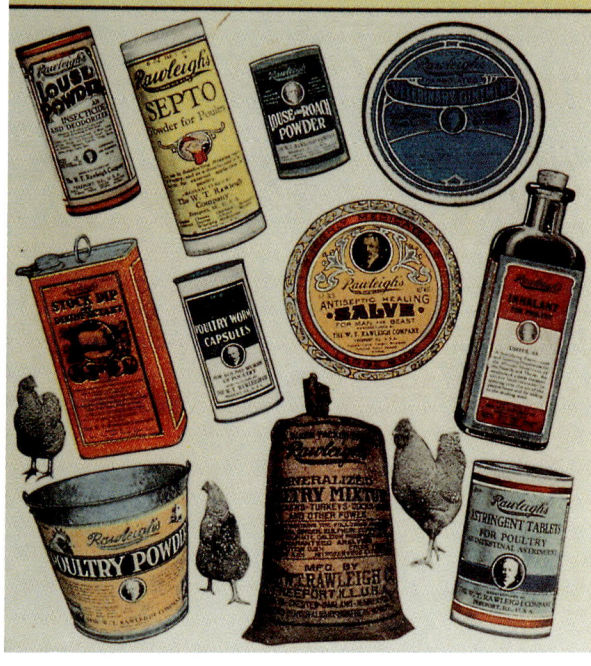

Rawleigh's Poultry Raisers' Supplies used extensively throughout the United States, Canada, and Australia. This original advertisement appeared in bulletin No. 252 ©1931 The Rawleigh Veterinary Service by the veterinarian of the Rawleigh Industries.

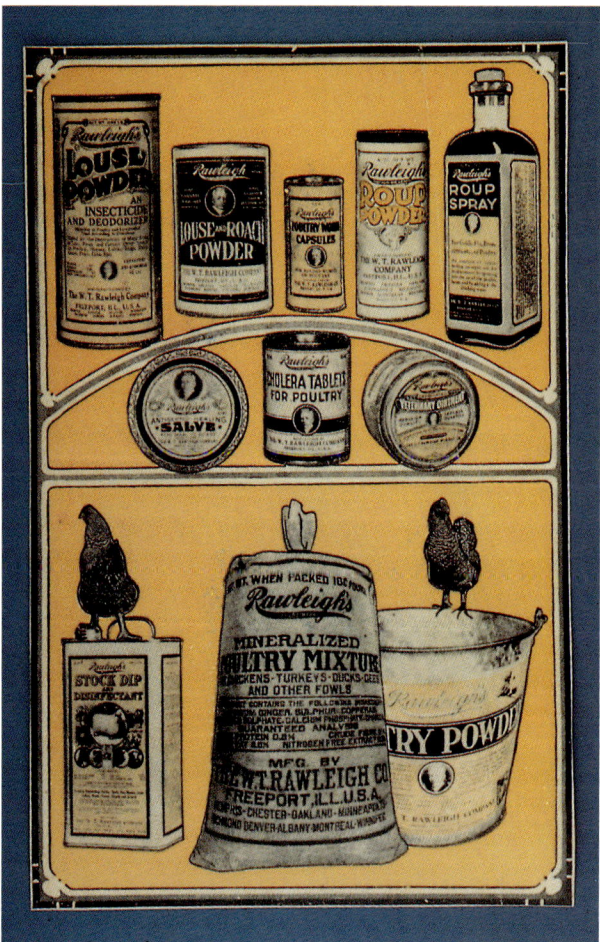

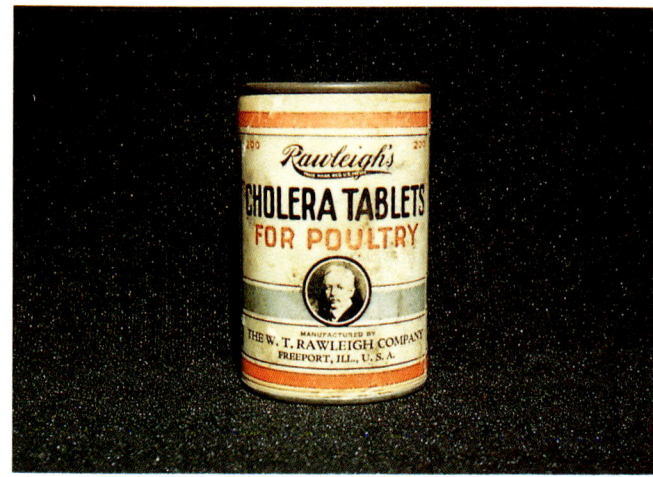

Rawleigh's Cholera Tablets For Poultry. Manufactured by The W.T. Rawleigh Company Freeport, Ill., U.S.A. Cholera Tablets for poultry consisted of a treatment that was approved by experimental stations, agricultural colleges, and poultry experts. It was a non-poisonous intestinal antiseptic of great value for intestinal ailments of all kinds in poultry. Recommended for diarrhea, white diarrhea, coccidiosis, fowl cholera and fowl typhoid, and intestinal infections. $10-$15.

Rawleigh's leading poultry preparations included Rawleigh's Louse Powder, Louse and Roach Powder, Poultry Worm Capsules, Roup Powder and Spray, Rawleigh's Salve, Cholera Tablets, Veterinary Ointment, Rawleigh's Dip and Disinfectant, Poultry Mixture, and Poultry Powder. ©1929 Rawleigh's Poultry Book.

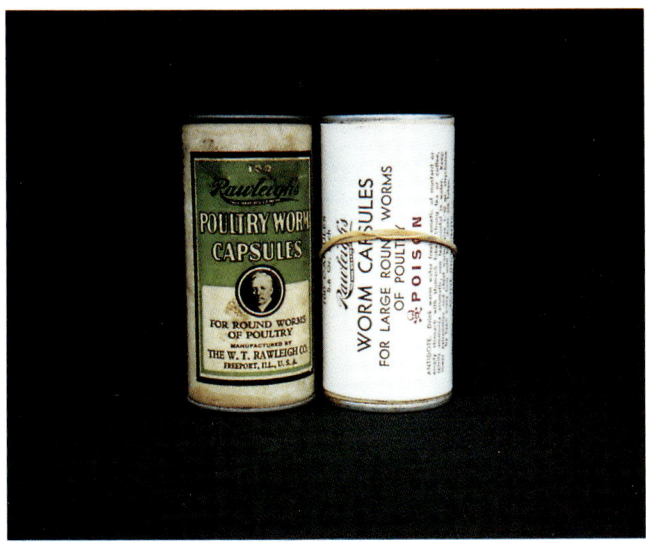

Two different variations of Rawleigh's Poultry Worm Capsules. Poultry Worm Capsules were a proven and reliable treatment for removing round worms from poultry. Flock treatment for poultry was unsatisfactory. Rawleigh's belief was to secure the best results by treating each bird individually. Rawleigh's Poultry Worm Capsules did not decrease production through fasting as was the case with other worm treatments. Manufactured by The W.T. Rawleigh Co., Freeport, Ill., U.S.A. and packed 100 capsules to the package. $10-$15 ea.

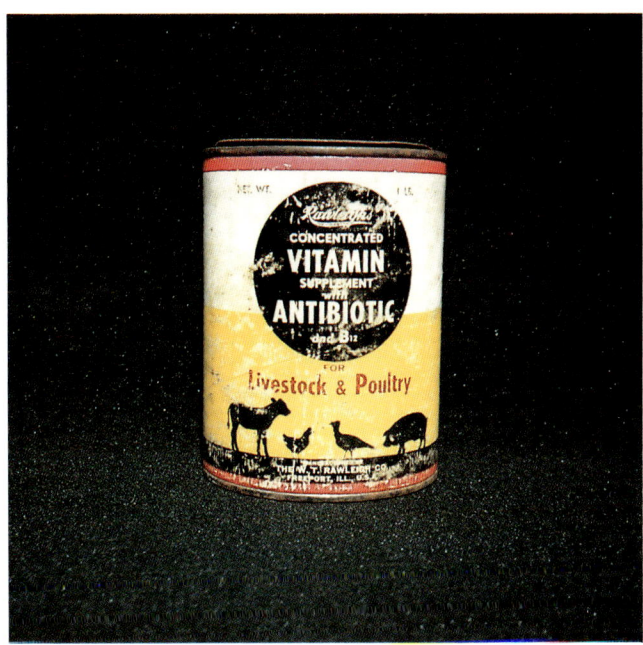

Rawleigh's Concentrated Vitamin Supplement with Antibiotic for livestock and poultry. Manufactured by The W.T. Rawleigh Co., Freeport, Ill., U.S.A. This product contained nine vitamins including the newly-discovered B-12 and the antibiotic, procaine penicillin. Bulletin No. 265 is believed to have come with this Supplement. Supplement $25-$30. Bulletin $20-$25.

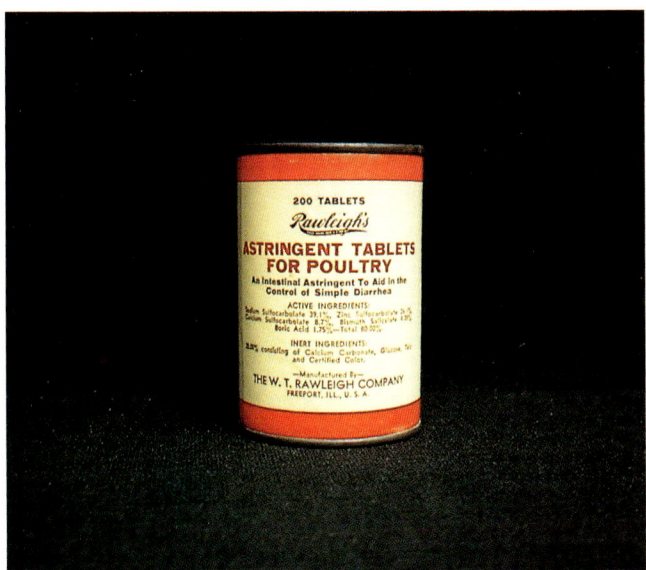

Rawleigh's Astringent Tablets For Poultry. An intestinal astringent to aid in the control of simple diarrhea. Manufactured by The W.T. Rawleigh Co., Freeport, Ill., U.S.A. $10-$15.

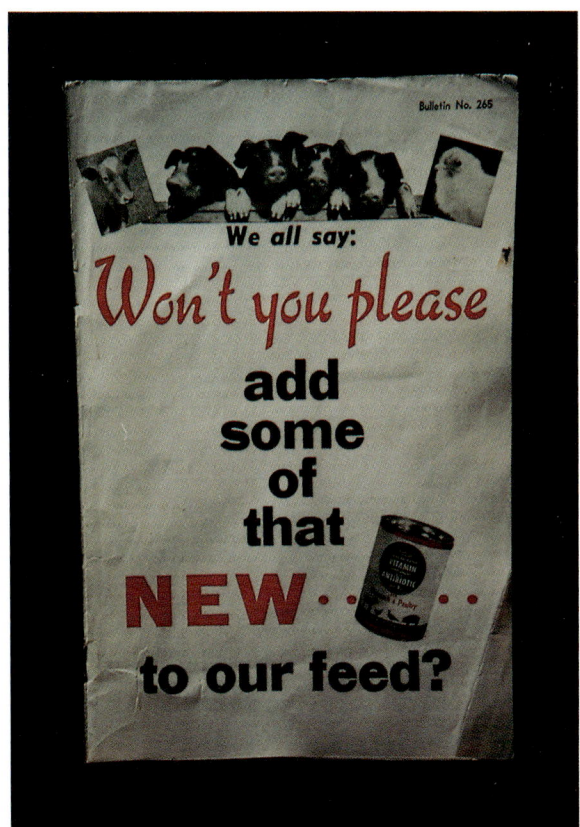

Seven page Bulletin No. 265 "We all say: Won't you please add some of that NEW Rawleigh's Concentrated Vitamin Supplement with Antibiotic to our feed?" Circa 1954. The W.T. Rawleigh Co., Freeport, Ill., U.S.A. $20-$25.

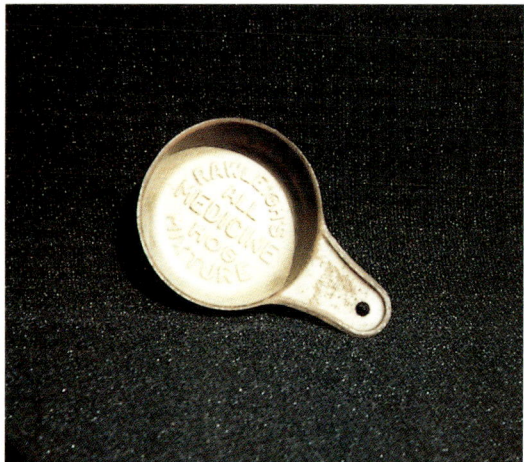

A metal scoop embossed inside "RAWLEIGH'S ALL MEDICINE HOG MIXTURE." *Dupler Collection.* $40-$50.

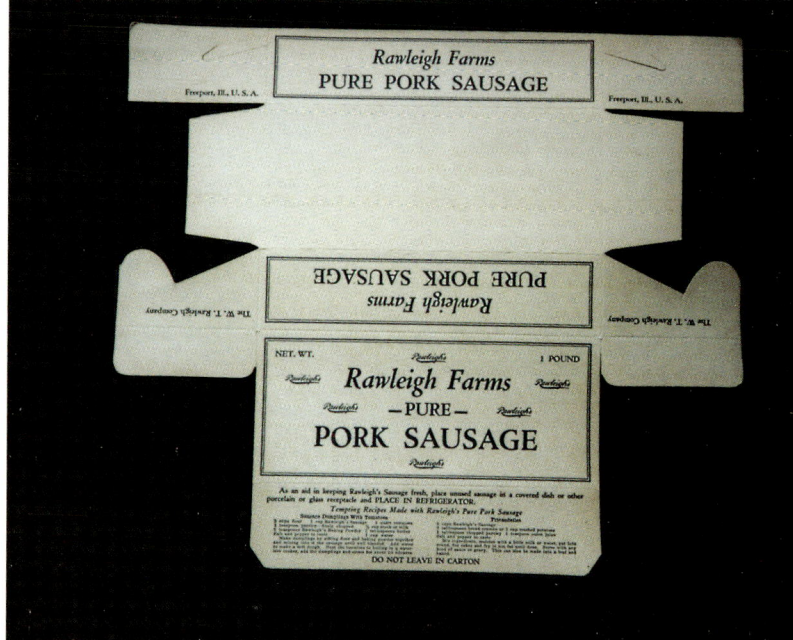

A 1 pound carton of Rawleigh Farms Pure Pork Sausage. Two recipes were provide using Rawleigh's Pure Pork Sausage. The flatten carton is marked The W.T. Rawleigh Company Freeport, Ill., U.S.A., and has not been formed into a carton. *Dupler Collection.* $50-$60.

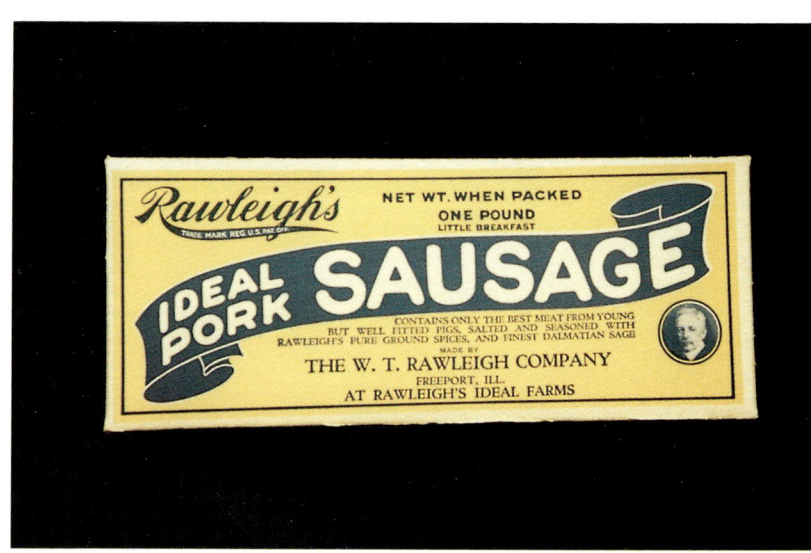

Rawleigh's Good Health Milk in half pint and one pint bottles. Each bottle is embossed "Rawleigh Farms Freeport, Ill Sealed BB48". Also available is a one quart liquid milk bottle. Photograph not available. Half pint: $25-$50. Pint: $50-$75. Quart $75-$100.

A 1 pound Rawleigh's Ideal Pork Sausage carton folded with W.T. Rawleigh's picture. The carton is marked "The W.T. Rawleigh Company Freeport, Ill., At Rawleigh's Ideal Farms." *Dupler Collection.* $50-$60.

Rawleigh's Pork Sausage was made of a combination of top-quality hog meat and the best grade of spices manufactured by the Rawleigh factory. Rawleigh's Sausage was produced during four months of operation from November through February. As there was never enough sausage to meet customers' demands, this packaging will require time in locating.

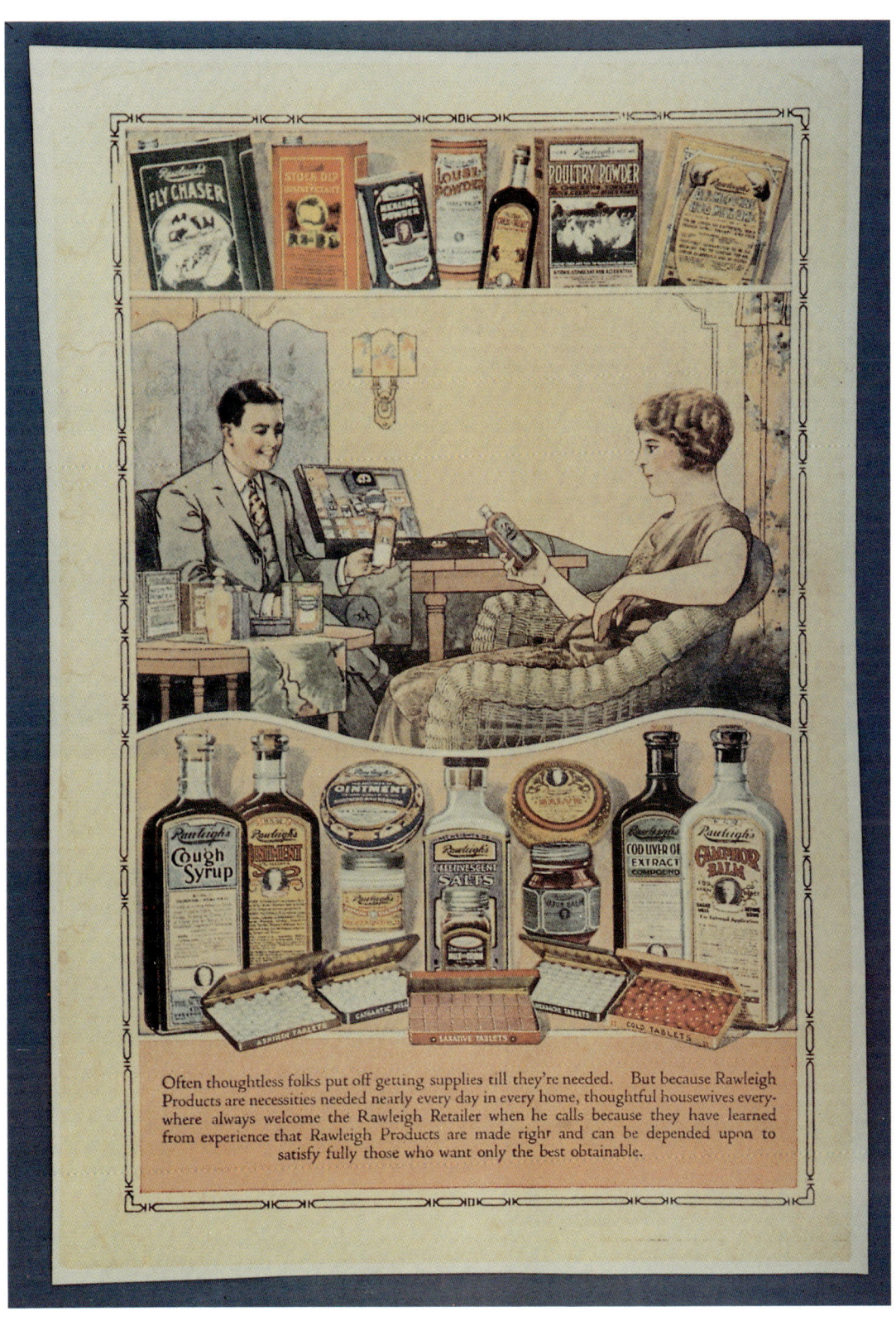

An original 1927 advertisement for various Rawleigh products. Farmers to housewives welcomed their Rawleigh Retailer.

Bibliography

GOLDEN PRIDE/RAWLEIGH "Good Health Starts With Nature & Nutrition" © 1995 by Golden Pride/Rawleigh, Inc., a Florida Corporation.

History of Stephenson County 1970. Freeport, Illinois.

Horlick, Bill. *The Rawleigh Man Murray Barron "A Life That Mattered".* Canada: Newmarket Printing Ltd., October 1994.

Rawleigh Almanac and Family Guide 1961. The W.T. Rawleigh Company.

Rawleigh Almanac and Family Guide 1962. The W.T. Rawleigh Company.

Rawleigh Almanac and Family Guide 1963. The W.T. Rawleigh Company.

Rawleigh Almanac and Family Guide Diamond Anniversary 1964. The W.T. Rawleigh Company.

Rawleigh Almanac and Family Guide Our 77th Year 1966. The W.T. Rawleigh Company.

Rawleigh's Complete Skin Care Program. The W.T. Rawleigh Company Chapin, SC 29036 U.S.A.

Rawleigh's Almanac Cook Book and Medical Guide 1914. The W.T. Rawleigh Medical Co. Freeport, Ill. U.S.A. Memphis, Chester, Winnipeg

Rawleigh's Almanac Cook Book and Medical Guide 1915. The W.T. Rawleigh Medical Co. Freeport, Ill. U.S.A. Memphis, Chester, Winnipeg

Rawleigh's Almanac Cook Book and Medical Guide 1916. The W.T. Rawleigh Medical Co. Freeport, Ill. U.S.A.

Rawleigh's Good Health Guide Cook Book Almanac 1922. The W.T. Rawleigh Co., Freeport, Ill U.S.A.

Rawleigh's Good Health Guide Cook Book Almanac 1924. © 1923 The W.T. Rawleigh Company Freeport, Ill., U.S.A.

Rawleigh's Good Health Guide Cook Book Almanac 1926. © 1925 The W.T. Rawleigh Company Freeport, Ill., U.S.A.

Rawleigh's Good Health Guide Cook Book Almanac 1927. © 1926 The W.T. Rawleigh Company Freeport, Ill., U.S.A.

Rawleigh's Good Health Guide Cook Book Almanac 1931. The W.T. Rawleigh Company Freeport, Ill., U.S.A.

Rawleigh's Good Health Guide Cook Book Year Book 1932. © 1931 The W.T. Rawleigh Company.

Rawleigh's Good Health Guide Cook Book Year Book 1933. © 1932 The W.T. Rawleigh Company.

Rawleigh's Good Health Guide Almanac Catalog 1935. © 1934 The W.T. Rawleigh Company.

Rawleigh's Good Health Guide Almanac Catalog 1936. The W.T. Rawleigh Company.

Rawleigh's Good Health Guide Almanac Cook Book 1937. The W.T. Rawleigh Company.

Rawleigh's Good Health Guide Almanac Cook Book 1938. The W.T. Rawleigh Company.

Rawleigh's Good Health Guide Almanac Cook Book 1939. The W.T. Rawleigh Company.

Rawleigh's Good Health Guide Almanac Cook Book 1941. The W.T. Rawleigh Company.

Rawleigh's Good Health Guide Almanac Cook Book 1942. The W.T. Rawleigh Company.

Rawleigh's Good Health Guide Almanac Cook Book 1944. The W.T. Rawleigh Company.

Rawleigh's Good Health Guide Almanac Cook Book 1946. The W.T. Rawleigh Company.

Rawleigh's Good Health Guide Almanac Cook Book Our 59th Year 1948. The W.T. Rawleigh Company.

Rawleigh's Good Health Guide Almanac Cook Book 1950. The W.T. Rawleigh Company.

Rawleigh's Good Health Guide Almanac Cook Book 1951. The W.T. Rawleigh Company.

Rawleigh's Good Health Guide Almanac Cook Book 1952. The W.T. Rawleigh Company.

Rawleigh's Good Health Guide Almanac Cook Book 1953. The W.T. Rawleigh Company.

Rawleigh's Good Health Guide Almanac Cook Book 1954. The W.T. Rawleigh Company.

Rawleigh's Good Health Guide Almanac Cook Book 1955. The W.T. Rawleigh Company.

Rawleigh's Good Health Guide Almanac Cook Book 1956. The W.T. Rawleigh Company.

Rawleigh's Good Health Guide Almanac Cook Book 1957. The W.T. Rawleigh Company.

Rawleigh's Good Health Guide Almanac Cook Book 1958. The W.T. Rawleigh Company.

Rawleigh's Good Health Guide Almanac Cook Book 1959. The W.T. Rawleigh Company.

Rawleigh's 1986 Family Shopping Guide. The W.T. Rawleigh Company.

Rawleigh's 60th Anniversary Good Health Guide 1949. The W.T. Rawleigh Co., Ltd. Printed in Canada.

Rawleigh's 60th Anniversary Good Health Guide 1949. The W.T. Rawleigh Company Freeport, Illinois.

Remembrances by Rawleigh © 1979 The W.T. Rawleigh Co.

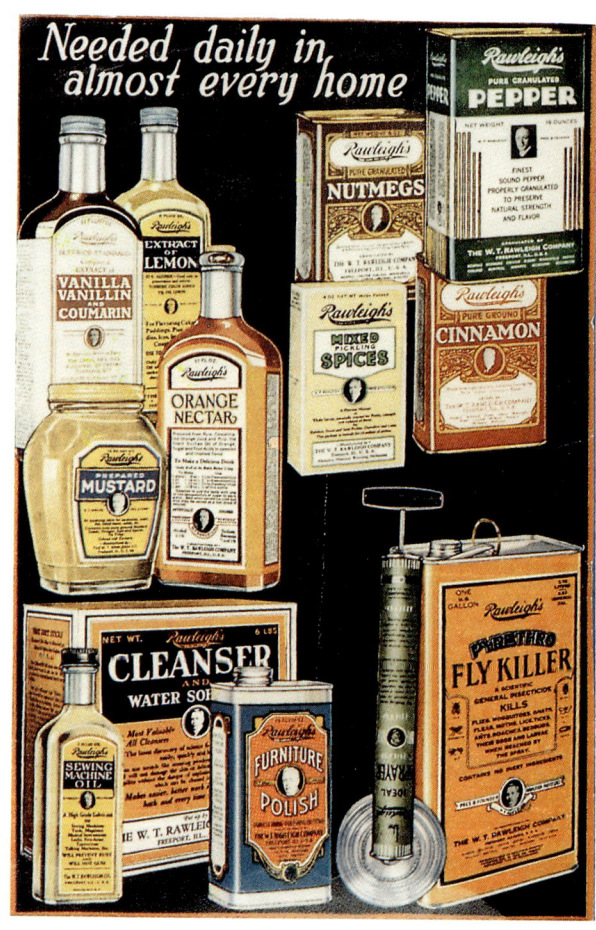

Index

A

add (**A**utomatic **D**ishwashing **D**etergent), 148
Advertisement, 4, 6, 8, 14, 16, 20, 22, 23, 24, 33, 34, 35, 36, 37, 38, 39, 40, 41, 42, 44, 45, 48, 49, 50, 88, 91, 94, 95, 100, 102, 116, 118, 119, 122, 123, 124, 125, 126, 127, 128, 132, 133, 136, 137, 139, 144, 145, 148, 151, 160, 161, 162, 163, 167, 170, 173
Aerosol Insecticide, 166
Africa, 19
Air Freshener, 149, 149, 150
Alabama, 15
Albany, 66, 67, 90, 104, 130, 169
Alexander, Mrs., 23
All-Medicine Mixtures, 19
All-Spice, 99, 100
Almanac and Cook Book, 72, 73
Almanac and Family Guide, 70, 71
American Institute of Conservation, 51
Analytical Laboratory, 11, 19
Anniversary, 59, 63, 64, 81
Annual Conferences, 25
Anti-Pain Oil, 7, 33, 42, 43
Antiseptic Solution, 35, 155
Arizona, 17, 26
Arkansas, 15, 16, 23
Asafen, 37, 38
Aspirin, 37
Astringent Tablets for Poultry, 171
Atlantic, 4
Australia, 7

B

Baking Powder, 89, 90, 151
Balm, 40, 41, 45, 46, 48
Balsa-wood Paddle, 101
Balsam, 42
Bandiseptic, 35
Barron, Charles and Delilah, 23
Barron, Murray C., 23
Baseball Hat, 115
Bath Salt, 142
Bee Pollen, 50
Bee Propolis, 50
Blair Medical Company, 9
Bleach, 147, 156
Bowl Cleaner, 156
Breed, Dwight B., 11
Brightener, 156
Brushes, Mops and Dusters, 60, 154, 155
Bubble Bath, 143
Bulletin No. 265, 171
Bulletin No. 1967, 167
Bushue Garry & Betty, 153

C

Calendars, 75, 76
California, 16
Camphor Balm, 165
Canada, 5, 6, 15, 23
Candy & Cookie Kit, 112
Canisters, 112, 113
Carolinas, 16
Castoria, 34, 41
Catalog, 81, 82, 83
Cattle and Barn Spray, 164, 166
Celery Salt, 34, 96
Central Location, 6
Chester, Pennsylvania, 11, 19, 44, 66, 67, 90, 100, 103, 104, 130, 131, 140, 169
China, 19
Cholera Tablets for Poultry, 170
Christmas Candy, 112
Cinnamon, 97, 98, 99
Citizen's Commercial Association, 10
Cleanser, 146, 151, 152
Cloves, 98, 99, 100
Cocoa, 90
Coconut, 93
Cologne, 140, 141, 142
Combs, 25
Commons, J.R., 26
Compound, 37, 42, 46
Conditioner, 135
Cookbooks and Recipes, 74, 75
Corkscrew, 25
Cosmetics, 4
Cough Lozenges, 43
Cough Syrup, 32, 41, 42, 48
Countryside, 12, 15
Cowley, James R., 11
Crate, 10, 116
Cream of Tartar, 95
Cutting Board, 114

D

Dealer, 21, 24, 25
Dealer Sign, 115
Decongestant, 41
Deeds of Daring by Blue and Gray, 9
Delicious Foods, 91
Delivery Bag, 76
Della Buttercup, 159
Deluxe Pre Electric, 142
Dental Cream, 143, 155, 156
Denver, 44, 66, 67, 90, 100, 104, 130, 131, 140, 169
Deodorant Block, 150
Dip and Disinfectant, 170
Diseases of Poultry, 167
Disinfectants, 4
Douglas Avenue, 10
Drink Mix, 92, 95
Drops Nose & Throat, 49
Dust Mop Spray, 154
Dustmaster Mop, 154
Dutch East Indies, 7, 19

E

Effervescent Salt, 34, 40, 42, 46
East Exchange Street, 9
East Main Street, 13
Evans, Dale, 27
Experimental Farms, 12, 157, 158, 159
Extracts, 4, 106, 110, 111, 133

F

Family Medicine Cabinet, 35
Family Shopping Guide, 77, 78
Farm Line Service Bulletin, 166
Flavoring, 109, 110, 111, 133
Floor Shine, 150
Floor Wax, 150
Floral Mist, 148
Florencia, 122, 124
Florida, 26, 27
Fly Bait, 163, 166
Fly Control Strip, 163
Fly Fluid, 168
Fly Killer, 151, 165, 168, 169
Flyers, 80
Fogmaster Sprayer, 164
Foot Spray, 134, 135
Foreign Countries, 84, 85
France, 7, 15
Freeport Standard, 11
Freeport, Illinois, 4, 5, 7, 10, 13, 14, 18, 19, 20, 38, 39, 41, 42, 43, 44, 45, 46, 47, 48, 49, 52, 53, 54, 55, 56, 57, 58, 59, 60, 61, 62, 63, 64, 65, 66, 67, 72, 73, 74, 76, 77, 89, 90, 92, 93, 94, 95, 96, 97, 98, 99, 100, 101, 102, 103, 104, 105, 106, 107, 108, 109, 112, 120, 127, 130, 131, 133, 134, 138, 139, 140, 142, 143, 146, 147, 149, 150, 151, 152, 153, 161, 168, 169, 170, 171, 172
Freeport's Oakland Cemetery, 10
Fruit Cake Tin, 111
Furniture Polish, 150, 152, 153

G

Gelatine, 92
Georgia, 15
German, 53
Gift Sets, 113
Ginger, 98, 99, 100
Glass Cleaner, 149
Golden Pride International, (Golden Pride/Rawleigh, Inc.) 23, 26, 27, 75
Good Health Chart, 31
Good Health Service Bulletins, 28, 29
Good Health Guide, 20, 22, 23, 51, 52, 53, 54, 55, 56, 57, 58, 59, 60, 61, 62, 63, 64, 65, 66, 67, 68, 69, 73
Good Health Rules, 20
GPI, 27
Grand Comore Island, 7
Great Western, 6
Gulf of Mexico, 4, 16

H

Hair Dressing, 135
Hair Rinse, 143, 153
Hair Set, 143
Hamilton, 18
Hand Cleaner, 153
Hand Cream, 143
Health Chart, 116
Hersey, Harry W., 13, 27
Hibbard, B.H., 26
Hoppock, Harland H., 15
Hoppock, Yvonne, 15
Hot Plaque, 114
House of Rawleigh, 5
House of Service, 12, 14
How To Build Good Blood, 83
Hudson Bay, 4, 16
Humpty Dumpty, 132

I

Idaho, 16
Ideal Oil, 144, 151
Illinois, 5, 6
Illinois Central, 6
India, 19
Insect Dust, 152, 165
Insect Powder, 152
Insect Spray, 163
Institution of Unusual Utility, 12
Invitational Conference, 153
Iowa, 5, 16
Ironing Cover, 156

J

Japan, 7

K

Kalender, 53, 54
Keith, Walter, 23
Kentucky, 6

Kreo, 152

L

La Jaynees, 120, 121, 122, 123, 124, 125, 141
Lady Love Skin Care Company, 27
Larger Bottles, 60
Laxative, 50
Leaflet No. 297, 75
Lemon Lotion, 140
Library of Congress, 51
Life Style, 80
Liniment, 34, 44
Liquid Wax, 152
London, 131, 140
Los Angeles, 17, 66

M

Madagascar, 7
Madison Tariff Committee, 26
Magnetic Broom, 155
Maine, 16
Mapleon Colantha Segis Aaltje, 159
Marseilles, France, 15
Massachusetts, 16
Mayor of Freeport, 10, 11
Medicated Vaporizer, 50
Medicines, 4, 40
Melbourne, 66, 67, 90, 100, 104, 130, 131, 169
Memphis, Tennessee, 5, 15, 16, 18, 19, 44, 66, 67, 90, 100, 103, 104, 140, 169
Michigan, 6
Milk Bottles, 172
Milk Magnesia, 40, 45
Mineral Point, Wisconsin, 9
Minneapolis, Minnesota, 17, 18, 44, 66, 67, 90, 104, 130, 131, 140, 169
Mint Sweets, 140
Mississippi, 15
Missouri, 16
Montana, 17
Montreal, 5, 44, 66, 90, 100, 104, 130, 131, 169
Morton, W.A., 26
Moth Crystals, 152, 153
Mountain Herb Liniment, 7
Mustard, 100, 101, 102, 151

N

Nail Brush, 154
National Archives, 51
Nebraska, 16
Necessities, 37, 119
Nectar, 91
New Brunswick, 16
New Factories, 60
New Hampshire, 16
New York, 16
New Zealand, 7

Northwestern, 6
Note Cards, 76
Nova Scotia, 16
Nutmeg, 99, 100

O

Oakland, California, 16, 18, 44, 66, 67, 90, 100, 104, 130, 131, 140, 169
Occupations and Professions, 14, 15
Ohio, 6
Oil, 39, 133
Ointments, 4, 18, 35, 40, 46, 47, 48, 49
Ontario, 16
Order Forms, 79
Oregon, 16

P

Pacific, 4
Pectin, 34, 92, 151
Pefferlaw, Ontario, 23
Pennsylvania, 16
People's Legislation Service, 26
Pepper, 27, 97, 98, 99, 100, 103, 104, 105, 106
Perfumes, 139, 140, 142
Pickling Spices, 98, 100
Pie Baker, 113, 114
Pie Fillings and Dessert, 93, 94
Pine Oil, 149, 150
Plant Food, 165
Pleasant Relief, 27, 44, 45
Pocket Guide, 79
Pomade, 18
Postcards, 81
Poultry Book, 166
Poultry Diseases, 167
Poultry Worm Capsules, 171
Powder, 122, 123, 124, 125, 126, 127, 132, 134, 135
Powell Street, 10, 11
Prince Edward Island, 16
Printing Department, 51, 52
Products 110
Professional Picture Framers' Association, 51

Q

Quality, 33
Quebec, 16, 106

R

Rawleigh
  Analytical Department, 4
  Anna May, 9
  Band, 12
  Charles, 9
  Glass Factory, 13, 60
  Laboratories, 30

  Lucille, 9
  Medical Company, 4, 5, 9, 10, 19, 20, 21, 22, 52, 53, 54, 103
  Modern Brush Factory, 154
  Report, 80
  Retailer, 22
  Sarah Babcock, 9
  Standard of Quality, 20
  Tariff Bureau, 26
  Wilbur Thomas, 9
  W.T. (also William Thomas), 5, 6, 7, 9, 10, 11, 12, 13, 14, 26
Rawleigh-Schryer Company, 10, 12, 18
Razor Blade, 137, 138
Ready Relief (RRR), 38, 41
Recruiting Opportunity, 25
Rectal Ointment, 34
Red Color, 111
Refrigerator Deodorizer, 148
Registered Trademark, 28
Remembrances, 79
Research Work, 60
Richmond, Virginia, 17, 44, 66, 67, 90, 100, 104, 130, 131, 169
Rogers, Roy, 27
Royal Jelly, 50
Ru-Mex-Ol, 32, 42, 45
Rubendall, Willard, 12
Rug & Upholstery Shampoo, 151

S

Sage, 27, 98, 99
Salad Dressing, 106
Sales Aids, 81
Sales Kit, 24
Salve, 18, 35, 47
Sausage, 105, 172
Schneider, Marguerite, 9
Schryer, Paul F., 12
Scoop, 25, 172
Scrubber, 152
Seasoning, 96, 102
Secrets of Loveliness, 124
Sewing Machine Oil, 4
Shampoo, 136, 137, 138, 139
Shaving, 137
Shopping Guides, 76
Silcone Spray, 149
Silver Polish, 34
Sir Ormsby Fobes Dictator, 159
Skin Care Program 79
Soap, 131, 132, 136
Spice, 4, 95, 133
Spice Rack, 114, 115
Sprayer, 152, 164, 165
St. Paul, 6
Starch, 144, 146, 147, 151, 156
Starch-Aid, 34, 144
Stephenson County, Illinois, 5, 9
Stock Feed, 4
Subs, 148
Sweet Clover, 140

T

Tablets, 30, 32, 34, 37, 38, 39, 40, 41, 42, 45, 48
Talcum, 127, 128, 129, 130, 131, 132, 142
Tapioca, 95
Tasting Party, 77
Tennessee, 15
Tenth Avenue, 17
Territory Vacant and Taken, 21
Texas, 15, 27
The American Legion Monthly, 23
The Country Home, 23
Third Street North, 17
Tonic, 19
Tooth Brushes, 155
Toronto, 16
Tariff Staff, 26
Trade School for Boys, 13
Transport Service, 60
Trevere, 119, 142
Trevillian, Minnie B, 9
Truck, 115

U

United States, 7
United States Post Office, 7
University of Wisconsin, 26
Utah, 16, 22

V

Vanilla, 27, 107, 108, 109
Vermont, 16
Veterinary Ointment, 161
Virginias, 16
Vitamin Supplement for Livestock and Poultry, 171
Vitamins, 144

W

Washington, 16, 26
Watkins, J.R. Medical Company, 9
Watkins, J.R., 9
Wellington, 66, 67, 90, 104, 130, 169
West Indies, 7
Wet Mop, 154
Will Power, 147
Winnipeg, 5, 16, 18, 19, 44, 66, 90, 100, 103, 104, 131, 140, 169
Wisconsin, 5, 17, 26
Witch Hazel, 34
World War I, 15
Writing Fluid, 34